MONICA ALEMAN.

Aleman.

Metabolic and Endocrine Problems of the Horse

Metabolic and Endocrine Problems of the Horse

Edited by Tim D G Watson

W B Saunders
London Edinburgh New York Philadelphia Sydney Toronto

W. B. Saunders is an imprint of Harcourt Brace and Company Limited

Harcourt Brace and Company Ltd
24–28 Oval Road, London NW1 7DX

The Curtis Center
Independence Square West
Philadelphia, PA 19106-3399, USA

Harcourt Brace & Company
55 Horner Avenue
Toronto, Ontario M8Z 4X6, Canada

Harcourt Brace & Company, Australia
30–52 Smidmore Street
Marrickville, NSW 2204, Australia

This book is printed on acid free paper

A catalogue record for this book is available from the British Library

ISBN 0-7020-2241-1

Typeset by Blackpool Typesetting Services Limited, Blackpool
Printed in Great Britain by Cambridge University Press, Cambridge

The cover illustration is based on Figure 1, p. 26, Figure 2, p. 27 and Figure 4, p. 109. Figure 4, p. 109, is used with permission from the *Canadian Veterinary Journal*.

Contents

Editorial Advisors

Contributors

Michelle Henry Barton
DVM, PhD
University of Georgia
Department of Large Animal Medicine
College of Veterinary Medicine
Athens, GA
USA

Jill Beech
VMD, Dip ACVIM
Professor of Medicine
University of Pennsylvania
School of Veterinary Medicine
New Bolton Center
Kennett Square, PA
USA

Thomas J Divers
DVM, Dip ACVIM
Associate Professor of Medicine
Cornell University College of Veterinary Medicine
Ithaca, NY
USA

Patricia A Harris
MA, VetMB, PhD, MRCVS
Waltham Centre for Equine Nutrition and Care
Waltham on the Wolds
Melton Mowbray
Leicestershire
UK

Derek C Knottenbelt
BVM&S, DVM&S, MRCVS
University of Liverpool
Division of Equine Studies
Department of Veterinary Clinical Science and Animal Husbandry
Leahurst
Merseyside
UK

Han van der Kolk
DVM, PhD
Utrecht University
Department of Large Animal Medicine and Nutrition
Faculty of Veterinary Medicine
Utrecht
The Netherlands

David S Kronfeld
PhD, DSc, MVSc, DipACVIM, DipACVN, MRCVS
Paul Mellon Distinguished Professor
Virginia Polytechnic Institute and State University
Blacksburg, VA
USA

Leopoldo Sosa León
BVSc, PhD
University of Sydney
Department of Veterinary Clinical Sciences
Sydney, NSW
Australia

Celia M Marr
BVMS, MVM, PhD, DEIM, MRCVS
Royal Veterinary College
Department of Farm Animal and Equine Medicine and Surgery
University of London
North Mymms
Hertfordshire
UK

James N Moore
DVM, PhD
University of Georgia
Department of Large Animal Medicine
College of Veterinary Medicine
Athens, GA
USA

Jonathan Naylor
MRCVS, PhD, DipACVIM, DipACVN
University of Saskatchewan
Department of Veterinary Internal Medicine
Western College of Veterinary Medicine
Saskatoon
Saskatchewan
Canada

Christopher M Riggs
BVSc, PhD, DEO, MRCVS
University of Liverpool
Division of Equine Studies
Department of Veterinary Clinical Science and Animal Husbandry
Leahurst
Merseyside
UK

Reuben J Rose
Professor of Veterinary Clinical Sciences
Rural Veterinary Centre
Department of Veterinary Clinical Sciences
University of Sydney
Camden, NSW
Australia

Tim D G Watson
BVM&S, PhD, MRCVS
Waltham Centre for Pet Nutrition
Waltham on the Wolds
Melton Mowbray
Leicestershire
UK

Preface

As its name indicates, this book is devoted to metabolic and endocrine diseases of horses and is timely given advances that have been made in understanding such problems in recent years. Texts on equine medicine have traditionally concentrated on those disorders of the respiratory and alimentary tracts that are common in horse practice, with emphasis on parasitic and infectious diseases. This was particularly true of the books that I used as a student just over a decade ago – I know this because I recently exhumed them, along with my course notes, from the attic. To be fair, newer texts do contain information on metabolic and endocrine diseases, a reflection of increasing awareness of such conditions in equine practice.

The primary purpose of this book is to supply to anyone with an interest the most contemporary knowledge on conditions such as laminitis, hyperlipaemia, disorders of the pituitary, adrenal and thyroid glands, and skeletal, hepatic and renal diseases. Additional chapters deal with endotoxaemia, the role of fluid therapy in the exercising horse, and the clinical assessment of nutritional status. Two criteria were employed in soliciting contributions for the book: the authors should be recognised as contemporary experts and an international perspective should be maintained. The authors were given the difficult task of reviewing the often complex pathophysiology and therapy of metabolic and endocrine problems, and yet making the information relevant to the practitioner.

Did we meet our objective – does this book supply in one volume the most contemporary information on equine metabolic and endocrine diseases? Some will argue that there are other diseases with metabolic components, as well as rare endocrinopathies, which are not included in this book. This may be true, but we have chosen to focus on diseases for which there have been significant advances in understanding pathophysiology and hence tailoring therapies. More important to me, however, is whether the book truly reflects the current state of the art. With the progress that science makes and the interval between completion of the chapters and publication of the text, there is always the concern that certain theories are about to be disproved, alternative therapies proposed, and new diseases recognised. While such progress may be unfortunate in terms of the lifespan of this particular book, it undoubtedly enhances our ability to diagnose and treat disease, and hence improve the health of our patients.

Tim D G Watson

1

Acute and Subacute Laminitis

Christopher M Riggs and Derek C Knottenbelt

Key Points

- Laminitis is a common disease that affects all types of domesticated Equidae world wide.
- Certain systemic diseases predispose to laminitis, especially those in which endotoxaemia is a feature. However, the aetiopathogenesis of the condition is still incompletely understood.
- Laminitis primarily involves a metabolic disturbance of the laminae of the hoof, which can cause their mechanical dysfunction. In severe cases the laminar disruption may be so extensive that the third phalanx separates from the hoof capsule.
- There is good evidence for a primary vascular component to the disease, which causes ischaemia of the laminae. However, experimental data remain confusing and there is support for other disease processes, including inappropriate activation of enzymes within the hoof causing autodegradation of the basement membrane and abnormalities of keratinocyte metabolism.
- Severe pathophysiological changes develop rapidly in laminitis and treatment of acute cases may be ineffective. Therefore, animals considered to be at risk of developing the disease should be treated with prophylactic measures.
- Drug therapies are based on reducing the risk of endotoxaemia, maintaining or improving perfusion of the digit, countering the effects of inflammatory mediators and providing pain relief.
- Physical therapies are a crucial adjunct to treatment and are aimed at reducing loads on the laminae. This may be achieved by severely limiting all exercise, providing a firm, supportive bedding, and applying temporary frog support.
- A proportion of cases will be refractory to all treatment and will require humane destruction.
- Severity of clinical signs and response to treatment are the most reliable prognostic indicators in the acute case.

Introduction

Laminitis describes a condition that involves metabolic disturbance in the laminae of the digit and the consequent compromise of their biochemical integrity. If the condition is severe or prolonged then continued loading of the laminae during weight-bearing and locomotion may result in their mechanical disruption. Although laminitis can occur in the absence of any other signs it frequently arises secondary to a primary systemic abnormality. It is, therefore, generally considered to reflect the local manifestation of a systemic disease [1, 2]. Several metabolic, haemodynamic and inflammatory changes have been recorded in the digits of affected animals. The rapidity with which subtle pathology develops, coupled with the absence of clinical signs for up to 3 days from an initiating cause of the disease, has made differentiation of primary from secondary pathological changes difficult. Models of laminitis, such as oral carbohydrate overload [3, 4] and induced black walnut toxicosis [5, 6] have been developed in an attempt to overcome such problems. However, there must remain some concern whether these models genuinely reflect naturally occurring forms of the disease.

Laminitis is a common and important disease, which occurs throughout the domesticated equine population of the world. Acute laminitis is often a cause of extreme suffering and its chronic sequelae frequently result in permanent disability [7, 8]. A recent study of racing Thoroughbreds suggested a higher than expected incidence of subclinical laminitis, which may be responsible for chronic poor performance of affected racehorses [9]. The range of severity of the clinical condition and variability in its progression and response to treatment make it a difficult and often frustrating challenge in equine practice. Increased understanding of systemic metabolic and hormonal abnormalities and their association with laminitis are essential if effective treatments and preventative strategies are to be developed.

Aetiology

Laminitis has been associated with a number of different predisposing factors (Table 1). It is well established that horses affected by some forms of systemic disease are particularly at risk of developing laminitis. A large number of studies have concentrated on determining possible links between systemic disease and the precipitation of an acute laminitic crisis. However, such studies are fraught with difficulties and the subject remains the focus of continued investigation. The field is complicated by the controversy that still exists over the precise pathogenesis of the condition.

Horses or ponies suffering from enteritis, pleuritis, endometritis or any other toxic condition are particularly prone to laminitis [10–12]. Correlation between high systemic levels of endotoxins and the onset of laminitis in affected animals [4, 13], has led to the implication of these substances in the disease process. However, laminitis may occur in cases in which there is no clinical evidence of endotoxaemia [14, 15]. Also, correlation between endotoxaemia and clinical laminitis has been inconsistent and attempts to induce the disease experimentally by intravenous infusion of bacterial endotoxins have failed [16–18]. This may be due to inappropriate administration of endotoxins in these experiments [4] or may reflect the presence of other mediators, such as vasoactive amines, in these disease states. Histamine has been implicated as a mediator of the disease on account of changes in digital vascular permeability recorded in laminitis [19]. However, more recent evidence suggest this is a secondary feature of the disease rather than a cause [15]. It has been suggested that inappropriate activation of the renin-angiotensin-aldosterone system [20] may be responsible for some of the early pathophysiological changes recorded in laminitis. Whether systemic changes in these factors are the cause or effect of disease remains to be determined.

It is well recognized that overweight ponies are at high risk of developing laminitis. Various studies have suggested an endocrinological basis for this predisposition. Coffman and Colles [21] and Field and Jeffcott [22] identified evidence of insulin insensitivity in laminitic ponies compared with normal animals. It was proposed that the reduction of insulin effectiveness may lead to elevation in thromboxane A2 activity causing vascular changes within the digit. Insulin insensitivity may also be the explanation for an association between hyperlipaemia and laminitis in overweight ponies [23].

Hypothyroidism [24] has also been connected with laminitis although more recent studies suggest that changes in systemic triiodothyronine are a consequence of the disease rather than a cause [25]. Hyperadrenocorticism is frequently associated with laminitis [26]. The mechanism behind this link is not completely understood but glucocorticoids are known to potentiate the vasoconstrictive effects of catecholamines [27], which may predispose to laminitis [2]. The observation that exogenous corticosteroids may precipitate an acute laminitic crisis provides some support for this hypothesis [28, 29]. High levels of endogenous corticosteroids may also contribute via exacerbation of insulin insensitivity.

Mechanical influences, such as excessive work on hard surfaces, extreme and persistent loadbearing due to contralateral limb lameness and severe or inappropriate foot paring have been linked with the onset of acute laminitis [30]. The aetiopathogenesis of the disease in such circumstances is uncertain. The fact that often only one digit is affected suggests that local trauma may be involved.

***Table 1.* Factors associated with the onset and/or development of laminitis**

- Gastrointestinal diseases
  - enteritis
  - strangulating intestinal lesions
  - carbohydrate overload
- Infectious and toxic conditions
  - septic pleuritis
  - endometritis
- Obesity
- Endocrine disorders
  - hyperadrenocorticism
  - hypothyroidism
- Mechanical influences on the foot

This may operate through a direct mechanical affect or be secondary to vaso-active processes, similar to changes seen in humans exposed to severe vibration [31].

Less common factors that have been implicated as possible causes of laminitis include selenium toxicosis [32], microembolism secondary to endocarditis [33] and high dietary oestrogen [34]. There is also recent evidence of a genetic predisposition to laminitis [35].

Pathogenesis

The similarity in the clinical signs of laminitis, regardless of the apparent primary cause, suggests that a common pathophysiological mechanism is involved in all cases. However, as in most other aspects of this disease, there remains a low level of agreement over its pathogenesis. Current theories may be divided into three broad groups (Figure 1).

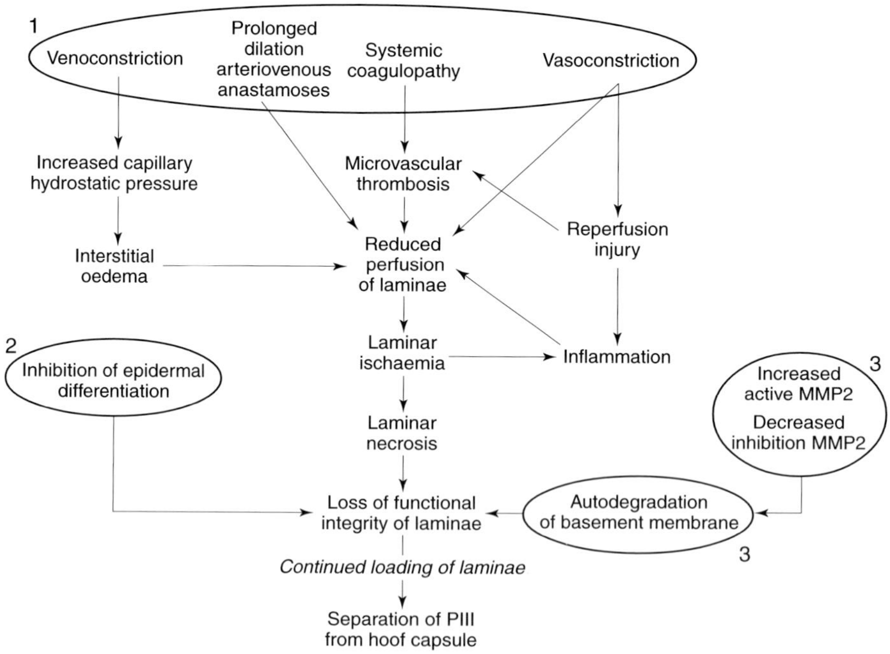

Figure 1. The pathogenesis of laminitis. Pathophysiological processes which have been implicated can be grouped into three broad categories: 1. Vascular abnormalities; 2. Disturbance in keratinocyte metabolism; 3. Autodegradation of the basement membrane. *MMP2 (Matrix metalloproteinase 2; collagenase 4); P III (third phalanx).*

1. Hypoperfusion of the Digit

A plethora of clinical and experimental data exist to show that significant alterations in blood flow to the digit are associated with the onset, and occur during the development, of acute laminitis [2, 36, 37]. Gross and microscopic studies of corrosion casts reveal loss of blood supply to the dermis [38, 39] and histopathological examinations have revealed morphological changes consistent with congestion and obstruction of the laminar capillaries [2]. In acute experimental laminitis with severe clinical signs, Roberts and co-workers [40] found evidence of oedema of some secondary laminae and necrosis of adjacent secondary epidermal laminae. More recent studies using near infrared spectroscopy demonstrated evidence of haemostasis in affected feet in acute laminitis [41, 36]. These findings have led to the commonly held view that the primary pathology in laminitis involves disturbance in the blood supply to the laminar corium, which results in localized ischaemia and, if sufficiently severe and prolonged, necrosis of the laminae. Several hypotheses exist to explain possible causes of reduced perfusion of the digit:

(a) Hunt [42] and Eaton [15] favour a primary venoconstriction (in response to one of several possible agonists), which results in a marked increase in intradigital capillary pressure and subsequent hydrostatic-mediated movement of fluid into the digital interstitium. Support for this hypothesis is provided by the observation that digital veins show greater reactivity to vasoconstrictive mediators than digital arteries [43]. Blood flow to the laminae is impeded when tissue pressures exceed the critical closing pressure of capillaries [15]. Indeed, laminitis has been likened to a manifestation of the compartmental syndrome, the situation exacerbated by the relatively inflexible confines of the hoof capsule [44]. Secondary changes, including diversion of blood from the laminar capillary bed via arteriovenous shunts and microvascular thrombosis, further contribute to an ischaemic crisis [14].

(b) Others have placed greater emphasis on the importance of a systemic coagulopathy and microthrombotic compromise of the digital vasculature as a primary event in laminitis [45, 46]. Recent gamma-scintigraphic studies of experimental ponies with radiolabelled platelets, combined with histopathological examination of post mortem material from the same animals, revealed evidence of microvascular thrombosis at the onset of acute laminitis [47]. However, analysis of serial blood samples from 15 horses during the prodromal stages of acute laminitis induced by carbohydrate overload failed to reveal any evidence of a significant imbalance in coagulation or fibrinolysis in association with the onset of laminitis [48]. This work was in agreement with the findings of an earlier study [49]. The evidence suggests that while microvascular thrombi may develop during acute laminitis an imbalance in haemostasis is not pathognomonic for the disease.

(c) Arteriovenous anastamoses are densely distributed throughout the equine digit [50, 51]. There is evidence that these vascular structures can divert the circulation of blood away from capillaries of the submural laminae [52]. It has been hypothesized that inappropriate, prolonged dilation of arterio-venous anastamoses, stimulated by the systemic and local release of vaso-active peptides, is primarily responsible for the laminar ischaemia seen during the development of laminitis [50, 51, 53]. Such a redistribution of blood would also explain the apparently paradoxical observations of ischaemic change of the laminae in the face of increased total blood flow to the digit [37]. However, attempts to confirm this hypothesis have been frustrated by technical difficulties. Moreover, dynamic radionuclide angiograms and static blood pool images obtained by gamma-scintigraphic studies failed to reveal any evidence of reduced blood flow to the laminae during either the acute or developmental phases of laminitis [54].

(d) Hood and co-workers [2] contend that while laminar ischaemia may occur as a consequence of a temporary peripheral vasospasm during the prodromal phase of laminits, it is the biochemical reactions that occur during the subsequent reperfusion of the ischaemic tissues that cause the majority of pain and tissue damage. Oxygen radicals and other cytotoxic molecules are formed during a period of reactive hyperaemia following ischaemia and these, coupled with neutrophil influx, an impaired haemorrheological status and microthrombosis, can more severely damage the digit than the period of ischaemia [2]. A large number of vasoactive substances capable of causing a temporary vasoconstriction have been identified [2]. In addition, there is increasing evidence that damage to the endothelium of affected vessels, by agents such as endotoxins, may impair their ability to autoregulate blood flow as part of the disease process [36, 55, 56]. The fact that only the blood vessels of the digit should be affected is not unique to the horse. Raynaud's phenomenon, a peripheral vascular disease of humans of unknown aetiopathogenesis, shows many similarities to laminitis [57].

(e) Inconsistencies recorded concerning variation in blood flow to the digit during the onset of laminitis have prompted others to speculate that such changes are secondary to some other primary event [58–60]. Elongation of secondary lamellae has been documented as an early histopathological change in laminitis. Even slight disruption of the laminar structure may be expected to lead to a degree of mechanical deformation of the surrounding tissues, which will have a rapid and profound effect on the patency of capillaries and fine veins within them. Other recent histopathological investigations have failed to reveal evidence of oedema of the laminar interstitium or significant abnormalities affecting blood vessels and capillaries in the lamellar region early in the onset of the disease [61].

2. Autodegradation of the Basement Membrane

The importance of the basement membrane in the functional anatomy of the equine hoof has been well illustrated: it provides the connection between the heavily keratinized hoof wall and the dense connective tissue of the distal phalanx [62]. Pollitt [62] identified this as a potential weakness, hypothesizing that injury to the basement membrane would lead to mechanical disruption of the bond between these two tissues. In studies of material from experimental horses with carbohydrate-induced laminitis. Pollitt demonstrated progressive disruption of the lamellar basement membrane, which correlated well with clinical signs of the disease [62]. Disintegration of the basement membrane and failure of its attachment to the basal cells of the epidermis was one of the earliest pathological events recorded in the tissues studied. Such change may occur following enzymatic autodegradation of the affected tissues. Increased production and, or, activation of collagenase IV in the laminar tissues, stimulated by circulating cytokines such as tumour necrosis factor (elevated in severe gastrointestinal disease [63]) was proposed as one potential mechanism for this process [61].

3. Inhibition of Epidermal Differentiation

Histopathological studies by Obel [64, 65] identified structural abnormalities of the epidermis of the lamellar region at a very early stage of acute laminitis. In cases with severe deformation of the secondary epidermal lamellae there was also oedema and infiltration of leucocytes in the laminar corium. Similar epidermal changes were recorded in non-weight bearing regions of the foot and in the chestnuts from the same animals, although the corium of these regions appeared normal even in advanced stages of laminitis. A more recent study of tissues obtained from a horse that suffered peracute laminitis following large bowel torsion provided similar findings [60]. The histopathological changes were located at the border between the basal and suprabasal cells of the secondary epidermal lamellae. This observation, together with an absence of pathological changes in the deeper part of the laminar corium, provides some support for the concept that the putative laminitis-causing agents act primarily on the epidermis. Close analysis of epidermis from the chestnuts of the affected horse revealed absence of keratohyalin granules indicating inhibited differentiation of the keratinocytes [60]. Several substances, such as retinoids, corticosteroids and bacterial toxins, are known to inhibit differentiation of keratinocytes and have all been linked with the aetiology of laminitis.

Chronic Laminitis

Whatever the pathophysiological process underlying acute laminitis, once the laminar bond between the epidermis and dermis has become sufficiently compromised then biomechanical forces acting on the components of the digit predispose to distal displacement of the third phalanx within the hoof capsule [66] (Figure 2). Most commonly this takes the form of dorso-distal rotation of the

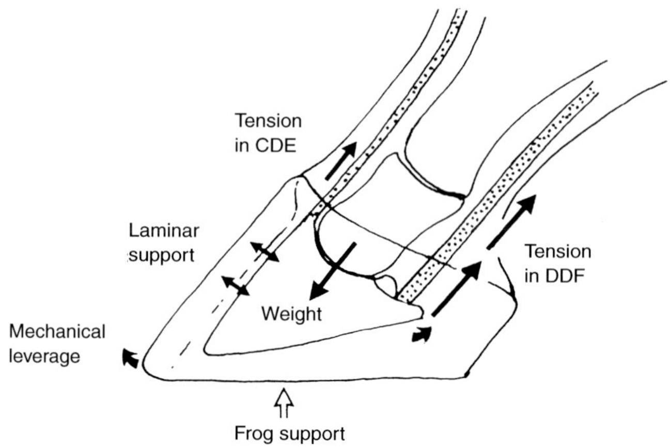

Figure 2. Functional loads on the equine digit. Forces imposed by the weight of the animal, mechanical leverage on the toe of the hoof during locomotion and tension in the deep digital flexor tendon are opposed by the laminae. The last two may contribute to rotation of the third phalanx.

third phalanx, presumably owing to a combination of biomechanical forces and predisposition of the dorsal laminae to more severe injury during acute laminitis [67]. However, occasionally the third phalanx will sink evenly within the hoof capsule, disruption of the laminar bond having occurred around its circumference [68]. Once such irreversible macroscopic pathology has occurred in laminitis the condition is considered to be chronic.

Clinical Features of Acute Laminitis

Pain

The most prominent sign in acute laminitis is foot pain. The extent of pain and alteration of gait (lameness) has been used to provide a classification of the disease [64]:

- Obel Grade 1: the least severe grade is characterized by a mild but continuous shifting of weight from one foot to the other.
- Obel Grade 2: lameness is more obvious. The animal is willing to walk but with a heel–toe action. A limb may be lifted without difficulty.
- Obel Grade 3: lifting of a limb is vigorously resisted and the horse usually refuses to move unless strongly encouraged.
- Obel Grade 4: the horse is often recumbent. High circulating catecholamine concentrations result in tachycardia, tachypnoea, sweating and hypertension.

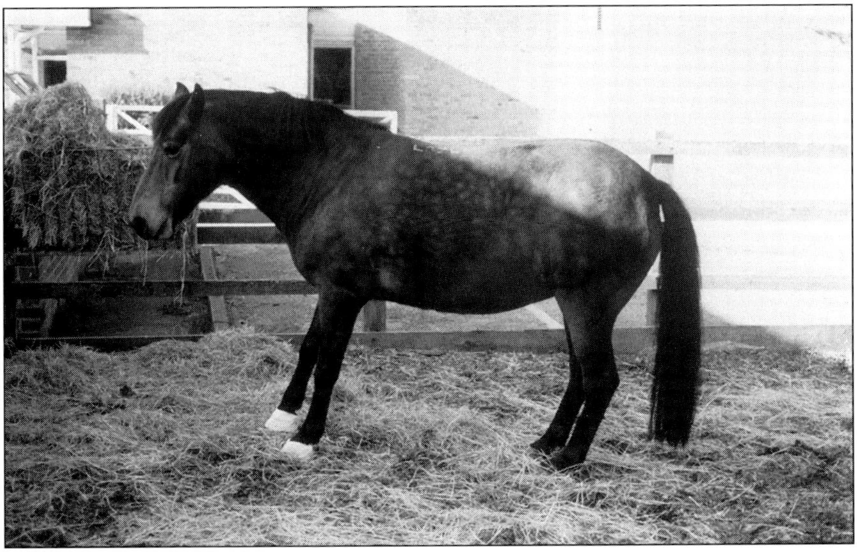

Figure 3. Typical stance of a horse with severe, acute laminitis.

Detection of lesser Obel Grades is often difficult for lay owners and so most cases of acute laminitis are presented at Grade 3 or 4. The greater severity of the pain usually present in the front feet encourages the horse to lean back in an effort to equilibrate the load bearing or more particularly to transfer weight to lesser affected and less painful hind feet. This results in a typical 'saw-horse' posture with an obvious 'leaning backwards' stance (Figure 3). A few cases show more severe hind foot pain and bias the stance accordingly towards the front [38].

Foot Signs

The underlying acute changes in the perfusion of the digit characteristically produce palpable heat at the surface of the hoof and increased amplitude of the pulses in the medial and lateral palmar or plantar digital arteries of the affected feet. While these features are typical of the disease they are also characteristic of any inflammatory lesion of the digit. Also, there is evidence that the blood supply to the foot is restricted during first stages of the disease [2] and hence laminitis cannot be ruled out if the hoof temperature and pulse amplitude are normal or reduced.

Structural Changes of the Foot

As mechanical disruption of the laminae occurs, the solar corium tends to lose its normal concave shape and become progressively flatter and then convex. This is associated with disto-palmar/plantar rotation of the third phalanx. The convexity is centred on the sole immediately cranial to the point of the frog and, if the rotation is severe, the pedal bone may prolapse through the sole at this point. Bruising of the sole in this region is sometimes evident before the sole perforates.

In other cases, palpation of the coronary band reveals oedema, or that the coronet has moved distally within the capsule of the insensitive laminae, producing an indentation between the top of the hoof wall and the surface of the pastern. This depression may indicate disruption of the laminae circumferentially around the hoof, and the subsequent 'sinking' of the pedal bone distally without rotation. Sinking may also be accompanied by haemorrhage or serous exudate from the coronary band [68]. In extreme cases the insensitive laminae separate completely from the sensitive laminae, so that the keratinized part of the hoof sloughs.

Further Diagnostic Tests

The diagnosis of laminitis is often based solely on the characteristic stance of the animal, pain associated with weight bearing and locomotion and signs relating to the feet. Horses with milder pain (Obel grade 1) will usually show increased sensitivity to the application of hoof testers cranial to the point of the frog. The use of hoof testers should be avoided when the horse is reluctant to pick up one or more feet, as the increased loading of the contralateral feet may predispose to further mechnical damage. If the pain is severe, the horse may show signs suggestive of abdominal pain, becoming recumbent and intermittently rolling (Obel grade 4). In this situation abdominal disease should be ruled out by a thorough physical examination before it is concluded that laminitis is the only condition present. Occasionally, horses with exertional rhabdomyolysis may present in a similar manner. This can usually be distinguished from laminitis by the history combined with the lack of pain associated with the feet, myoglobinuria and myoglobinaemia. An affected animal's stance and movement is sometimes such as to suggest a more proximal source of pain. Diagnostic perineural anaesthesia may be useful in confirming the feet as the source of lameness in such cases. However, nerve blocks should be used with caution as the pain relief they effect will alter the animal's distribution of weight which may predispose to further trauma to the laminae.

Infrequently a single foot is affected by laminitis and in these cases other lesions affecting the digit, such as subsolar abscessation and fractures of the third phalanx, must be excluded by a thorough clinical examination and, if necessary, radiography. Well positioned lateral radiographs of the digits will demonstrate the relationship between the third phalanx and the hoof capsule and will reveal their separation following extensive disruption of the laminae [69, 70]. They also facilitate the detection of fluid or gas pockets which may form in the laminar interface. These radiographic signs are consistent with the chronic stage of the disease. There are no radiographic signs associated with acute and subacute cases unless there has been a previous chronic episode.

Treatment

Treatment of any disease where the underlying aetiopathogenesis is poorly understood is likely to be at best speculative, and at worst counterproductive. That laminitis is no exception to this is demonstrated by the range of idiosyncratic remedies which have been in and out of favour over centuries [1, 30].

Effective therapy is also hampered by the inescapable lag phase during which there is ongoing biochemical and biomechanical disruption and laminar damage without obvious clinical signs [3, 4]. One would anticipate that therapy may be more effective if instigated during the critical period when the disease is incipient rather than once the condition has become established. It therefore behoves us as clinicians to be especially vigilant in those cases where laminitis may reasonably be expected to occur, for example those likely to develop, or showing signs of, endotoxaemia. Prophylactic treatment of these cases with chemotherapeutic agents designed to modify the effective circulation to the digit is logical if the theories of laminitis developing following vascular compromise are correct. At the other end of the spectrum, those horses that have recovered from the subacute or acute episode, and those that have progressed to the chronic stage, also deserve careful management to alleviate the physical consequences of the disease and reduce the risk of future attacks.

Medical Management of the Subacute Case

Horses presenting with any condition likely to produce endotoxaemia fall into this category. Animals with strangulating intestinal lesions, colitis, enteritis, carbohydrate overload, septic pleuritis and endometritis should always be regarded as on the brink of acute laminitis. Treatment is initially aimed at the primary condition (Table 2). This may involve surgical resection of the source of the endotoxin as well as systemic treatment to support the circulation with intravenous fluid therapy. Systemic antibacterial agents and appropriate non-steroidal anti-inflammatory drugs are also important to reduce circulating levels of endotoxin and counter its effects on tissues. Flunixin meglumine at low doses is reported to reduce the effects of endotoxin in experimental animals [71]. More recently, anti-endotoxin antibodies and vaccination have been used (see Chapter 10).

Various agents have been advocated to decrease the absorption of endotoxins from the gastointestinal tract or to limit their production within it. Animals known to have consumed excess carbohydrate should be dosed with mineral oil by nasogastric intubation to minimize absorption of endotoxins [34]. It has

Table 2. **Treatment of subacute laminitis**

- Treat primary condition(s), where appropriate
  - prevention and treatment of endotoxaemia
  - limitation of carbohydrate overload
- Vasodilator therapy
  - warm water foot baths
  - acetylpromazine
  - phenoxybenzamine
  - isoxsuprine
  - glyceryl trinitrate
- Prevention of microvascular thrombosis
  - heparin
  - aspirin
- Reduction of reperfusion injury
  - dimethyl sulphoxide
- Physical therapy
  - rest
  - deep, comfortable bedding
  - frog support

recently been demonstrated that a formulation of virginiamycin (Founderguard™) fed prophylactically to horses significantly reduced the incidence of laminitis following experimental carbohydrate overload [72]. Virginiamycin is effective against lactic acid producing bacteria in the equine digestive tract, and may prevent lactic acidosis associated with carbohydrate overload. Reducing the acidity of the intestinal contents may prevent the release of endotoxin from Gram-negative bacteria.

The use of vasodilators was prompted by theories that the digital circulation is compromised in laminitis by vasospasm, or the shunting of blood away from the periphery via arteriovenous anastomoses [2, 14]. Traditionally, laminitis was treated by standing the horse in tubs of cold water [30]. This can have a marked analgesic effect, but it is also likely to cause profound vasoconstriction which may exacerbate the laminar ischaemia. The majority of clinicians now favour warm water therapy [73], which is more likely to cause peripheral vasodilation and hence improve circulation to the digit.

Acetylpromazine has been shown to increase blood flow in the palmar digital artery in the conscious standing horse [74], although the effects on blood flow at the level of the laminar capillaries are unknown. The duration of any vasodilator effect has not been reported in laminitic animals. The dose regime which has been used in acute laminitis is 0.03–0.06 mg/kg BW, IM, q6–8h [75].

Other drugs that have been suggested in an attempt to increase laminar perfusion are phenoxybenzamine, isoxsuprine hydrochloride and glyceryl trinitrate [34, 36]. Phenoxybenzamine and isoxsuprine reduce peripheral resistance in the same manner as acetylpromazine, by acting as adrenergic receptor agonists. Phenoxybenzamine can provide vasodilation for 12–24 hours [76], but it is difficult to use in the horse as a solution for intravenous administration has to be made from capsules designed for the the oral route. Isoxsuprine has been used at a dose rate of 0.6 mg/kg BW, po, q12h [71]. All these drugs have hypotensive effects and should only be used in normovolaemic horses.

Glyceryl trinitrate has recently been used topically in the treatment of naturally occurring laminitis in ponies [16]. This compound acts as an endothelium-independent donor of nitric oxide, a potent smooth muscle relaxant. The effect may be to improve pedal circulation by mediating the dilation of the digital vasculature [77]. Glyceryl trinitrate is applied to the skin overlying the medial and lateral palmar or plantar digital arteries in the form of a 2% ointment covered by a dressing, or as commercially available adhesive patches (Nitro-Dur, Schering-Plough Ltd). The hair overlying the neurovascular bundles at the level of the pastern is clipped, shaved and dried, and the patches are taped onto the skin and replaced q24h. The total dose used experimentally for 250 to 300 kg ponies equated to approximately 60 mg q24h for 2 days followed by 40 mg q24h for a further 2 days and 20 mg q24h for a final 2 days. It has not been possible to measure the effective dose at the level of the arterial wall as the absorption of glyceryl trinitrate via the transcutaneous route is unknown. The experimental dose regime was varied depending on the improvement in lameness and reduction in systemic systolic and diastolic blood pressure [36]. It should be noted that there is a potential contra-indication of using alpha-2 agonists in laminitic animals, as xylazine has been shown experimentally to cause a reduction in digital arterial flow in healthy horses [74]. Although the effect was transient and has not been measured in horses with laminitis, it could exacerbate any pre-existing ischaemia associated with the disease.

A second group of chemotherapeutic agents aims to reduce the coagulability of the blood, based on the premise that laminitis is initiated by a coagulopathy. Heparin was found to reduce the prevalence of laminitis when used in the carbohydrate overload model of the disease [78]. A retrospective study of the incidence of laminitis in cases of surgical colic due to a small intestinal lesion compared two groups of horses, those that received heparin therapy and those that did not [79]. The groups were otherwise similar in terms of the diagnosis at surgery, the white blood cell and total protein concentrations in the peritoneal fluid and the postoperative management. Although the number of horses that developed laminitis in the treated group was smaller, this difference was not statistically significant. The different results of the two studies may be because laminitis in colic cases is mediated via a different mechanism from that in carbohydrate overload. Alternatively, it could be that the heparin was given to the colic cases too late in the development of the disease, whereas heparin treatment in the carbohydrate overload model was given earlier in the disease process. A third possibility is that antithrombin III, the activity of which is increased by heparin, is less plentiful in cases of small intestinal colic [79]. A recent study found a significant effect of heparin prophylaxis in cases of duodenitis/proximal jejunitis [80], which emphasizes our currently inadequate understanding of the aetiopathological mechanisms at work in this disease. The recommended dose rate for heparin is 40–80 iu/kg BW, IV or SC, q8–12h [79, 80].

An alternative antithrombotic agent is aspirin. The relatively poor anti-inflammatory effect of aspirin in the horse is due to the short half-life and weak inhibition of cyclo-oxygenase by the active metabolite, salicylate [81]. In contrast, the relatively potent antithrombotic effect is mediated by irreversible inhibition of platelet cyclo-oxygenase by the parent drug. Bleeding time was significantly increased in healthy ponies for at least 24 hours after a dose of 4 mg/kg BW, IV [81]. The intravenous route was used in this study, as the degree and rate of absorption after oral dosing in the horse is so variable [82]. However, doses of 5, 10 and 20 mg/kg BW, po, have been shown to significantly reduce serum thromboxane B_2, a product of cyclo-oxygenase activity, for over 7 days [83] and a single dose of 20 mg/kg BW, po prolonged bleeding time for several days [84]. In practice, 10–20 mg/kg BW, po, q48h has been used in cases of laminitis. The anti-inflammatory effect of aspirin at this low dose is negligible, so that it may safely be combined with another non-steroidal anti-inflammatory agent. Bleeding times and serum concentrations of thromboxane B_2 after aspirin administration have not been reported for horses with laminitis. The effects of aspirin on the circulation of the digit are also not known. The more prolonged antithrombotic effect of warfarin has been described in the long term treatment of chronic cases of laminitis [85].

Damage caused to the laminae during reperfusion may be more significant than ischaemia itself [2]. In this case there may be a role for the use of dimethyl sulphoxide to reduce reperfusion injury in its capacity as a free radical scavenger. However, dimethyl sulphoxide also acts as an anti-inflammatory, analgesic, endothelial cell protector and inhibitor of platelet aggregation [85]. Any of these properties may account for its perceived beneficial effect. The reported dose range is from 0.1 to 1 g/kg BW, IV, q8–24h for 2–4 days.

If evidence for a role of endogenous metalloproteinases in the primary pathogenesis of the disease [61] is substantiated in future studies then the use of inhibitors of these enzymes [86] may be of great benefit as a new treatment for laminitis.

Physical Therapy for the Subacute Case

Physical therapies are an important adjunct to the management of the subacute laminitic. The majority are aimed at reducing the loads born by the laminae and hence decreasing the risk of severe laminar disruption occuring. Whereas exercise used to be encouraged in the hope that it may increase circulation within the digit, strict rest is now generally advocated in order to minimize the loading on the feet [73]. A deep, comfortable bedding should be supplied, ideally of a material that provides firm support to the sole such as sand or peat, in order to encourage the horse to lie down and to partially redistribute loads from the laminae. Additional support may be provided in the form of pads (either rolled gauze swabs or Lily Pads, Therapeutic Equine Products) carefully applied to the caudal third of the frog [34, 67, 87]. Recent work indicates that frog support can cause increased discomfort in chronic cases of laminitis [88]. This emphasizes the importance of assessing each individual case to determine the beneficial or detrimental effects that a particular treatment may have and the need to be prepared to reverse that treatment if necessary.

Medical Management of the Acute Case

These are animals in which the presenting complaint is the laminitis itself, although this may be secondary to an underlying problem that has been overlooked. Alternatively, acute cases develop from subacute cases where the prophylactic measures have failed. In both cases, the therapeutic principles outlined for subacute laminitis should be applied. A complete physical examination is essential to identify any underlying disorders, which must be treated (Table 3). Therapy with vasodilators and anticoagulants is initiated or continued, on the basis that the disease is an ongoing process and that it is important to prevent further damage to as yet unaffected laminae. Similarly, support for the feet should be provided, but at the acute stage two further areas must also be addressed, namely the treatment of acute inflammation and the relief of pain.

As the feet become painful, catecholamines are released into the circulation, and these may be partially responsible for peripheral vasoconstriction and the systemic hypertension measured in animals with laminitis [36]. Providing effective analgesia may contribute to an improvement in the pedal circulation by lowering the concentration of circulating catecholamines [85].

The non-steroidal anti-inflammatory drugs phenylbutazone and flunixin meglumine and, to a lesser extent, ketoprofen have been widely used in the treatment of acute cases for both their anti-inflammatory and analgesic effects [75]. Both effects are mediated in part via inhibition of the cyclo-oxygenase enzyme. Phenylbutazone is considerably less expensive than flunixin and ketoprofen and may be superior in its analgesic effects [34, 75]. However, there is evidence that phenylbutazone causes more significant adverse effects than the other drugs [89]. In acute laminitis, flunixin meglumine has been used at its anti-inflammatory dose of 1.1 mg/kg BW, q24h. Goetz [85] describes the combined use of

***Table 3.* Treatment of acute laminitis**

- Continuation of therapies for subacute laminitis, where appropriate
- Analgesia
  - phenylbutazone
  - flunixin meglumine
  - ketoprofen
- Physical therapy
  - surgical farriery
  - corrective shoeing

phenylbutazone, for its superior analgesic effect, with flunixin meglumine in cases that are endotoxaemic. The dose rate for phenylbutazone is 4.4 mg/kg BW, IV or po, q12h [85], although milder cases may respond well to lower doses, with less potential for adverse effects. In severe cases higher doses have been used, although this carries a greater risk of toxicity. Animals receiving non-steroidal anti-inflammatory agents should be well hydrated to reduce the risk of nephrotoxicity. These drugs may be combined with aspirin used at anti-thrombotic doses [34].

As corticosteroids have been implicated as contributory factors in the development of laminitis [27, 29], their use as anti-inflammatory agents in suspected cases of laminitis is contraindicated [85]. Local analgesia of the digit may be useful to facilitate radiographic procedures, but should not be used as the primary analgesic treatment, as increased weight bearing and locomotion while the feet are desensitized may disrupt the laminae [73].

Physical Therapy for the Acute Case

Physical management of acute laminitis follows principles identical to those described for the subacute case. Like many other aspects of the disease the role of surgical farriery in acute laminitis remains controversial [90]. There are advocates of an aggressive early approach, involving dorsal wall resection and application of heart bar shoes within days of the onset of clinical signs [91]. However, there is concern that the act of performing such procedures causes the animal physical and physiological stress, which outweigh any potential benefits. There is also debate whether either procedure leads to significant improvements. In general, extensive foot trimming and corrective shoeing should be delayed until the initial digital pain and inflammation have subsided [34]. Immediate farriery attention should address correction of marked abnormalities of foot balance, such as trimming excessively long toes to reduce the leverage effect on the dorsal laminae (Figure 2). The use of an elevated heel shoe has been advocated in the treatment of acute laminitis [92]. Partial flexion of the distal interphalangeal joint will decrease tension in the deep digital flexor tendon, thereby reducing the main force responsible for the distoplamar/plantar rotation of the third phalanx (Figure 2). A more extreme method for achieving a similar goal is deep digital flexor tenotomy [93]. The technique may decrease pain associated with the acute refractory stage of laminitis but there is little evidence that the long-term survival rate of affected horses is improved [94]. Application of some form of external fixation to transfer loads from the ground to the third metacarpal or metatarsal bone has been considered as a means of negating all distracting forces on the laminae during the acute stages of the disease [95] although there are currently no published reports of the successful use of such a device in this context. A wide range of shoes and shoeing techniques has been recommended for the longer term management of chronic laminitis [67].

The Refractory Acute Case

A proportion of cases will not show a positive response to the combination of medical and physical therapies described above. No alternative medical therapy has been reported to be successful in these refractory cases. The more radical surgical techniques may be justified in these animals as an alternative to euthanasia.

Management of the Recovered Acute and Subacute Case

Animals that appear to have recovered may still have acquired significant damage to the laminae of the hoof and should be treated with care during the convalescent period, which lasts until the damaged areas have been replaced with new hoof horn [34]. This may take several months. During this time exercise should be restricted. Feed additives, such as methionine and biotin are beneficial for hoof repair. Biotin has been shown to increase the growth rate and hardness of hooves in normal horses [96]. Horses recovering from a bout of laminitis are prone to develop subsolar abscessation and infection at the white line. The dose of anti-inflammatory drugs should be tapered and stopped as soon as possible, so that any lameness due to sepsis will become apparent.

Prognosis

The majority of horses and ponies affected with acute laminitis will recover [87]. However, a proportion remain refractory to all forms of treatment and develop severe complications that ultimately necessitate humane destruction of the animal. The speed with which developing laminitis is recognized and appropriate therapy instituted will have some bearing on the severity of the acute disease, however, not infrequently even aggressive therapy at an early stage seems to have no significant effect on the outcome.

A reliable prognostic indicator, which could be assessed objectively early in the course of the disease, would facilitate decisions regarding the choice of whether to pursue more radical treatments or to destroy the animal. Treatment of severe laminitis inevitably involves prolonged suffering of the animal and considerable expense to the client and hence there is merit in an early decision to terminate a hopeless case. There have been several studies documenting objective features of laminitic cases which may help determine the prognosis for each case. However, none has proved entirely reliable.

It is generally considered that the most important factor affecting the outcome of an individual case is the initial severity of laminar damage [8]. This is consistent with the observation that the functional outcome correlates well with severity of clinical signs (Obel grade) in a significant proportion of cases [7]. Lack of response to therapy, persistent, uncontrollable pain and rapid development of phalangeal displacement are all poor prognostic indicators in the acute case. Size and body weight have been related to outcome, with larger, heavier animals carrying a worse prognosis [68].

In more chronic cases Stick and co-workers [97] related the degree of rotation of the third phalanx (determined radiographically by measuring the angle between the dorsal wall of the hoof and that of the third phalanx) to future athletic activity. Rotations <5.5° had a favourable outcome, those between 6.8° and 11.5° a guarded prognosis and those >11.5° an unfavourable prognosis. However, this must be interpreted with caution. In some cases, especially those in which the foot has been poorly balanced, the dorsal hoof wall may be long and form a relatively flat angle to the ground, giving the radiographic impression of its divergence relative to the third phalanx. A more reliable indicator of true rotation of the third phalanx is to measure its angle relative to that of the first and second phalanges. The degree of distal displacement of the third phalanx relative to the hoof capsule (determined from radiographs by measuring the distance between the extensor process and the coronary band) has been used as a prognostic indicator [98]. However, there is considerable variation in this distance between normal animals and hence serial radiographs demonstrating an increase over time are often required for it to be of most use in assessing laminitic cases.

Acknowledgements

The authors are grateful to Elizabeth Riggs for her contribution towards the writing of this chapter.

References

1. Baxter GM. Laminitis. In: Robinson NE (ed) *Current Therapy in Equine Medicine*, 3rd edn. Philadelphia: WB Saunders 1992; 154–160.
2. Hood DM, Grosenbaugh DA, Mostafa NB *et al.* The role of vascular mechanisms in the development of acute equine laminitis. *J Vet Int Med.* 1993; **7**, 228–234.
3. Garner HE, Coffinan JR, Hahn AW *et al.* Equine laminitis of alimentary origin: an experimental model. *Am J Vet Res.* 1975; **36**, 441–444.
4. Sprouse RF, Garner HE & Green M. Plasma endotoxin levels in horses subjected to carbohydrate induced laminitis. *Equine Vet J.* 1987; **19**, 25–28.
5. Minnick PD, Brown CM, Braselton WE *et al.* The induction of equine laminitis with an aqueous extract of the heartwood of black walnut (*Juglans nigra*). *Vet Hum Toxicol.* 1987; **29**, 230–233.
6. Galey ID, Twardock AR, Goetz TE *et al.* Gamma scintigraphic analysis of the distribution of perfusion of blood in the equine foot during black walnut (*Juglans nigra*) -induced laminitis. *Am J Vet Res.* 1990; **51**, 688–695.
7. Hunt RJ. A retrospective evaluation of laminitis in horses. *Equine Vet J.* 1993; **25**, 61–64.
8. Moyer W & Redden RR. Chronic and severe laminitis: a critique of therapy with heart bar shoes and hoof wall resection. *Equine Vet J.* 1989; **21**, 317–318.

9. Linford RL, O'Brien TR & Trout DR. Qualitative and morphometric radiographic findings in the distal phalanx and digital soft tissues of sound Thoroughbred racehorses. *Am J Vet Res.* 1993; **54**, 38–51.
10. Moore JN, Garner HE & Berg JN. Intracaecal endotoxin and lactate during the onset of laminitis. *Am J Vet Res.* 1979; **40**, 722–723.
11. Carroll CL, Hazard G, Coloe PJ & Hooper PT. Laminitis and possible enterotoxaemia associated with carbohydrate overload in mares. *Equine Vet J.* 1987; **19**, 344–346.
12. Blanchard TL, Elmore RG, Vamer DD *et al.* Dystocia, toxic metritis and laminitis in mares. *Proc Am Ass Equine Practnr.* 1987; **33**, 641–648.
13. Weiss DJ Geor RJ, Johnston G, & Trent, AM. Microvascular thrombosis associated with the onset of acute laminitis in ponies. *Am J Vet Res.* 1994; **55**, 602–612.
14. Hunt RJ. The pathophysiology of acute laminitis. *Comp Continuing Educ.* 1991; **13**, 1003–1010.
15. Eaton SA, Allen D, Eades SC & Schneider DA. Digital Starling forces and haemodynamics during early laminitis induced by an aqueous extract of black walnut (*Juglans nigra*) in horses. *Am J Vet Res.* 1995; **56**, 1338–1344.
16. Hood DM. Endotoxaemia as a direct cause of laminitis. *Am Ass Equine Pract.* 1995; **41**, 245–247.
17. Stephens KA. Studies on sublethal endotoxaemia in the horse. *Southwestern Vet.* 1984; **36**, 27–37.
18. Fessler JF, Bottoms GD & Rossel OF. Endotoxin induced change in haemograms, plasma enzymes and blood chemical values in anaesthetised ponies: Effects of flunixin megulamine. *Am J Vet Res.* 1982; **43**, 140–143.
19. Robinson NE & Dabney JM. Vascular response in the equine digit. *Am J Vet Res.* 1975; **36**, 1249–1253.
20. Amoss MS, Hood DM, Williams JD *et al.* Concentrations of plasma catecholamines, serum aldosterone and plasma renin activity following induced laminitis in the horse. *Southwest Vet.* 1988; **36**, 16–25.
21. Coffman JR & Colles CM. Insulin tolerance in laminitis ponies. *Can J Comp Med.* 1983; **47**, 347–351.
22. Field JR & Jeffcott LB. Equine laminitis – another hypothesis for pathogenesis. *Med Hypoth.* 1989; **30**, 203–210.
23. Watson TDG, Murphy D & Love S. Equine hyperlipaemia in the United Kingdom: clinical features and blood chemistry of 18 cases. *Vet Rec.* 1992; **131**, 48–51.
24. Colles CM & Jeffcott LB. Laminitis in the horse. *Vet Rec.* 1977; **100**, 262–264.
25. Hood DM, Hightower D, Amoss MS *et al.* Thyroid function in horses affected with laminitis. *Southwestern Vet.* 1987; **38**, 85–91.
26. Love S. Equine Cushings disease. *Br Vet J.* 1993; **149**, 139–153.
27. Eyre P, Elmes PJ & Strickland S. Corticosteroid-potentiated vascular response of the equine digit: a possible pharmacological basis for laminitis. *Am J Vet Res.* 1979; **40**, 135–138.
28. Muylle E & Oyaert E. Lung function tests in obstructive pulmonary disease in horses. *Equine Vet J.* 1973; **5**, 37.
29. Slone DE, Purohit RC & Ganjam V. K. Effects of dexamethasone and triamcinolone that may predispose to laminitis in horses. *Proc Am Ass Equine Pract.* 1981; **27**, 469–471.
30. O'Connor JJ. Affections of the feet. In: *Dollar's Veterinary Surgery*. London: Baillière, Tindall and Cox 1930; 912–917.
31. Bovenzi M, Giansante C, Fiorito A *et al.* Relation of haemostatic function, neurovascular impairment, and vibration exposure in workers in different stages of vibation-induced white finger. *Br J Ind Med.* 1985; **42**, 253–259.
32. Pascoe RR. Environmental skin disease. In: *Colour Atlas of Equine Dermatology*. London: Wolfe 1990; 18–33.
33. Dedrick P, Reef VB, Sweeney RW & Morris DD. Treatment of bacterial endocarditis in a horse. *J Am Vet Med Assoc.* 1988; **193**, 339–342.
34. Baxter GM. Equine Laminitis. *Equine Pract.* 1992; **14**, 13–22.

35. Hood DM, Beckham AS, Walker MA & Morgan SJ. Genetic predisposition to chronic laminitis in horses. *Proc Am Ass Equine Pract.* 1994; **40**, 45–46.
36. Hinkley KA, Feam S, Howard BR & Henderson IW. Nitric oxide as treatment for grass induced laminitis in ponies. *Equine Vet J.* 1996; **28**, 17–28.
37. Robinson NE. Digital blood flow, arteriovenous anastamoses and laminitis. *Equine Vet J.* 1990; **22**, 381–383.
38. Pollitt CC. Laminitis. In: *The Horse's Foot.* London: Wosby-Wolf 1995; 169–205.
39. Hood DM, Grosenbaugh DA & Slater MR. Vascular perfusion in horses with chronic laminitis. *Equine Vet J.* 1994; **26**, 191–196.
40. Roberts ED, Ochoa R & Haynes PF. Correlation of dermal-epidermal laminar lesions of equine hoof with various disease conditions. *Vet Pathol.* 1980; **17**, 656–666.
41. Hinkley KA, Feam S, Howard BR & Henderson IW. Near infrared spectroscopy of pedal haemodynamics and oxygenation in normal and laminitic horses. *Equine Vet J.* 1995; **27**, 465–470.
42. Hunt RJ. The pathophysiology of acute laminitis. *Comp Continuing Educ.* 1991; **13**, 1003–1010.
43. Baxter GM, Laskey RE, Tackett RL *et al. In vitro* reactivity of digital arteries and veins to vasoconstrictive mediators in healthy horses and in horses with early laminitis. *Am J Vet Res.* 1989; **50**, 508–517.
44. Allen D, Clark ES, Moore JN & Prasse KW. Evaluation of digital Starling forces and haemodynamics during early laminitis. *Am J Vet Res.* 1990; **51**, 1930–1934.
45. Hood DM, Gremmel SM, Arnoss MS *et al.* Equine laminitis III: Coagulation dysfunction in the developmental and acute disease. *J Equine Med Surg.* 1979; **3**, 355–360.
46. Johnstone IB & Blackwell TE. Disseminated intravascular coagulation in a horse with post partum ulcerative colitis and laminitis. *Can Vet J.* 1984; **25**, 195–198.
47. Weiss DJ, Geor RJ, Johnston G & Trent AM. Microvascular thrombosis associated with onset of acute laminitis in ponies. *Am J Vet Res.* 1994; **55**, 606–610.
48. Prasse KW, Allen D, Moore JN & Dubcan A. Evaluation of coagulation and fibrinolysis during the prodromal stages of carbohydrate-induced acute laminitis in horses. *Am J Vet Res.* 1990; **51**, 1950–1955.
49. Kirker-Head CA, Stephens KA, Toal RL *et al.* Circulatory and blood gas changes accompanying the development and treatment of induced laminitis. *Equine Vet Sci.* 1987; **6**, 293–301.
50. Pollitt CC & Molyneux GS. A scanning electron microscopic study of the dermal microcirculation of the equine foot. *Equine Vet J.* 1990; **22**, 79–87.
51. Molyneux GS, Haller CJ, Mogg K & Pollitt CC. The structure, innervation and location of arteriovenous anastomoses in the equine foot. *Equine Vet J.* 1994; **26**, 305–312.
52. Hood DM, Amoss MS, Highwater D, *et al.* Equine laminitis I: Radioisotope analysis of the foot during the acute disease. *J Equine Med Surg.* 1978; **2**, 439–444.
53. Robinson NE, Scott JB, Dabney JM & Jones GA. Digital vascular responses and permeability in equine alimentary laminitis. *Am J Vet Res.* 1976; **37**, 1171–1176.
54. Trout DW, Hornof WJ, Linford RL & O'Brien TR. Scintigraphic evaluation of digital circulation during the developmental and acute phases of equine laminitis. *Equine Vet J.* 1990; **22**, 416–421.
55. Cogswell AM, Johnson PJ & Adams HR. Evidence for endothelial-derived relaxing factor/nitric oxide in equine digital arteries. *Am J Vet Res.* 1995; **56**, 1637–1641.
56. Baxter GM. Alterations of endothelium-dependent digital vascular response in horses given low-dose endotoxin. *Vet Surg.* 1995; **24**, 87–96.
57. Hood DM, Amoss MS & Grosenbaugh DA. Equine laminitis: a potential model of Raynaud's phenomenon. *Angiology.* 1990; **41**, 270–277.
58. Ekfalck A, Jones B & Obel N. Possible importance for laminitis research of recent studies on substances influencing the differentiation of cultured keratinocytes. *J Vet Med Assoc.* 1991; **38**, 721–727.
59. Funkquist B. Aspects of studies on the pathogenesis of equine laminitis. *Equine Vet J.* 1992; **24**, 253–255.

60. Ekfalck A, Rodriguez H & Obel N. Histopathology in post-surgical laminitis with a peracute course in a horse. *Equine Vet J.* 1992; 24, 321–324.
61. Pollitt CC. Basement membrane pathology: a feature of acute equine laminitis. *Equine Vet J.* 1996; **28**, 38–46.
62. Pollitt CC. The basement membrane at the equine hoof dermal epidermal junction. *Equine Vet J.* 1994; **26**, 399–407.
63. May SA, Spiers S, Carter SD *et al.* Identification of tumour necrosis factor in the blood and peritoneal cavity of horses with colic. *Equine Vet J.* 1992; **Suppl. 13**, 19–21.
64. Obel N. Studies on the histopathology of acute laminitis. 1948. Dissertation, Stockholm.
65. Ekfalck A, Funkquist B, Jones B & Obel N. Incorporation of L-^{75}Se-cysteine in tissue fragments from the matrix of the hoof and the claw – a tool for studying the pathogenesis of laminitis? *Equine Vet J.* 1985; **17**, 377–380.
66. Coffman JR, Johnson JH, Finocchio EJ & Guffy MM. Biomechanics of pedal bone rotation in equine laminitis. *J Am Vet Med Assoc.* 1970; **156**, 219–221.
67. Goetz TE. Anatomic, hoof, and shoeing considerations for the treatment of laminitis in horses. *J Am Vet Med Assoc.* 1987; **190**, 1323–1332.
68. Baxter GM. Equine laminitis caused by distal displacement of the distal phalanx: 12 cases (1976–1985). *J Am Vet Med Assoc.* 1986; **189**, 326–329.
69. Eustace RA. Equine laminitis. *In Practice.* 1990; **12**, 156–161.
70. Koblik PD, O'Brien TR & Coyne CP. Effect of dorsopalmar projection obliquity on radiographic measurement of distal phalangeal rotation angle in horses with laminitis. *J Am Vet Med Assoc.* 1988; **192**, 346–349.
71. Semrad SD, Haedee GE, Hardee MM & Moore JN. Low dose flunixin meglumine: effects on eicosanoid production and clinical signs induced by experimental endotoxaemia in horses. *Equine Vet J.* 1987; **19**, 201–206.
72. Rowe JB, Lees MJ, Pethick DW *et al.* Prevention of laminitis resulting from carbohydrate overload in horses. *Aust Equine Vet J.* 1994; **1**, 29.
73. Redden RF. Minimizing complications of laminitis in horses. *Mod Vet Pract.* 1986; **67**, 446–450.
74. Hunt RJ, Brandon Cl & McCann ME. Effects of acetylpromazine, xylazine and vertical load on digital arterial blood flow in horses. *Am J Vet Res.* 1994; **55**, 375–378.
75. Baxter GM. Acute laminitis. *Vet Clin North Am.* 1994; **10(3)**, 627–642.
76. Stick JA. Laminitis. In: Robinson NE (ed.) *Current Therapy in Equine Medicine* 2nd edn. Philadelphia: WB Saunders 1987; 277–281.
77. Elliot J, Bryant CE & Soydan J. The role of nitric oxide in the response of equine digital veins to vasodilator and vasoconstrictor agents. *Equine Vet J.* 1994; **26**, 378–384.
78. Hood DM. Current concepts of the pathophysiology of laminitis. *Proc Am Assoc Equine Pract.* 1979; **25**, 13–20.
79. Belknap JK & Moore JN. Evaluation of heparin for prophylaxis of equine laminitis: 71 cases (1980–1986). *J Am Vet Med Assoc.* 1989; **195**, 505–507.
80. Cohen ND, Parson EM, Seahorn TL *et al.* Prevalence and factors associated with laminitis in horses affected with duodenitis/proximal jejunitis: 116 cases (1985–1991). *J Am Vet Med Assoc.* 1994; **204**, 250–254.
81. Cambridge H, Lees P, Hooke RE & Russel CS. Antithrombotic actions of aspirin in the horse. *Equine Vet J.* 1991; **23**, 23–27.
82. Davis LE & Westfall BA. Species differences in biotransformation and excretion of salicylate. *Am J Vet Res.* 1972; **33**, 1253–1262.
83. Baxter GM & Moore JN. Ellect of aspirin on *ex vivo* generation of throboxane in healthy horses. *Am J Vet Res.* 1987; **48**, 13–16.
84. Judson DG & Barton M. Effect of aspirin on haemostasis in the horse. *Res Vet Sci.* 1981; **30**, 241–242.
85. Goetz TE. The treatment of laminitis in horses. *Vet Clin North Am. Equine Practice.* 1989; **5**, 73–108.

86. Beckett RP, Davidson AH, Drummond AH, *et al.* Recent advances in matrix metalloproteinase inhibitor research. *Drug Discovery Today.* 1996; **1**, 16–26.
87. Redden RF. Complicated laminitis. *Proc Am Ass Equine Pract.* 1988; **34**, 311–320.
88. Hood DM, Beckham AS, Chaffin MK, *et al.* Comparison of phenylbutazone, Lily Pads and trimming on expressed pain in horses with chronic laminitis. *Proc Am Ass Equine Pract.* 1995; **41**, 248–250.
89. MacAllister CG, Morgan SJ, Boine AT *et al.* Comparison of adverse effects of phenylbutazone, flunixin meglumine and ketoprofen in horses. *J Am Vet Med Assoc.* 1993; **202**, 71–76.
90. Moyer W & Redden RR. Chronic and severe laminitis: a critique of therapy with heart bar shoes and hoof wall resection. *Equine Vet J.* 1989; **21**, 317–318.
91. Perenans K, Verschooten F, DeMoor A & Desmet P. Laminitis in the pony: conservative treatment vs dorsal hoof wall resection. *Equine Vet J.* 1991; **23**, 243–246.
92. Redden RR. 18° elevation of the heel as an aid to treating acute and chronic laminitis. *Proc Am Ass Equine Pract.* 1992; **38**, 375–379.
93. Allen D, White NA, Foemer JF & Gordon BJ. Surgical management of chronic laminitis in horses: thirteen cases. *J Am Vet Med Assoc.* 1986; **189**, 1604–1606.
94. Hunt RJ, Allen D, Baxter GM *et al.* Mid-metacarpal deep digital flexor tenotomy in the management of refractory laminitis in horses. *Vet Surg.* 1991; **20**, 15–20.
95. Hunt RJ, Kobluk CN & Steckel RR. Diseases of the foot. In: Kobluck, CN, Ames, TR & Geor RJ (eds) *The Horse. Diseases and Clinical Management.* Philadelphia: WB Saunders 1995; 669–678.
96. Buffa EA, Van Den Berg SS, Verstraete FJM *et al.* Effect of dietary biotin supplement on equine hoof-horn growth rate and hardness. *Equine Vet J.* 1992; **24**, 472–474
97. Stick JA, Jann HW, Scott EA & Robinson NE. Pedal bone rotation as a prognostic sign in laminitis of horses. *J Am Vet Med Assoc.* 1982; **180**, 251–253.
98. Eustace RA. *Explaining Laminitis and its Prevention.* Bristol: JW Arrowsmith Ltd 1992; 65–71.

2

Equine Hyperlipaemia

Tim Watson

Key Points

- Hyperlipaemia is a disorder of lipid metabolism that primarily affects ponies, donkeys and miniature horse and donkey breeds.
- Predisposing factors include breed type, sex, obesity, pregnancy and lactation.
- The condition is precipitated in animals at risk by anorexia, malnutrition, stress, or disease.
- Clinical signs are initially vague but patients rapidly deteriorate as fatty infiltration of body tissues results in organ failure.
- Plasma triglycerides in excess of 5 mmol/L are diagnostic. Animals with triglycerides between 1 and 5 mmol/L are in immediate risk of developing hyperlipaemia.
- A therapeutic programme should treat any concurrent disease, correct dehydration, electrolyte and acid–base imbalances, offer symptomatic treatment and nutritional support, and normalize lipid metabolism.
- Preventive strategies should address preventable risk factors, such as obesity, stress, malnutrition, intestinal parasitism, and pregnancy/lactation.

Introduction

Hyperlipaemia is a disease of equidae characterized by hypertriglyceridaemia and fatty infiltration of body organs. It was first described in the Netherlands in 1969 [1] and has subsequently been reported world wide [as reviewed in 2]. The condition primarily affects ponies and donkeys, including miniature types of each, and is associated with high mortality rates. The incidence of hyperlipaemia in such animals has been reported as 3–5% in population studies [3, 4] and 11–18% in surveys of animals presented to veterinary hospitals [5, 6]. A similar condition has also been reported in camelids [7]. The clinical course of hyperlipaemia is rapid and successful therapy is dependent upon early diagnosis and initiation of therapy.

Epidemiology

Several reports have indicated that hyperlipaemia is most commonly seen in small pony breeds, particularly Shetland ponies [1, 3, 8, 9]. By no means should the disease be considered exclusive to the Shetland, as Welsh mountain ponies [3, 9], Australian ponies [3] and pony crossbreeds [9] also feature in case reports. Hyperlipaemia is also a significant cause of mortality in donkeys, with a prevalence [4] similar to that in ponies [3]. Two retrospective studies have reported the occurence of hyperlipaemia in miniature ponies and donkeys; hyperlipaemia was diagnosed in 11% [5] and 18% [6] of such animals presented to veterinary hospitals in the USA. Hyperlipaemia is uncommon in horse breeds, although it has been reported in a Paso Fino mare [10] and a Quarter Horse with acorn poisoning [11]. Hyperlipaemia was also documented in three Standardbred colts, a Thoroughbred colt and mare, and an Arabian, all of which had severe multiorgan failure [12].

The incidence of hyperlipaemia is higher in mares than stallions and geldings [3, 8, 9]. This was recently borne out in a retrospective survival analysis, which showed that female donkeys were at significantly greater risk for developing hyperlipaemia than their male counterparts [4]. The hazard ratio associated with being female in that study was 2. The predisposition of mares to hyperlipaemia has previously been explained by the high incidence in pregnant or lactating mares [2]. In Reid and Mohammed's study [4], however, the risk posed by being female was independent of reproductive status.

Although hyperlipaemia is not commonly seen in animals less than 18 months of age, it has been described as a congenital condition in a Shetland pony foal born to a hyperlipaemic dam [13], and in three severely compromised foals of 1, 3.5 and 7 months of age [12]. Hyperlipaemia was also reported in four miniature horse foals and one miniature donkey foal by Moore *et al.* [5] and the minimum age at admission in the series of miniature horses reported by Mogg and Palmer [6] was 2 months. It is not clear, however, whether this represents a truly higher occurrence of hyperlipaemia in foals of miniature breeds compared with ponies and donkeys. In the analysis reported by Reid and Mohammed [4], older animals were at higher risk of hyperlipaemia than younger animals. It is conceivable that this reflects an age-related decline in insulin sensitivity (see section on *Pathophysiology*), as occurs in other species [14].

Some reports indicate a seasonal pattern to the occurrence of hyperlipaemia with peaks in the spring, between February and May in the northern hemisphere [1] and December and January in the southern hemisphere [8]. These patterns are consistent with the breeding season in each hemisphere and the predilection of the disease for the last trimester of gestation. However, the occurence of the hyperlipaemia in non-breeding animals, together with extended breeding seasons, mean that hyperlipaemia can be seen at any time of the year [9].

Hyperlipaemia is often seen as a complication of a primary disease process. In the published cases reports, concurrent or underlying disease was identified in 27–100% of cases [1, 3, 5, 6, 8, 9, 12]. Gastrointestinal diseases, specifically intestinal parasitism [1, 5, 8, 9], enteritis/colitis [1, 5, 6] and gastric and large intestinal impactions [1, 5, 6] are commonly identified. Other disease include dysphagia [9], oesophageal obstruction and ulceration [5, 6], intestinal lymphosarcoma [9], septicaemia [5, 12], hyperadrenocorticism [5, 12], peritonitis [6], metritis [8], laminitis [9], renal failure [12], hepatopathy [6], and hypocalcaemic tetany [6].

Many affected animals have a history of anorexia in the period immediately prior to the onset of clinical signs. In some cases this is directly attributable to the effects of the underlying disease process. In other cases food intake may have been reduced by inadequate pasture availability, insufficient supplementary feeding, following a change of environment or diet, or enforced starvation as part of the management of laminitis, oesophageal or intestinal disease. With the increased nutritional requirements of pregnancy, particularly in the last 90 days, and lactation, there is greater opportunity for malnutrition, especially when foods of inappropriate energy density are fed.

Two other important risk factors for hyperlipaemia are obesity and stress. As many as 90% of affected ponies were defined as being obese prior to the onset of hyperlipaemia in one survey [3], whereas other surveys reported 60% [8] and 67% [9] of cases as obese. The predisposition of obese donkeys to hyperlipaemia was confirmed in the survival analysis study, in which being obese was associated with hazard ratio of 1.5 [4]. The prevalence of obesity in the two retrospective studies of hyperlipaemia in miniature horses and donkeys was lower than in other surveys of ponies, at 11% [5] and 22% [6]. Stress factors implicated in the disease process include transportation, change of environment or diet, inclement weather, nutritional stress, and the stress of pregnancy/lactation and disease.

Risk Factors For Hyperlipaemia

The cases series and epidemiological studies clearly identify a number of risk factors for hyperlipaemia, which can be grouped as (a) preventable or unpreventable, and alternatively as (b) precipitating or predisposing factors (Table 1). The group of preventable risk factors includes obesity, stress, malnutrition, intestinal parasitism and pregnancy/lactation, whereas breed type, being female, anorexia and concurrent disease could be considered as unpreventable. In the

Table 1. **Two methods for the classification of risk factors for hyperlipaemia, which help identify animals at risk for implementation of preventive strategies and early initiation of therapy**

(a)		(b)	
Preventable	*Unpreventable*	*Precipitate*	*Predispose*
Obesity	Breed type	Anorexia	Breed type
Stress	Being female	Malnutrition	Being female
Malnutrition	Anorexia	Stress	Obesity
Intestinal parasitism	Disease	Disease*	Pregnancy/lactation
Pregnancy/lactation			

*Including intestinal parasitisim

alternative view, breed type, being female, obesity and pregnancy/lactation are seen as predisposing animals to hyperlipaemia, and anorexia, malnutrition, stress and disease precipitate disease. Although these schemes represent a generalization and oversimplification of what is a complex disease, they are consistent with what is known of pathophysiology of hyperlipaemia. Importantly, they do help to identify animals at risk of hyperlipaemia for implementation of preventive strategies, as well as the early detection and effective treatment of hyperlipaemia.

Pathophysiology

Energy is stored in adipose tissue in the form of triglycerides which are broken down to release non-esterified fatty acids (NEFA) when the body needs to draw upon its reserves, for example, when energy intake does not match energy expenditure. The hydrolysis of triglycerides is mediated by glucagon activating the enzyme hormone sensitive lipase (HSL) in the presence of low insulin and glucose concentrations, which normally inhibit HSL and counteract hydrolysis by promoting esterification of free fatty acids (Figure 1). The activity of HSL can also be induced by hormones associated with the response to stress (adrenocortotrophic hormone, glucorticoids, catecholamines) and pregnancy/lactation (progesterone and growth hormone), which in effect antagonize the inhibitory action of insulin.

Activation of HSL results in the release of NEFA into the circulation from where they can be taken up by tissues for oxidation as a source of energy. The majority of NEFA are taken up by the liver where they are used for the synthesis

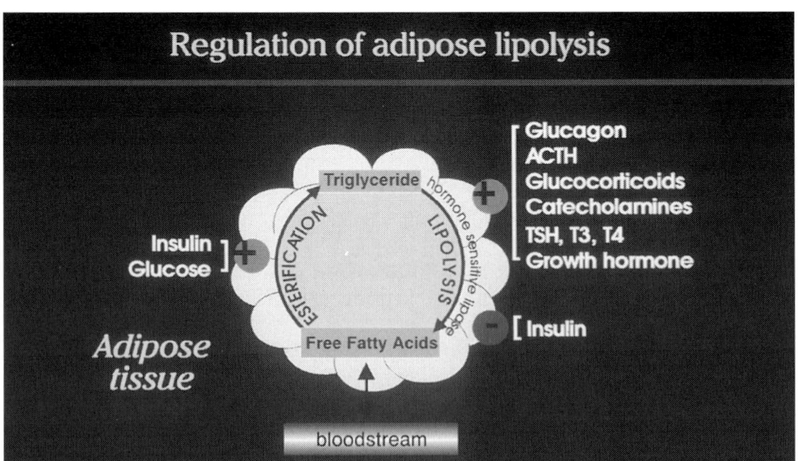

Figure 1. Schematic representation of the regulation of adipose triglyceride lipolysis. ACTH = adrenocorticotrophic hormone, TSH = thyroid stimulating hormone, T3 = tri-iodothyronine, T4 = thyroxine (N.B. free fatty acids = non-esterified fatty acids).

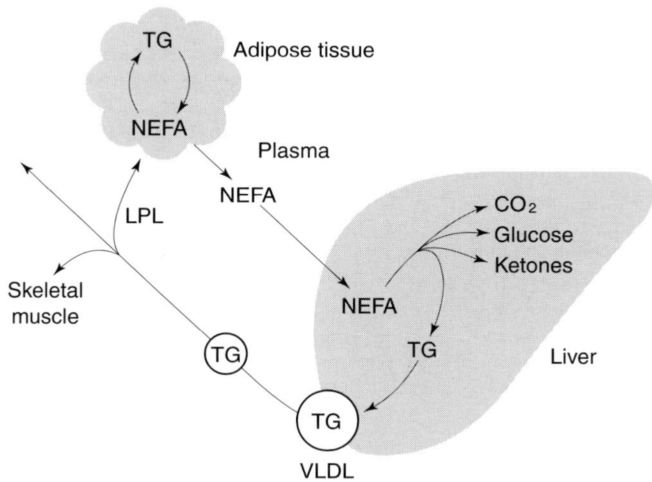

Figure 2. Schematic representation of the metabolic fate of non-esterified fatty acids mobilized from adipose tissue (NEFA = non-esterified fatty acids; TG = triglycerides; VLDL = very low density lipoproteins; LPL = lipoprotein lipase).

of ketones and glucose, or esterified to form triglycerides (Figure 2). The horse appears to have limited capacity for ketogenesis, as demonstrated by the fact that animals fasted for prolonged periods do not develop ketonaemia or ketonuria [15]. Triglycerides are exported from the liver in the form of very low density lipoproteins (VLDL) for transport to skeletal muscle and adipose tissue where they are used as a source of energy or stored.

When food is withheld from ponies, plasma NEFA concentrations rise [12, 15, 16, 17] consistent with the activation of HSL. The NEFA, however, appear to overwhelm the liver's oxidative, gluconeogenic, and limited ketogenic pathways and are channelled into triglyceride synthesis. This results in greater export of triglycerides in the form of VLDL, such that plasma VLDL [18–20] and hence triglyceride concentrations rise [12, 15, 17–20]. This same sequence of events occurs in animals with hyperlipaemia, albeit at a greater magnitude [12, 21]. A kinetic study [22] has shown that the greatly elevated plasma NEFA and triglyceride concentrations in these animals are due to an increased flux of NEFA to the liver and increased synthesis and secretion of VLDL triglycerides (Figure 3). However, the increased VLDL synthesis does not match the rate of triglyceride synthesis as triglycerides accumulate within the liver. The pathophysiology of hyperlipaemia in camelids differs in that these animals appear to have increased ketogenic capacity and develop ketonaemia and ketonuria in association with hyperlipaemia [7].

There has been some speculation that the raised plasma triglyceride might reflect reduced clearance of VLDL triglycerides from the circulation [18–20]. In one study, serum triglyceride and creatinine concentrations were correlated [12], suggesting that azotaemia may inhibit peripheral removal of triglycerides and

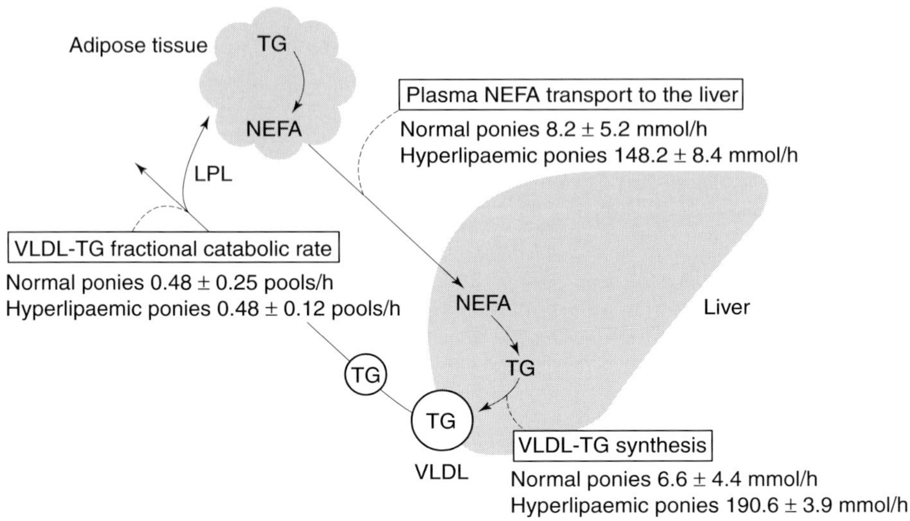

Figure 3. Schematic representation of non-esterified fatty acid (NEFA) and very low density lipoprotein (VLDL) metabolism in ponies with hyperlipaemia. Kinetic data are shown for NEFA transport to the liver, hepatic VLDL-triglyceride synthesis, and VLDL-triglyceride fractional catabolic rate in normal and hyperlipaemic ponies [22].

exacerabate hyperlipaemia [23]. There is also the possibility that endotoxaemia and the production of cytokines, particularly tumour necrosis factor, could reduce the activity of lipoprotein lipase [24], the enzyme responsible for the clearance of VLDL triglycerides. Clinical [21] and kinetic [22] studies have shown, however, that activity of lipoprotein lipase is increased, rather than reduced, in ponies with hyperlipaemia and that the fractional catabolic rate of VLDL is the same as that in normal ponies (Figure 3). Direct uptake of VLDL, by cells of the reticulo-endothelium system [25], may explain the widespread fatty infiltration seen in ponies with hyperlipaemia.

How do the Risk Factors for Hyperlipaemia Relate to the Pathophysiology?

Elucidation of the biochemical pathways responsible for the hypertriglyceridaemia in ponies with hyperlipaemia has helped explain the role of various risk factors for the disease. Tissue resistance to the action of insulin is a common feature of the risk factors for hyperlipaemia and results in ability to regulate the activity of HSL. Studies have shown that ponies are relatively insulin resistant compared with larger types of horses and that this is accentuated by obesity [26]. In other species, insensitivity to the action of insulin results in higher rates of adipose lipolysis, increased plasma NEFA, VLDL synthesis and secretion, and hypertriglyceridaemia [27]. Insulin resistance would, therefore, explain why plasma VLDL and triglyceride concentrations are higher in Shetland ponies than Thoroughbred horses [28], and why, in donkeys, plasma NEFA and triglycerides are positively correlated with body condition [29]. In addition, in donkeys with hyperlipidaemia/hyperlipaemia, plasma triglyceride and insulin concentrations were correlated and greater insulin values tended to occur in animals that were overweight [30]. Insulin resistance is also a feature of the equine pregnancy that becomes more pronounced towards term [31], when it is associated with increases in plasma NEFA and triglycerides [32, 33]. The increased risk associated with greater age [4] is consistent with an age-related decline in insulin sensitivity, as occurs in other species [34].

Thus multiple factors – breed, obesity, pregnancy/lactation – appear to act to diminish the ability of insulin to regulate HSL. Then, when the enzyme is activated in response to a negative energy balance or as a consequence of stress or concurrent disease, lipolysis progresses in an exaggerated and uncontrolled fashion. Non-esterified fatty acids are released in amounts that overwhelm the liver's oxidative, gluconeogenic and ketogenic capacity, such that triglycerides are produced resulting in hypertriglyceridaemia and hyperlipaemia.

Clinical Presentation and Signs

The clinical signs of hyperlipaemia usually reflect the existence of hepatic and, or, renal failure, resulting from fatty infiltration, and may be complicated by the manifestations of concurrent or underlying disease and by metabolic acidosis. Early symptoms are commonly anorexia and lethargy. At this stage, animals may also appear weak when walking (Table 2). Rapid progression of the disease is associated with the development of profound depression and eventual coma. Other neurological signs include reluctance to walk, incoordination and ataxia,

Table 2. **Major clinical signs of equine hyperlipaemia**

Initial signs
- anorexia
- lethargy
- weakness

Signs of progression
- reluctance to move, uncoordination, ataxia, muscular fasciculations
- Sham drinking, dysphagia
- Head pressing, circling
- Recumbency, padding of legs, nystagmus, champing
- Convulsions
- Profound depression, coma

Other signs
- weight loss
- ventral oedema, ascites
- mild, intermittent abdominal pain
- reduced intestinal motility and faecal output

muscular fasciculations after exercise, head pressing and circling. The appearance of sham drinking and dysphagia may be due to encephalopathy or primary oesophageal disease. In the agonal stages of the disease, the animal will become recumbent and show champing, nystagmus, and convulsions.

Some animals may have experienced rapid weight loss prior to presentation for veterinary attention and ventral oedema and ascites may be obvious in patients with hypoalbuminaemia. Mild, intermittent, abdominal pain may be exhibited as restlessness, flank watching and rolling. This may reflect primary gastrointestinal tract disease, such as an impaction, or enlargement of the liver and stretching of the hepatic capsule. Intestinal motility and faecal output are often reduced, which could be a factor in the prevalence of colonic impaction and enteroliths in animals with hyperlipaemia. Rectal examination often reveals a few hard, mucus-coated, faecal balls. Other clinical signs reported include pyrexia, tachycardia and tachypnoea, congested mucous membranes, icterus and halitosis. Pregnant mares may abort spontaneously or go into premature labour.

The clinical course of hyperlipaemia is rapid. In one study, the mean duration of signs prior to presentation at a veterinary hospital was 2.4 days, with a range of 1–7 days [6]. In another study, the affected ponies had been anorectic for 2–7 days (mean 5 days) prior to hospitalization [5]. The interval between first appearance of signs and death or euthanasia is typically 6–10 days; it is rarely greater than 3 weeks and can be as short as 3 days.

Diagnosis

The definitive method for the diagnosis of hyperlipaemia is the measurement of plasma triglyceride concentrations. Plasma triglycerides in excess of 5 mmol/L (~500 mg/dL) in ponies with clinical signs consistent with hyperlipaemia are diagnostic. In many cases the triglycerides are many fold in excess of this value, often in the range 20–80 mmol/L. In contrast to other species, in horses there is no requirement to withhold food in the 12–16 hours before sampling, as plasma triglyceride concentrations are not significantly increased following a meal in adult horses.

Triglyceride concentrations of less than 5 mmol/L, but greater than the upper limit of normality (1 mmol/L), may be found in ponies without clinical signs or evidence of hepatic lipid infiltration. This has been termed *hyperlipidaemia* [12] by certain authors and it has been suggested that these animals, if untreated, will go on to develop hyperlipaemia, particularly if food intake is insufficient and, or, the animal is pregnant/lactating [23]. This may not, however, always be the case as plasma triglycerides of 3–5 mmol/L are occasionally found in pregnant pony mares that do not go on to develop hyperlipaemia [TDG Watson, unpublished observations]. Regardless, it is best to assume that any horse with raised plasma triglycerides is at risk of developing hyperlipaemia and so managed to avoid precipitating factors such as stress or undernutrition.

The normal range of plasma triglycerides is higher in suckling foals because of their relatively high daily fat intake and concentrations greater than 1 mmol/L may be found [TDG Watson, unpublished observations]. The diagnostic criteria for donkeys are also slightly different in that plasma triglycerides in healthy, non-pregnant animals may be as high as 3.5 mmol/L [29]. There is, at present, no evidence to indicate that plasma triglyceride concentrations in miniature horses or donkeys differ from their full-size relatives.

Historically, hyperlipaemia was diagnosed by the recognition of gross lipaemia in blood samples centrifuged or left to stand so that the red cells sediment, or by the bluish surface colour of blood poured on to a dark surface [1]. Although these are characteristic features of gross lipaemia, lipaemia may not be obvious in animals with plasma triglycerides in the critical range of 1–5 mmol/L. Also, these tests do not give an accurate estimate of the severity of hyperlipaemia, on which the prognosis or response to therapy could be assessed. Plasma concentrations of other lipids, notably cholesterol, phospholipids and NEFA, are also raised [1, 12, 21, 35, 36]. However, the increases are not as marked as for triglycerides, making these parameters less useful for diagnostic purposes. Demonstration of lipid infiltration of the liver by examination of percutaneous biopsies is diagnostic, but should never be required given the ease, speed and diagnostic sensitivity and specificity of plasma triglyceride concentrations.

Clinical Chemistry

A number of blood chemistries are deranged in animals with hyperlipaemia, reflecting both the metabolic disorder and any concurrent or underlying disease. Chemistry panels are useful to assess the metabolic status of the patient and detect the presence and severity of organ failure. This is particularly important in deciding upon the patient's precise requirements for supportive therapies. A selective panel appropriate for this purpose is outlined in Table 3.

***Table 3.* Blood panel for the investigation and monitoring of patients with hyperlipaemia**

Metabolic status
- triglycerides
- glucose
- hydration – albumin, packed cell volume
- electrolytes – Na^+, K^+, Cl^-, Ca^{++}
- acid/base status – pH, HCO_3, pCO_2

Liver function
- gamma-glutamyl transferase, alkaline phosphatase
- bile acids
- ammonia

Kidney function
- urea, creatinine

Blood glucose concentrations may be normal, low, or increased depending upon the duration of anorexia, the previous use of oral or intravenous glucose preparations, and the presence of Cushing's disease. Neither ketonaemia [35] nor ketonuria [8] are seen in ponies or donkeys with hyperlipaemia, reflecting the low equine capacity for ketogenesis and the role of hyperinsulinaemia in the disease process. Metabolic acidosis is a consistent clinical feature with decreased arterial pH, carbon dioxide partial pressure and bicarbonate, and a base deficit of 0–24 mEq/L [8, 13, 36].

Fatty infiltration of the liver is associated with increased plasma activities of gamma-glutamyl transferase, alkaline phosphatase, lactate dehydrogenase and sorbitol dehydrogenase. Liver function may be reduced, as measured by plasma total bilirubin and bile acids concentrations, clotting times, and sulfobromophthalein sodium clearance. Blood ammonia concentrations are increased in some cases, but these require immediate analysis following collection and do not always correlate well with the degree of hepatic encephalopathy.

Urea and creatinine concentrations may be normal on presentation [11, 35], but tend to increase as the disease progresses when there is significant renal failure. Impairment of hepatic function may limit the reliability of blood urea nitrogen as an indicator of early renal failure. Increases in serum creatinine may simply reflect dehydration and return to normal following oral or intravenous rehydration.

Plasma albumin concentrations may be normal, increased in dehydrated patients, or reduced in patients with intestinal parasitism or chronic hepatopathy. Plasma protein electrophoretic patterns may be altered by concurrent diseases, such as intestinal parasitism. Although pancreatitis is a recognized complication of hyperlipaemia, serum amylase and lipase activities are not generally raised. This may reflect poor correlation between pancreatic pathology and plasma enzyme activities or be a consequence of interference by lipaemia in the analytical mathods [37]. This latter concern can be overcome by clearing the plasma or serum of lipaemia prior to analysis by ultracentrifugation or chemical precipitation [38].

Pathology

The significant post mortem findings in animals with hyperlipaemia relate to the deposition of excessive lipid (triglycerides) in body tissues. The liver and kidneys are most severely affected, appearing pale and swollen with a greasy texture. In severe instances, there may be fissuring of the liver or even rupture with catastrophic intra-abdominal haemorrhage. Skeletal muscle, the adrenal cortices, and myocardium may also be affected. Pancreatitis, with oedema and adhesions to surrounding organs, is also found in some cases. Nonspecific findings include focal haemorrhages, pulmonary oedema, myocardial infarction, renal infarcts and thrombosis of the caudal vein.

Histology confirms the presence of widespread lipid infiltration and reveals occasional venous thrombosis in a number of body tissues. A proliferative glomerulitis has been reported in conjunction with lipid infiltration of the kidneys [8]. Other histological findings include hyaline degeneration of skeletal muscle, nutritional atrophy of the exocrine pancreas and depletion of lymphoid follicles in the spleen and lymph nodes. Other gross and histological changes will reflect any concurrent disease.

Treatment

Therapy for animals with hyperlipaemia should be directed at (a) treating any underlying or concurrent disease, (b) correction of dehydration, electrolyte and acid-base imbalances, (c) symptomatic treatment, (d) nutritional support, and (e) normalization of lipid metabolism (Table 4).

Treatment of Underlying Disease

Given the high prevalence of intestinal parasitism in some reports of hyperlipaemia, it is prudent to treat all cases with an appropriate anthelminthic even though the worming history may appear adequate. Treatment of Cushing's disease with pergolide has been shown to alleviate hyperlipaemia [5] and septicaemia and bacterial infections should be treated with vigorous antibiotic therapy.

Supportive Therapy

Fluid therapy is essential for restoration and maintenance of circulatory volume, correction of electrolyte abnormalities and reversal of metabolic acidosis. Intravenous polyionic fluids, containing lactate or pyruvate as precursors of

***Table 4.* Objectives for the treatment of equine hyperlipaemia**

1. Treat any underlying or concurrent diseases
2. Fluid therapy
   - restore and maintain circulatory volume
   - correct electrolyte abnormalities
   - reverse metabolic acidosis
3. Symptomatic therapy
   - non-steroidal anti-inflammatories, analgesics, anti-ulcer preparations
   - reduce hepatic encephalopathy
   - plasma for hypoalbuminaemia, endotoxaemia, failure of passive transfer
4. Nutritional support
   - maintain positive energy balance
5. Normalization of lipid metabolism
   - reduce mobilization of plasma triglycerides – insulin and glucose
   - increase clearance of plasma triglycerides – heparin?

bicarbonate, should be used initially. These may, however, be ineffective in acidotic patients with severe liver failure, where intravenous bicarbonate should be administered. Bicarbonate should be used with caution as too rapid an increase in blood pH may exacerbate any hepatic encephalopathy and over-dosing can lead to persistent metabolic alkalosis and respiratory depression, as well as hypokalaemia in anorectic animals. For these reasons, bicarbonate is best reserved for patients with metabolic acidosis confirmed by blood gas analysis and the initial dose should not exceed 2 L of 5% sodium bicarbonate for an adult horse [39]. Dextrose should be included in the regimen for animals with hypoglycaemia, either supplementing the polyionic solution with dextrose or alternating with 5% dextrose. The latter may need to be supplemented with potassium chloride or calcium gluconate depending upon the patient's electrolyte status. Overdosing with dextrose will lead to transient or prolonged periods of hyperglycaemia associated with diuresis, dehydration and hypo-natraemia.

Symptomatic Therapy

Considerations for symptomatic therapy include non-steroidal anti-inflammatory drugs (inflammation, pyrexia, endotoxaemia), anti-ulcer preparations (ranitidine, sucralfate), and analgesics. Horses with hepatic encephalopathy may benefit from oral administration of neomycin and/or lactulose to reduce ammonia production and absorption (see Chapter 8). Long-term use of neomycin should be avoided because of the risk of antibiotic-induced enteritis. Plasma transfusions have been given to hyperlipaemic patients with hypo-albuminaemia, endotoxaemia, or foals with failure of passive transfer.

Nutritional Support

Nutritional support programmes are arguably the most important component of the therapeutic plan. The objective is to achieve and maintain a positive energy balance to limit the mobilization of NEFA from adipose tissue. Animals that are still eating should be offered fresh, highly palatable foods, such as newly cut grass, leafy hay, rolled grains, or meals with molasses added that have a relatively high energy density. This is particularly important in those animals identified as at risk of developing hyperlipaemia on the basis of raised plasma triglyceride concentrations. Given the rapid progression of the disease, I prefer not to rely upon voluntary food intake in animals with clinical signs and plasma triglycerides in excess of 5 mmol/L. In these cases, enteral feeding should be instituted using a nasogastric tube. There is then the option of using glucose and electrolyte solutions, commercial enteral formulations, or slurries made from hay or pelleted feeds.

Various oral glucose regimens have been used for the management of hyper-lipaemia, which generally equate to 100 g dextrose per day for miniature horses and small ponies. Because of concerns that excessive glucose administration may cause or exacerbate metabolic acidosis, it has been suggested that 100 g of galactose is substituted for glucose on alternate days [40]. Plasma glucose concentrations should be monitored on a daily basis as overzealous glucose administration, in combination with concurrent insulin insensitivity, can result in hyperglycaemia.

Wherever feasible, it is preferable to use more nutritionally complete formulations. Recipes for the formulations of tube feeds are available; these typically consist of a solution of water, dextrose, casein or dehydrated cottage cheese, dehydrated grass meal (e.g. lucerne or alfalfa) and electrolyte/vitamin mixes [41, 42]. Hyperlipaemia was successfully managed in five miniature horses using commercially available enteral formulations designed for horses [5]. The authors suggested that commercial preparations are advantageous in being relatively low residue, thereby avoiding any exacerbation of colitis, readily available, easy to store and administer, and associated with good clinical responses. A human enteral formula was successfully used to manage a miniature horse with hyperlipaemia [43].

The daily ration should be calculated and divided into a number (4–12) of smaller feeds so that the volumes does not exceed 3 L for miniature horses, 5 L for small ponies, and 7 L for larger ponies and horses. Moore *et al.* [5] outlined a regimen whereby daily digestible energy (DE) intake was calculated with respect to body weight (Mcal/day $= 0.975 + 0.021 \times$ body weight in kg), and then multiplied by a 'stress factor' of 1.2–2.0 to compensate for the increased metabolic rate associated with stress and hospitalization. These authors administered 75% of the basal DE on day 1, 100% of basal DE on day 2 and 75% of eventual DE on day 3 rising to 100% on day 4, to ensure gastrointestinal tolerance of the regime.

Some form of intravenous nutrition is indicated for patients with compromised gastrointestinal function (ileus, diarrhoea, reflux). In the majority of instances, this will take the form of constant intravenous infusion of 5% dextrose at 1–2 ml/kg BW.h. Although this will not completely meet the patient's energy requirements, it is generally of benefit. Overdosing with glucose may, however, cause diuresis, dehydration and hyponatraemia, and blood and urine glucose concentrations should be regularly monitored and balanced electrolytes added to the regime as required or, if dextrose, continued for more than 48 hours without enteral nutrition. The successful use of a human parenteral nutrition formulation in a miniature horse foal with hyperlipaemia has been reported [5]. The preparation was administered for 4 days and then reduced over 2 days as enteral feeding was introduced. Although this form of treatment is costly in terms of formulae costs, supportive care and monitoring, it is a viable option in miniature horses and small ponies for clients who are prepared for the expense.

Anabolic steroids and multivitamin preparations have been used to help stimulate appetite and assist hepatic function. Glucorticoids are strictly contraindictated on the basis that they stimulate HSL and may induce laminitis. The merits of aborting pregnant mares with hyperlipaemia is debatable. Abortion or premature labour is generally associated with a rapid recovery, presumably as a result of the reversal of a significant drain on the mare's energy supplies and the hormonal patterns that encourage insulin resistance. However, there is the associated risk of metritis and/or laminitis and the foal's chances of survival may be poor if the pregnancy is terminated prematurely. Foals should be weaned from lactating mares that develop hyperlipaemia.

Normalization of Lipid Metabolism

The goal is to return plasma triglyceride concentrations to normal. This can be achieved by (a) reducing the net release of NEFA from adipose tissue and (b) accelerating the removal of triglycerides from VLDL to adipose tissue and skeletal muscle.

The net release of NEFA reflects the activity of HSL and the rate of re-esterification of NEFA. Reversal of a negative energy balance, aversion of stress factors, and removal of the hormonal influence of pregnancy/lactation will limit the stimulus for lipolysis. The activity of HSL is inhibited by insulin, which is the basis for the widespread use of exogenous insulin the management of hyperlipaemia. Protamine zinc insulin has been used in the majority of case reports, with dosages ranging from 30 to 80 iu (0.1 to 0.3 iu/kg BW) by intramuscular injection once or twice daily. Insulin, in combination with oral or intravenous glucose, is also the primary mechanism by which re-esterification of NEFA can be promoted. The efficacy of insulin has been questioned because of the likelihood that hyperlipaemia patients are insulin resistant and there are no data from controlled studies. However, provided that insulin is administered only to patients that are normoglycaemic and receiving oral or intravenous glucose, there is no actual danger from the treatment. Nicotinic acid, which is an alternative inhibitor of HSL used in the management of certain hypertriglyceridaemias in humans, has not been evaluated in horses with hyperlipaemia.

Intravenous heparin (100–200 iu/kg BW, BID) has been used in a number of reports of hyperlipaemia in the belief that it increases the activity of lipoprotein lipase and hence the clearance of triglycerides from plasma. Heparin provides alternative binding sites for lipoprotein lipase molecules, thereby releasing the enzyme from its anchorage to capillary endothelium. The circulating lipoprotein lipase–heparin complexes become attached to VLDL, which has two potentially hazardous effects. First, there is continued lipolysis of triglycerides resulting in the release of NEFA into the circulation and to tissues other than the target adipose and skeletal muscle tissues. Second, there is recent evidence that presence of heparin directs the VLDL to direct uptake of these lipoproteins by the liver [44]. This would have the potentially detrimental effect of increasing the triglyceride content of an already lipidotic liver. Aside from these two theoretical drawbacks to heparin therapy, the rationale for its use has been questioned in the light of data suggesting that the activity of lipoprotein lipase is increased to its physiological maximum in ponies with hyperlipaemia [21]. Furthermore, there is a significant risk of inducing haemorrhagic episodes in animals with impaired clotting function.

Prognosis

The mortality associated with hyperlipaemia, including those animals that are euthanased, ranges in published reports from 57% to 85%. In animals that recover, the response to treatment is usually rapid, with plasma triglycerides returning to normal within 3–10 days [5]. The prognosis for some individuals is determined by the nature, extent and treatability of underlying or concurrent disease. It has been suggested that the prognosis is also dependent upon the severity of hyperlipaemia [1]. However, subsequent studies have shown that there is no difference in plasma triglycerides between those animals that recover from or succumb to hyperlipaemia [9, 36]. Animals with hyperlipidaemia, i.e. plasma triglycerides of less than 5 mmol/L, carry a much better prognosis once treatment is initiated [6].

Studies have also shown that blood chemistries cannot be reliably used to predict the outcome of the disease [9, 36]. However, favourable responses to treatment in terms of plasma triglycerides and other blood chemistries were associated with improvements in clinical demeanour and successful outcome. Daily use of the blood tests outlined in Table 3 is therefore recommended to monitor the efficacy of therapy. Failure of treatment to bring about rapid reductions in triglycerides in particular should be noted as a poor prognostic sign.

Prevention

The difficulties encountered in successfully treating hyperlipaemia place special emphasis on preventing the disease in animals at risk. The major focus will be on the preventable risk factors – obesity, exposure to stress factors, malnutrition, pregnancy/lactation, and some diseases, notably intestinal parasitism (Table 1). The anthelmintic programme should be reviewed and amended as appropriate. Pasture should be supplemented with good quality hay, if necessary, to maintain adequate nutrition, especially of pregnant mares. It is important to avoid 'clustering of risk factors', for example breeding from a grossly obese pony mare or subjecting a heavily pregnant, obese pony mare to transportation stress. Food intake and demeanour should be monitored carefully following changes in diet or environment and it may be worthwhile feeding high quality, energy-dense concentrates during this time to buffer any reduction in appetite or food intake. Drastic weight reduction programmes should be avoided. Exercise programmes, together with controlled feed intake, may improve insulin sensitivity in ponies and hence reduce the risk of hyperlipaemia [45].

As adjunct to these measures, plasma triglycerides can be monitored during pregnancy or following transportation to gain the earliest indication of hyperlipaemia. There are no data to suggest that pony mares that suffer hyperlipaemia during one pregnancy are at increased risk of developing hyperlipaemia in any subsequent pregnancies. Survival is improved significantly by early detection and treatment. Owners of animals at risk should therefore be advised to seek immediate veterinary attention for any animal that becomes dull, lethargic or anorectic.

References

1. Schotman AJH & Wagenaar G. Hyperlipemia in ponies. *Z Vet Med.* 1969; **A16**, 1–7.
2. Watson TDG & Love S. Equine hyperlipidemia. *Compend Contin Educ Pract Vet.* 1994; **16**, 89–97.
3. Jeffcott LB & Field JR. Epidemiological aspects of hyperlipaemia in ponies in southeastern Australia. *Austr Vet J.* 1985; **62**, 140–141.
4. Reid SWJ & Mohammed HO. Survival analysis approach to risk factors associated with hyperlipemia in donkeys. *J Am Vet Med Assoc.* 1996; **209**, 1449–1452.
5. Moore BR, Abood SK & Hinchcliff KW. Hyperlipemia in 9 miniature horses and miniature donkeys. *J Vet Intern Med.* 1994; **8**, 376–381.
6. Mogg TD & Palmer JE. Hyperlipidemia, hyperlipemia, and hepatic lipidosis in American miniatures horses: 23 cases (1990–1994). *J Am Vet Med Assoc.* 1995; **207**, 604–607.
7. Anderson DE, Constable PD, Yvorchuk KE, Anderson NV, St-Jean G & Rock L. Hyperlipemia and ketonuria in an alpaca and a llama. *J Vet Intern Med.* 1994; **8**, 207–211.
8. Gay CC, Sullivan ND, Wilkinson JS *et al.* Hyperlipemia in ponies. *Aust Vet J.* 1978; **54**, 459–462.
9. Watson TDG, Murphy D & Love S. Equine hyperlipaemia in the United Kingdom, Clinical features and blood biochemistry of 18 cases. *Vet Rec.* 1992; **131**, 48–51.
10. Murray M. Hepatic lipidosis in a post parturient mare. *Equine Vet J.* 1985; **17**, 68–69.
11. Field JR. Hyperlipemia in a quarter horse. *Compend Contin Educ Pract Vet.* 1988; **10**, 218–221.
12. Naylor JM, Kronfeld DS & Acland H. Hyperlipemia in horses: Effects of undernutrition and disease. *Am J Vet Res.* 1980; **41**, 899–905.
13. Gilbert RO. Congenital hyperlipaemia in a Shetland pony foal. *Equine Vet J.* 1986; **18**, 598–500.
14. Hirata A, Shimamoto K, Masuada A, Miyazaki Y, Fukuoka M & Imura O. Influence of ageing on insulin sensitivity in essential hypertensives and normotensives. *Hypertens Res.* 1995; **18**, 307–311.
15. Rose RJ & Sampson D. Changes in certain metabolic parameters in horses associated with food deprivation and endurance exercise. *Res Vet Sci.* 1982; **32**, 198–202.
16. Bauer JE & Ransone WD. Fatty acid composition of serum lipids in fasting ponies. Lipids. 1983; **18**, 397–401.
17. Baetz AL & Pearson JE. Blood constituent changes in fasted ponies. *Am J Vet Res.* 1972; **33**, 1941–1946.
18. Morris MD, Zilversmit DB & Hintz HF. Hyperlipoproteinemia in fasting ponies. *J Lipid Res.* 1972; **13**, 383–389.
19. Bauer JE. Plasma lipids and lipoproteins of fasted ponies. *Am J Vet Res.* 1983; **44**, 379–384.

20. Freestone JF, Wolfsheimer KJ, Ford RB *et al.* Triglyceride, insulin, and cortisol responses of ponies to fasting and dexamethasone administration. *J Vet Intern Med.* 1991; **5**, 15–22.
21. Watson TDG, Burns L, Love S *et al.* Plasma lipids, lipoproteins and postheparin lipases in ponies with hyperlipaemia. *Equine Vet J.* 1992; **24**, 341–346.
22. Watson TDG. Lipoprotein metabolism in the horse. PhD Thesis, University of Glasgow, Glasgow, UK 1991; 146–169.
23. Naylor JM. Hyperlipemia and hyperlipidemia in horses, ponies, and donkeys. *Compend Contin Educ Pract Vet.* 1982; **4**, 321–326.
24. Feingold KR, Marshall M, Gulli R *et al.* Effect of endotoxin and cytokines on lipoprotein lipase activity in mice. *Arterioscler Thromb.* 1994; **14**, 1866–1872.
25. Gianturco SH, Bradley WA, Gotto AM *et al.* Hypertriglyceridemic very low density lipproproteins induce triglyceride synthesis and accumulation in mouse peritoneal macrophages. *J Clin Invest.* 1982; **70**; 168–178.
26. Jeffcott LB, Field JR, McLean JG *et al.* Glucose tolerance and insulin sensitivity in ponies and Standardbred horses. *Equine Vet J.* 1986; **18**, 97–101.
27. Abbate SL & Brunzell JD. Pathophysiology of hyperlipemia in diabetes mellitus. *J Cardiovasc Pharmacol.* 1990; **16** (Suppl 9), S1–S7.
28. Watson TDG, Burns L, Love S *et al.* The isolation, characterisation and quantification of the equine plasma lipoproteins. *Equine Vet J.* 1991; **23**, 353–359.
29. Watson TDG, Packard CJ, Shepherd J *et al.* An investigation of the relationships between body condition and plasma lipid and lipoprotein concentrations in 24 donkeys. *Vet Rec.* 1990; **127**, 498–500.
30. Forhead AJ, French J, Ikin P *et al.* Relationship between plasma insulin and triglyceride concentrations in hypertriglyceridaemic donkeys. *Res Vet Sci.* 1994; **56**, 389–392
31. Fowden AL, Comline RS & Silver M. Insulin secretion and carbohydrate metabolism during pregnancy in the mare. *Equine Vet J.* 1984; **16**, 239–246.
32. Stammers JP, Silver M & Fowden AL. Effects of nutrition on uterine and umbilical venous plasma lipids in chronically catheterised mares in late gestation. *Equine Vet J.* 1989; **5** (Suppl), 37–40.
33. Watson TDG, Burns L, Packard CJ *et al.* Effects of pregnancy and lactation on plasma lipids and lipoprotein concentrations, lipoprotein composition and post-heparin lipase activities in Shetland pony mares. *J Reprod Fert.* 1993; **97**, 563–568.
34. Hirata A, Shimamoto K, Masuda A *et al.* Influence of aging on insulin sensitivity in essential hypertensives and normotensives. *Hypertens Res.* 1995; **18**, 307–311.
35. Eriksen L & Simesen MG. Hyperlipemia in ponies. *Nord Vet Med.* 1970; **22**, 273–284.
36. Wensing TH, Schotman AJH & Kroneman J. Various new clinical chemical data in the blood of normal ponies and ponies affected with hyperlipaemia (hyperlipoproteinaemia). *Tijdschr Diergeneeskd.* 1973; **98**, 673–680.
37. Alleman AR. The effects of hemolysis and lipemia on serum biochemical consitutents. *Vet Med.* 1990; **85**, 1272–1284.
38. Thompson MB & Kunze DJ. Polyethylene glycol-6000 as a clearing agent for lipemic serum samples from dogs and the effects on 13 serum assays. *Am J Vet Res.* 1984; **45**, 2154–2157.
39. Schmall LM. Fluid and electrolyte therapy. In: Robinson NE (ed) *Current Therapy in Equine Medicine*, 4th edn. Philadelphia: WB Saunders 1997; 727–731.
40. Wensing TH, Schotman AJH & Kroneman J. A new method in the treatment of hyperlipaemia (hyperlipoproteinaemia) in ponies. *Neth J Vet Sci.* 1973; **5**, 145–147.
41. Burkholder WJ & Thatcher CD. Enteral nutritional support of sick horses. In: Robinson NE (ed) *Current Therapy in Equine Medicine*, 3rd edn. Philadeliphia. WB Saunders 1992; 727–731.
42. Harris PA, Frape DL, Jeffcott LB *et al.* Nutritional aspects of metabolic disease (Hyperlipaemia). In: Higgins AJ & Wright IM (eds) *The Equine Manual.* London: WB Saunders 1995; 181–183.

43. Golenz MR, Knight DA & Yvorchuk St J. Use of a human enteral feeding preparation for treatment of hyperlipemia and nutritional support during healing of an esophageal laceration in a miniature horse. *J Am Vet Med Assoc.* 1992; **200**, 951–953.
44. Nykjaer A, Bengtsson-Olivecrona G, Lookene A *et al.* The alpha2-macroglobulin receptor/low density lipoprotein receptor-related protein binds lipoprotein lipase and β-migrating very low density lipoprotein associated with the lipase. *J Biol Chem.* 1993; **268**, 15048–15055.
45. Freestone JF, Beadle R, Shoemaker K *et al.* Improved insulin sensitivity in hyperinsulinaemic ponies through physical conditioning and controlled feed intake. *Equine Vet J.* 1992; **24**, 187–190.

3

Diseases of the Pituitary Gland, Including Hyperadrenocorticism

Han van der Kolk

Key Points

- Cushing's disease is a frequent diagnosis in aged horses, with a minimum age of 7 years, and is caused by adenoma of the pituitary pars intermedia.
- Common clinical signs include hirsutism, weight loss, lethargy, laminitis, polyuria and polydipsia, and hyperhidrosis.
- Cushing's disease cannot be ruled out in horses with normal plasma glucose concentrations.
- The measurement of corticoid: creatinine ratio in a morning urine sample is a useful screening test.
- Diagnosis is best confirmed using an overnight dexamethasone suppression test.
- Medical therapy with dopamine agonists (bromocriptine, pergolide) or serotonin antagonists (cyproheptadine) can be associated with improvements in clinical signs.

Introduction

A pituitary pars intermedia adenoma (PIA) was first described in horses in 1932 [1]. The first description of hirsutism associated with a PIA was in 1956 ("7 kg of hair was combed off a 18-year-old warmblood mare") [2]. Unfortunately, in 1966 PIA became firmly associated with hyperglycaemia [3] and, consequently, case reports of PIA deal almost exclusively with hyperglycaemia, weight loss [3–5], and polyuria/polydipsia [3, 6–13]. Although PIA without hyperglycaemia was in fact reported in 1982 [12], the condition was poorly recognized and, as a result, may have been rather underestimated.

This chapter is illustrated with data from 48 cases of equine PIA seen at the Large Animal Medicine Clinic, Utrecht University, which are hereafter referred to as 'the Utrecht cases'. The horses were presented between February 1990 and

October 1995 with PIA suspected on the basis of hirsutism. The diagnosis was confirmed at necropsy in all 48 cases.

Normal Equine Pituitary and Adrenal Anatomy

The pars distalis is surrounded by a large pars intermedia [14], and the former encloses the pars intermedia in a thin adherent layer [15]. In the horse, the diaphragma sella is poorly developed, thereby allowing dorsal expansion of the hypophysis [3]. The pars distalis and the pars intermedia were found to weigh 900 mg and 150 mg, respectively, in four normal horses [15]. Seventy normal pituitaries from Dutch warmblood horses comprising five stallions, 18 geldings and 47 mares, with an average age of 11 years, weighed 3.08 ± 0.53 g (mean ± standard deviation) and measured 22.8 ± 1.9 by 20.3 ± 2.1 mm in the transverse plane, and 11.3 ± 1.9 mm in the sagittal plane [van der Kolk, unpublished observations].

The secretory cells in the adenohypophysis are subdivided into acidophils, basophils and chromophobes. Basophils comprise cells that secrete both gonadotrophs and thyroid stimulating hormone (TSH). Chromophobes secrete adrenocorticotrophic hormone (ACTH) and melanocyte stimulating hormone (MSH). Approximately 10% of the pars distalis comprises corticotrophs and this region is rich in prolactin-positive cells [16].

Using the following procedure in an unrestrained horse, which has a 75% success rate, the intercavernous sinus near the outlet of the pituitary veins can be accessed, thereby facilitating collection of effluent for measurement of hormone secretion rates. A heparin-coated 50 cm silicone elastomer canula (internal diameter of 0.7 mm and outside diameter of 2.0 mm) with a 30° angle must be passed into the superficial facial vein, then into the deep facial vein, through the vena reflexa and into the ophthalmic vein. Next into and along the cavernous sinus until it reaches the posterior end, which is about 30 cm in a Standardbred horse [17].

The right adrenal gland lies against the caudal vena cava, and there are usually two short veins approximately 3 mm in diameter emptying directly into the vena cava. A vein emerging from the caudal pole of the left adrenal gland empties into the left renal vein. Many small arterial vessels approximately 1 mm in diameter were found supplying blood to each adrenal gland [18].

The Hypothalamic–Pituitary–Adrenocortical Axis

The inhibitory effect of cortisol on ACTH secretion was greater, when corticotrophin-releasing hormone (CRH) was the secretagogue instead of vasopressin in perfused equine anterior pituitary cells [19]. Equine CRH is a 41 amino acid peptide, probably identical in structure to human CRH [20]. Equine and human ACTH also have the same amino acid composition and biological activity [21]. In the pars intermedia, ACTH appears to be processed efficiently to α-MSH and corticotrophin-like intermediate lobe peptide [15].

Cortisol and corticosterone are the major plasma glucocorticoids in horses, with their ratio ranging from 8:1 in domesticated horses [22] to 168:1 in feral stallions [23]. In normal horses there is a diurnal rhythm of plasma cortisol [22, 24–28] with peak values in the morning. Cortisol concentrations do not appear to be affected by breed [26], age [24], sex [24, 26, 29] or pregnancy [24], but are elevated by exercise, during halothane anaesthesia [30], fasting [31], hypoglycaemia [26, 32], disease [33], and surgery [26]. The horse has relatively low concentrations of cortisol-binding globulin [34]. Consequently, a small increase in total plasma cortisol results in a large rise in bioactive free cortisol. The biological half-life of cortisol is approximately 2 hours [35].

Pituitary and Adrenocortical Pathology

When assessing pituitary dysfunction, it should be realized that exogenous glucocorticoids can have a prolonged effect on the hypophysis. For instance, the intramuscular administration of prednisolone acetate (0.6 mg/kg bodyweight (BW)) depressed adrenal gland responsiveness for 3 weeks [36]. Also, single intramuscular administration of 0.05 mg/kg BW of dexamethasone-21-isonicotinate suppressed cortisol production for 4–5 days [36]. Plasma cortisol concentrations returned to normal by 4 days after six intramuscular injections of dexamethasone alcohol (0.088 mg/kg BW) given at 5-day intervals [37]. Normal ACTH responses indicated that measurable adrenal atrophy did not develop. Daily intramuscular injections of 20 mg of dexamethasone alcohol resulted in death in one horse due to thromboembolic colic on the 22nd day and hypoadrenocorticism on the 11th day in another horse [33].

Pituitary pars intermedia adenoma is the most common disorder of the hypophysis. Other diseases of the pituitary include abscessation, which was reported in four horses with a history of fever and nasal discharge preceding acute neurological disease [38]. Multifocal corticotroph hyperplasia has also been reported as a frequent, although incidental, finding in the pars distalis of horses older than 9 years [16]. Cushing's disease usually results from adenoma in the intermediate lobe and only rarely from the anterior lobe [39]. In horses with PIA, 68% had macroadenomas that replaced most of the pars distalis. The other 32% of cases had microadenomas [16]. Hyperadrenocorticism associated with either adrenocortical tumours or ectopic ACTH production has not been reported in the horse. Although equine adrenocortical neoplasms have been reported, these do not appear to have been functional [40–43].

Pituitary pars intermedia adenoma grows by expansion, has a low mitotic index, does not metastasize, and usually involves chromophobes [3, 44]. However, the neurohypophysis can sometimes be infiltrated [3, 16]. Two PIA were classified as (potential) malignant transformations in one report [45]. The pituitaries of horses with Cushing's disease weigh approximately three to four times those of healthy animals [46]. In the reported cases, the PIA compressed the hypothalamus [3, 10, 44, 47], the pars distalis [3, 5, 6, 16, 39, 45, 47, 48], the optic chiasma [3, 44, 45, 47], and the pars nervosa [3, 5, 6, 39, 47]. In one other study no changes in the hypothalamus were observed [39].

Two different cell types are recognizable in PIA. The cells of the first type appear large and cylindrical, with a round to oval, sometimes indented, nucleus. In these cells, granules are dispersed throughout the cytoplasm. The cells of the second type are small and elongated. However, the occurrence of so-called Crooke's cells has been excluded [39]. The presence of ACTH-producing neoplastic cells in a PIA has been demonstrated [9]. The tumour cells were lacking in immunoreactivity to luteinizing hormone (when the human hormones were used), TSH, and growth hormone. Weak prolactin immunoreactivity was found in a few cells. Follicle stimulating hormone-immunoreactive cells occurred in tumours in follicle-like structures [39].

Immunocytochemical evaluation of PIA revealed a strong cytoplasmic reaction for pro-opiolipomelanocortin peptides (POMC), a moderate to strong reaction for α-MSH and β-endorphin, a weak reaction for ACTH, and negative immunostaining for prolactin (using equine prolactin), glial fibrillary acidic protein, and neurone-specific enolase [16]. However, the immunostaining of PIA was similar of that of non-neoplastic pars intermedia [16, 46, 49].

There is conflicting evidence over whether adrenal cortex hyperplasia occurs [4, 5, 12, 14, 47–50] or not [2, 6] in horses with PIA. In larger surveys, hyperplasia of the adrenal cortex was evident in about 20% of cases [16, 39].

Pathophysiology

The hypothesis that Cushing's disease or hyperadrenocorticism may result from a loss of the dopaminergic innervation of the pars intermedia is consistent with the finding that the dopamine concentration of PIA tissue was less than 12% of normal [46]. The disease is attributed to an over-production of POMC peptides in addition to space-occupying effects, resulting in dysfunction of the hypothalamus and neurohypophysis [16]. Horses with PIA are highly resistant to glucocorticoid negative feedback inhibition of plasma ACTH secretion as glucocorticoids inhibit pars distalis, but not pars intermedia, secretion of POMC peptides [12]. Although plasma ACTH is elevated, the levels of α-MSH, corticotrophin-like intermediate lobe peptide, β-MSH, and β-endorphin are disproportionately increased [12]. The overall post-translational processing of POMC peptides in PIA appears to be similar to that in normal pars intermedia [15], but adenomatous tissue secretes some ACTH that is biologically inactive [12, 49] and a higher proportion of opiate-active β-endorphin [46]. Plasma and cerebrospinal fluid immunoreactive β-endorphin concentrations were 60- and 120-fold higher, respectively, in horses with Cushing's disease [46].

Hirsutism, it is proposed, is related to either excessive testosterone secretion from the adrenal cortex [14] or excessive secretion of MSH [45]. The pathophysiology of laminitis in horses with PIA relates to the hypothesis that the hoof vasculature is under sympathic vasomotor tone, of both neurogenic (noradrenaline) and humoral (adrenaline) origin. Corticosteroids might create venous obstruction in the distal part of the limb by enhancing the venoconstrictor potency of adrenaline, noradrenaline and serotonin [51]. Although this hypothesis would be supported by a loss of the diurnal rhythm, there is conflicting evidence whether there is a loss of the diurnal rhythm in cortisol secretion [10, 12, 47, 52] or not [39] in horses with PIA.

Clinical Signs and Complications

Cushing's disease is a frequent diagnosis in aged horses, with a minimum age of 7 years [12, 16]. The prevalence in horses admitted to Utrecht University in 1991 was 0.5% [45]. The Utrecht cases comprised 23 Warmblood horses and 25 ponies. They ranged in age from 12 to 35 years (mean 21.1 years) and comprised 22 geldings and 26 mares. This average age is in agreement with previously reported means of 18.2 [39], 19 [16], 20.2 [53], and 21 years [46]. There is no apparent sex predisposition to the disease, although it has been suggested that it occurs more commonly in females than in males [16, 39]. In contrast, other authors have reported an apparent male predilection [49, 53]. An increased prevalence in ponies has been reported [53].

Initially, horses with PIA show a remarkable clinical sign, namely hirsutism, which is an excessively long and curly coat, often with a history of failure to shed (Figures 1 and 2). Incidentally, black and dark brown hair can change in colour to light (golden) brown. Other clinical signs include hyperhidrosis [3, 12, 14, 39, 47, 53], polyphagia [5, 6, 14, 48], and, in 12–60% of cases, bulging of supraorbital fat [39, 45, 53]. It is important to realize that horses with Cushing's disease do not always show signs of polyuria and polydipsia [45, 54].

The six most common clinical signs are hirsutism, weight loss, lethargy (e.g. poor performance), laminitis, polyuria and polydipsia, and hyperhidrosis (Table 1). The prevalence of these signs within individual horses with PIA ranges from three to all six, with an average of five being present [53]. The onset of the clinical signs is generally insidious over the preceding 18 months [12] to 4 years [8], and hirsutism has been traced back in a 23-year-old pony gelding to 10 years prior to presentation via yearly photographs.

The two major complications of PIA are diabetes mellitus with concurrent weight loss, and laminitis, which occur in approximately 38% and 24% of cases, respectively [45]. Other complications include secondary infections, infertility, pseudolactation, delayed wound healing, bilateral blindness, seizures, and

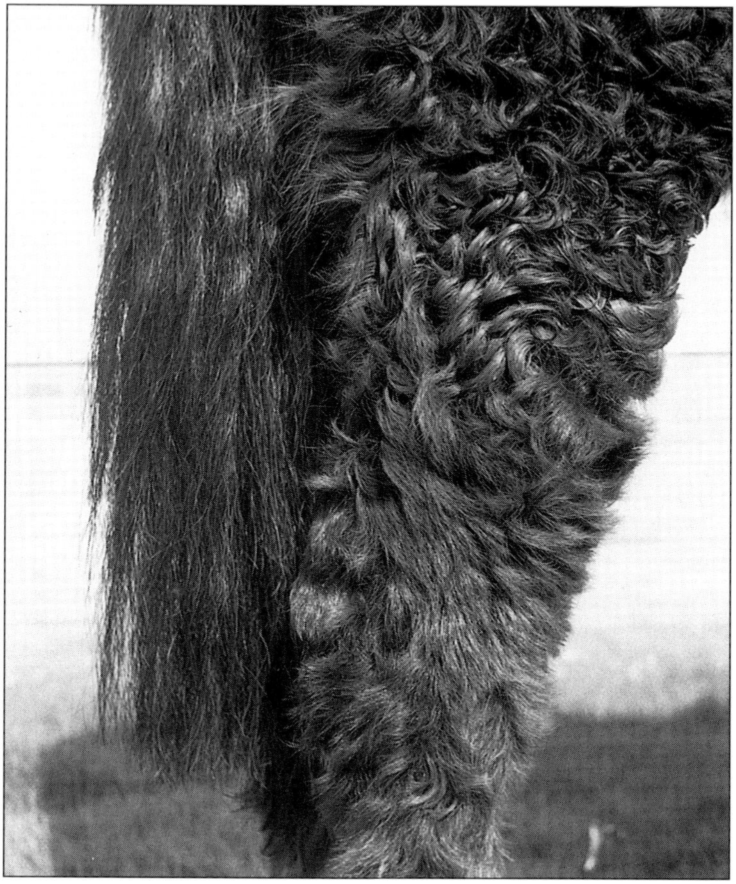

Figure 1. Hirsutism in a 20-year-old Warmblood mare.

diabetes insipidus. In cases where there is secondary diabetes mellitus or diabetes insipidus, polyuria and polydipsia can be seen. However, diabetes mellitus without apparent polydipsia has also been reported [4, 5, 45]. Seizures in combination with hyperglycaemia have been reported [45, 47]. Horses with PIA are particularly susceptible to secondary infection, such as alveolitis [39, 49], osteomyelitis [39], pneumonia [4, 53], mycotic pneumonia [44, 47, 49], bronchopneumonia [9, 39, 50], subsolar abscesses [55], abscesses in the wall of the colon [5], conjunctivitis [6, 9, 53], sinusitis [4, 45, 50], tibiotarsal synovitis [50], tendinitis [45], pleural abscesses [9], buccal and gingival ulcers [4, 9, 11], abscesses adjacent to the sternum [3], posthitis with paraphimosis [3], tongue abscess [49], parapharyngeal abscess [49], meningitis [45], peritonitis [45], mycotic encephalitis [49], cystitis [4, 53], and vaginitis [10]. Bacteria commonly isolated include *Klebsiella pneumoniae* [9], *Staphylococcus aureus* [4, 9], β-haemolytic streptococci [3, 9], *Rhodococcus equi*, and *Streptococcus zooepidemicus*. In one study,

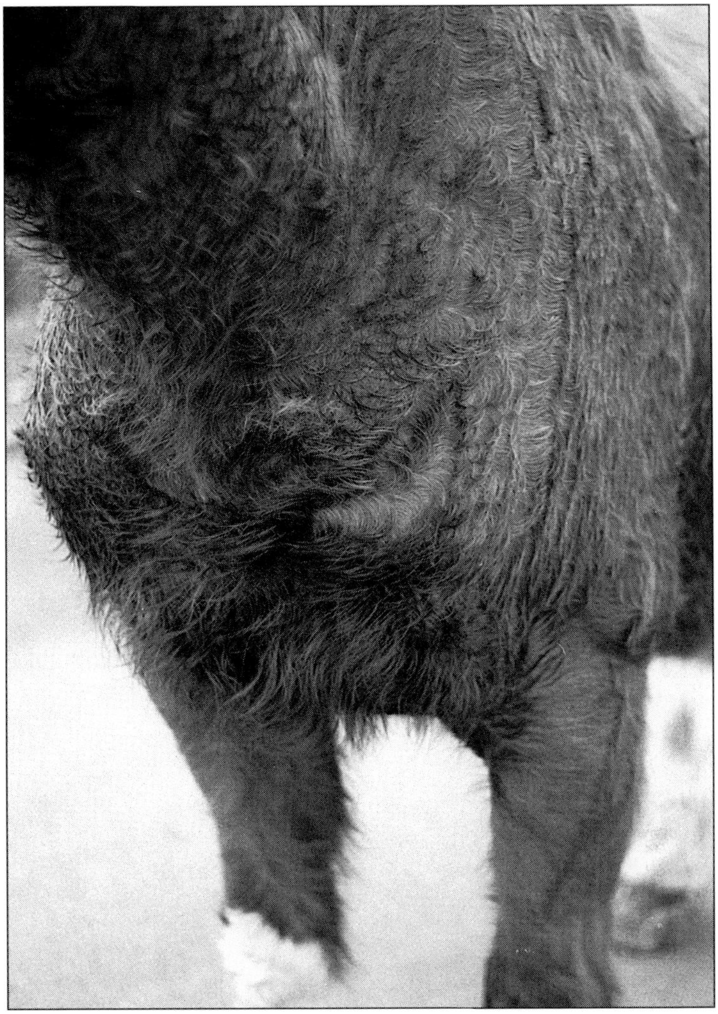

Figure 2. Hirsutism in a 22-year-old Warmblood gelding.

Table 1. Clinical presentation of Cushing's disease in horses

Common Clinical Signs	*Major Complications*
Hirsutism	Diabetes mellitus
Lethargy, poor performance	Laminitis
Hyperhidrosis	Secondary infections
Bulging of supraorbital fat	Reproductive dysfunction
	Delayed wound healing
	Bilateral blindness
	Seizures
	Diabetes insipidus

37% of horses suffering from PIA had bacterial and fungal infections suggested to be sequelae of immunosuppression, and 71% of these had hyperglycaemia [16].

Although infertility is well recognized as a complication of PIA, normal oestrous cycles [2, 47] and pregnancy do occur in horses with PIA (Figure 3). One out of 21 cases showed bilateral blindness associated with Wallerian degeneration of the optic tract [45]. Osteoporosis is not generally evident, although fractures have been reported of the lower jaw [39, 45], multiple ribs [3, 16], the pedal bone [48], and the pelvis following trauma [45]. Hypertrophic osteopathy has also been associated with PIA [56]. There is no evidence of multiple endocrine neoplasia, except for two horses with concurrent phaeochromocytomas, two horses with thyroid adenomas [16], and a horse with a thyroid follicular carcinoma with metastasis [57].

No relationship was found between relative pituitary weight in horses with Cushing's disease and symptoms (laminitis, bilateral blindness and seizures) or plasma concentrations of ACTH, cortisol, glucose and insulin [58].

A pars distalis hyperplasia has been described in a 25-year-old gelding suffering from anorexia, slight hirsutism, fat deposition in the neck region, and polyuria and polydipsia [39].

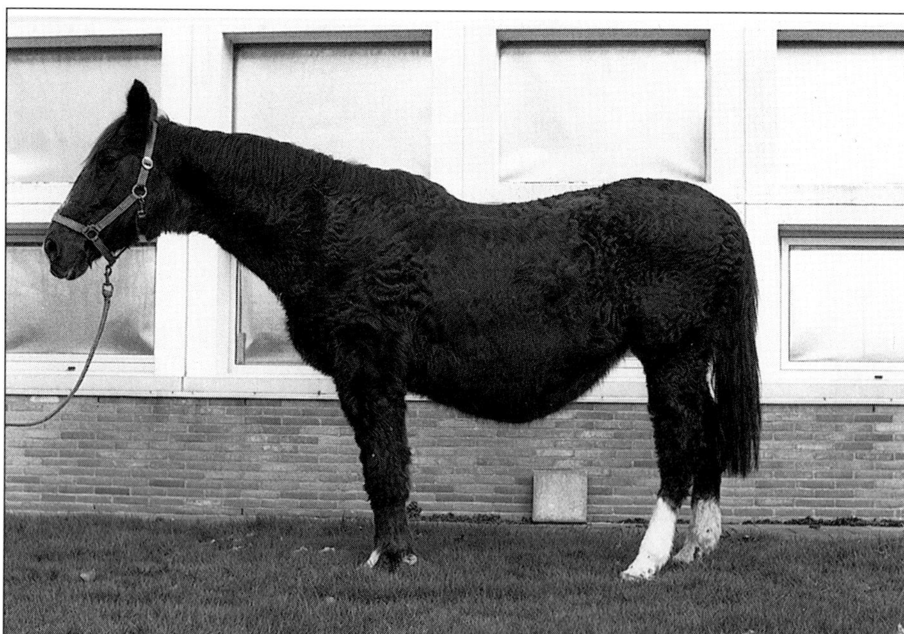

Figure 3. A 20-year-old pregnant Warmblood mare at term with a pituitary pars intermedia adenoma and secondary diabetes mellitus. The mare delivered a poorly grown foal, which died soon after birth.

Clinical Pathology

The laboratory findings from the Utrecht cases are summarized in Table 2. There was relative neutrophilia and relative lymphopenia, which was in agreement with the results reported by others [4, 10, 12, 39, 47, 59]. The mean alkaline phosphatase activity was higher than the upper reference value and this test had a sensitivity of 34%.

In addition to these findings, absolute neutrophilia and lymphopenia have been reported [9, 39], as has eosinopenia [9, 10, 47, 49, 59]. As the equine species is rather deplete in eosinophils in peripheral blood, the latter is difficult to interpret. In one case series, eosinopenia was present in 69% of cases, whereas eosinophilia was present in 12% [53]. A normal white cell distribution has also been described [8]. Haematology, therefore, offers little assistance in the diagnosis of PIA.

Increased serum activities of aspartate aminotransferase [4, 6, 8], creatine kinase [6], sorbitol dehydrogenase [4, 39], gamma-glutamyl transferase [11, 59], and alkaline phosphatase [6, 8, 11] have been reported. Normal alkaline phosphatase activity has also been found [59]. In a horse with PIA, bands 8 to 13 of alkaline phosphatase activity (when focused on agarose gels with a pH gradient of 3.5–9.5) were very prominent, but not specific for the disease [60].

Glycogen is the primary component of cytoplasmic vacuolation of hepatocytes caused by glucocorticoids [61], which leads to enlargement of liver cells [3] in horses with PIA. Other authors have reported marked hepatocyte swelling with cytoplasmic droplets containing fat [8]. However, on the basis of the

Table 2. **Selected clinical pathology data from horses with PIA presented to Utrecht University**

Parameter	*Units*	*n*	*Mean (SD)*	*Range*	*Normal Range*	*Diagnostic Sensitivity*
White cell count	g/L	33	8.5 (3.6)	1.3–19.1	7–10	39%
Eosinophils	%	20	0.95 (1.6)	0–5	< 4	ND
Neutrophils	%	20	78.8 (12.7)	46–94	35–60	ND
Lymphocytes	%	20	18.7 (11.7)	3–47	30–35	ND
Total protein	g/L	32	70.0 (7.9)	51–83	60–90	9%
Albumin	g/L	32	34.2 (6.0)	21.9–43.0	21–50	0%
Alpha-globulin	g/L	32	8.1 (2.4)	3.3–13.8	9–18	69%
Beta-globulin	g/L	32	16.5 (5.6)	6.6–38.4	< 20	19%
Gamma-globulin	g/L	32	11.0 (4.1)	3.0–18.6	< 23	0%
Alkaline phosphatase	U/L	35	512 (1342)	57–8290	140–300	34%
Glucose	mmol/L	36	7.4 (3.2)	4.2–17.3	3.9–5.6	64%
Urine specific gravity		18	1.036 (0.009)	1.022–1.047	> 1.025	17%
Plasma ACTH	pg/mL	19	427 (343)	58–> 1000	< 55	100%
Plasma insulin	μU/mL	17	122 (80)	30–260	< 57	77%

ND = not determined, SD = standard deviation, ACTH = adrenocorticotrophic hormone.

observation that steroid hepatopathy is not commonly associated with PIA in horses, the equine liver appears less sensitive to the effects of corticosteroids than that of other species. Corticosteroid-induced hepatopathy has been reported after three intramuscular injections of triamcinolone acetonide (412 mg in total) [61].

Plasma glucose concentrations were available for 36 of the Utrecht cases (Table 2) and in only 25% of the Utrecht cases of PIA did the concentrations exceed 9.0 mmol/L. The sensitivity of plasma glucose concentrations was 64%. The former was similar to the 26% prevalence of hyperglycaemia in another report [16]. Hyperglycaemia, defined as blood glucose >5.6 mmol/L, had a prevalence of 75% in another case series [53].

Urinalysis in 18 of the Utrecht cases revealed a normal mean specific gravity (Table 2), which is very similar to the results found by others [3, 4, 5, 9, 10, 48]. The urine specific gravity in normoglycaemic horses with PIA was not different from that in hyperglycaemic horses with PIA. Two very low values in the literature (1.005 [3] and 1.009 [8]) might have been due to central diabetes insipidus.

The mean basal concentrations of ACTH and insulin were increased in the Utrecht cases (Table 2). The maximal reported basal plasma ACTH concentration in a horse with PIA was 13 000 pg/mL [10]. Release of ACTH in horses with PIA is much larger than that observed in normal horses, although it is not as pronounced as release of the other POMC-derived peptides [12, 15]. Although an elevated basal plasma insulin concentration is a common finding in horses with Cushing's disease [6, 12, 13, 39], PIA cannot be ruled out in cases which have normal basal plasma insulin concentrations [9]. The mean insulin concentration in the Utrecht cases ($122 \pm 80\,\mu$U/mL) was very similar to that reported from 11 hyperglycaemic horses ($110.0 \pm 57.8\,\mu$U/mL) [62]. Basal concentrations of other hormones have been reported, including serum progesterone (0.795 nmol/L), testosterone (0.277 nmol/L), dehydroepiandrosterone (0.34 ng/mL), and androstenedione (0.09 ng/mL) [12]. Basal thyroxine (T_4) and tri-iodothyronine (T_3) concentrations have been reported as normal [13] or decreased [8].

Diagnosis

The diagnosis of hyperadrenocorticism remains a clinical challenge. Many tests have been used successfully, such as the dexamethasone suppression test (DST) [4, 10, 11, 13, 47, 52, 53], the ACTH stimulation test [4, 6, 9, 10, 12, 13, 47, 59], the combined DST/ACTH stimulation test [8, 9, 53], the insulin/glucose tolerance test [3, 5, 10, 12, 47], the oral glucose absorption test [8, 9], and the thyrotrophin releasing hormone (TRH) test [53, 62]. In addition, ventrodorsal radiography [63] and computed tomography [4] have been successful, as well as single samples for basal ACTH [6, 45, 54], insulin [45, 54, 62, 64], and the urinary corticoid:creatinine (c:c) ratio [54, 65]. In contrast, single samples for basal cortisol concentration are of no diagnostic value [6, 9, 10, 13, 16, 45, 47, 62], as they are within normal limits in 47% of cases [53].

The collection of a morning urine sample for the assessment of the c:c ratio can be useful as a screening test. The Utrecht cases had a mean c:c ratio of $67 \pm 110 \times 10^{-6}$ (range 8–500; sensitivity 83%) and an urinary corticoid concentration of 904 ± 849 nmol/l (sensitivity 83%). However, false negative and false positive cases were found [65]. In seven control horses the mean urinary c:c ratio was $11 \pm 4.3 \times 10^{-6}$ (range 4.7–16; critical value >20) [54, 65]. The urinary c:c ratio can be affected by other factors, such as exercise. For example, analysis of urine from two horses taking part in a Concours Sauter International event revealed urinary corticoid concentrations of greater than 1000 nmol/l and c:c ratios in excess of 35×10^{-6} [van der Kolk, unpublished observations]. There was no correlation between basal plasma cortisol concentration and the concentration of urinary corticoids in horses with PIA (Figure 4). This is in agreement with the finding that only 9.5% of variation in urinary cortisol could be explained by the influence of plasma cortisol [29].

In normal horses, the DST (Table 3) resulted in a 69% decrease in plasma cortisol 24 hours later [66]. A significant dose-related suppression in plasma cortisol concentrations was also observed in control horses 16 hours after dexamethasone administration (5, 10, 20, or 40 μg/kg BW, IM), with the 40 μg/kg BW dose causing maximal blockade, which was in contrast to horses with PIA [52]. There was no difference in plasma cortisol concentrations between DST initiated at either 9 am or 9 pm in healthy horses [67]. Using the overnight DST (Table 3), all healthy horses had plasma cortisol concentrations of less than 27.6 nmol/L 20–24 hours after dexamethasone administration. In contrast to

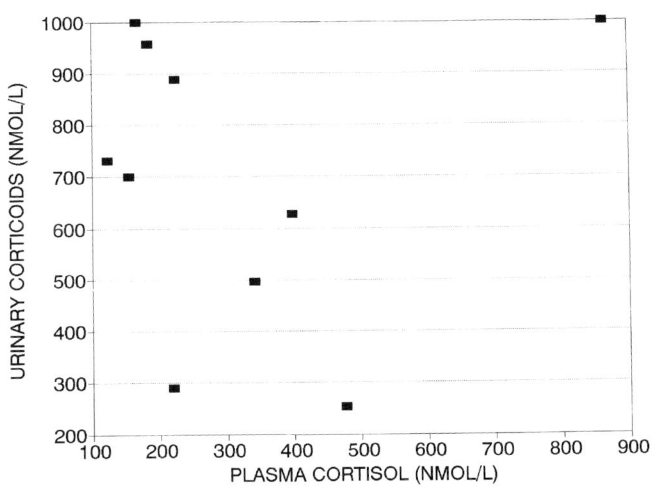

Figure 4. Plasma cortisol concentration (nmol/L) versus urinary corticoid concentration (nmol/L) in 10 horses with pituitary pars intermedia adenoma.

***Table 3.* Protocols for dynamic endocrinological function tests for the diagnosis of PIA in horses**

Dexamethasone suppression test
Assess plasma cortisol concentrations before and 24 hours after 10–20 mg dexamethasone i.m. at 09.00 hours [66].

Overnight dexamethasone suppression test
Blood sample for cortisol assessment are collected prior to and 20 hours after 40 μg of dexamethasone/kg BW i.m. at 17.00 hours [52].

ACTH stimulation test
Plasma cortisol concentrations are assessed before and 2 hours after 25 iu of synthetic $ACTH_{1-24}$ IV at 09.00 hours [45].

Combined dexamethasone suppression/ACTH stimulation test
Plasma cortisol concentrations are assessed immediately before and 3 hours after 10 mg dexamethasone i.m. at 09.00 hours. After collection of the 3-hour post-dexamethasone blood sample, 100 mg of synthetic ACTH is administered IV and a third blood sample is collected 2 hours later at 14.00 hours [69].

Thyrotropin-releasing hormone response test
1 mg of TRH is given IV and blood samples collected at 0 and 0.5 hours [62] for cortisol assessment.

TSH response test
After taking a basal blood sample in the morning, 5 iu of (bovine) TSH is administered IV. A blood sample is collected 4 hours later for measurement of T_4 and T_3 [62].

Intravenous glucose tolerance test
This can be done in nonfasted horses, using 50% dextrose at a dosage of 0.5 g/kg BW. Blood samples are taken 0, 0.25, 0.5, 1, 2, 3, 4, 5, and 6 hours after glucose administration [64].

Ventrodorsal radiography in combination with contrast venography
A 2 cm skin incision is made over the facial veins. Catheters are advanced into the deep facial veins and cavernous sinuses near the outflow tract of the pituitary gland. Their positions are confirmed with plain radiographs. Twenty millilitres of diatrizoate meglumine is then injected into both catheters [63].

the above, all horses with PIA ($n = 43$) had values >27.6 nmol/L at 20 and 24 hours [52]. The performance of the overnight DST is equivalent to the 24-hour DST, with maximal sensitivity (100% at 20 hours) and specificity [52].

There appear to be no major complications with the DST. Clinical evidence of acute laminitis or other complications was not observed in horses with PIA or control horses after a single dose of dexamethasone, and as a result the overnight DST is a reliable clinical test [52]. No laminitis was reported following other endocrine tests [53], although an acute episode of laminitis was observed on the day after a DST in a pony [47]. In addition, a false negative test result has been reported [6]. Dexamethasone alcohol administration to 12 pregnant mares (100 mg by intramuscular injection, on each of days 321 through 324 of gestation) shortened duration of gestation significantly by 12 days, without dystocia or retained placentas. Measurement of foal weights up to 13 weeks post partum indicated no detriment to growth [68].

An ACTH-stimulation test (Table 3) was performed on 17 of the Utrecht cases. The mean basal plasma cortisol concentration of 253 ± 181 nmol/L (range 74 to 864) increased to 557 ± 214 nmol/L (range 248 to 1083). The sensitivity of the test increased from 17% to 77% with a critical value of 413 nmol/L. Remarkably, in two cases the basal plasma cortisol concentration was low, but showed a normal response to ACTH (89–458 and 74–437). The sensitivity in this study was similar to the value of 75% reported by others [53]. A false negative test result has been reported [12].

The combined DST/ACTH stimulation test (Table 3) decreased plasma cortisol to undetectable concentrations (<27.6 nmol/L) 3 hours after dexamethasone. Following administration of synthetic ACTH, plasma cortisol increased to 252% of base line [69]. Neither the ACTH stimulation test nor the combined DST/ACTH stimulation test clearly differentiated horses with PIA from control horses [52]. In addition, the combined DST/ACTH stimulation test does not evaluate prolonged cortisol suppression to dexamethasone.

The TRH test (Table 3) significantly increased the plasma cortisol concentration in horses with PIA after 30 minutes in contrast to healthy horses [62]. No data on the sensitivity of this test are available and it has been suggested that this test is unsuitable for the diagnosis of PIA [70]. One hour after the administration of TRH the increase in T_3 and T_4 was similar in healthy horses and horses suffering from PIA [62]. There is an apparent diminution of the response to TRH by high basal cortisol concentrations [53].

Hyperglycaemic horses with PIA showed resting hyperinsulinaemia and were not capable of responding to acute glucose loading with a rapid increase in insulin, resulting in a delayed (>1.5 hours) return of glucose to base line [64]. Although delayed disappearance of glucose following oral or intravenous loading suggests insulin resistance, a diagnosis of PIA cannot be ruled out on the basis of normal results from glucose tolerance tests. All of the POMC peptides rose 1 hour after intramuscular injection of insulin (0.15 U/kg BW) to horses with PIA [12]. Plasma glucagon concentrations were decreased following intravenous administration of glucose (0.5 g/kg BW, as a 50% solution) to a pony with PIA [6]. The effects of various doses of insulin on plasma glucose concentrations in cases of secondary hyperglycaemia are generally negligible [3, 5, 6, 8, 9, 12, 48, 59], although some reductions in glucose concentrations have been reported [12, 13, 48, 59].

Computed tomography was performed using an intravenous iodinated contrast agent (meglumine iothalamate 0.45 ml/kg BW) [4]. However, as in ventrodorsal radiography, general anaesthesia is necessary and it should be borne in mind that in only 68% of horses with PIA is the pituitary enlarged [16] and amenable to imaging. In ventrodorsal radiography, a diagnosis can only be made when the lateral cavernous sinuses, which surround the hypophysis, are deviated laterally and impinge upon by the enlarged gland [63].

Differential Diagnosis

Persistent hyperglycaemia is most likely to be associated with a PIA. The differential diagnosis of persistent hyperglycaemia includes type 1 and type 2 diabetes mellitus, and phaeochromocytoma. Hirsutism has also been associated with meningioma located in the pituitary gland of a 6-year-old mare [71]. Monthly intramuscular injections of an anabolic steroid (stanozolol, 350 mg) for 8 years to an American Quarter Horse gelding was associated with failure to shed completely its winter haircoat [72]. With regard to the haircoat changes, it should be borne in mind that strongylosis is associated with long, but not curly, hair.

Metabolism

Compared with normal horses, horses with Cushing's disease have increased lipolysis and ketogenesis. No differences were found between horses with hyperadrenocorticism and normoglycaemia and horses with hyperadrenocorticism and hyperglycaemia with regard to rates of lipolysis and ketogenesis, and basal insulin concentrations. Urinalysis can reveal ketonuria in some [6, 8, 50], but not all [9, 48], cases of PIA. Hyperlipaemia is rare in horses with PIA [73], although it has been reported in two ponies [11, 50]. This is in agreement with the fact that the intramuscular administration of dexamethasone (0.04 mg/kg BW/IM) failed to increase plasma triglycerides in healthy ponies [74].

Treatment

Medical therapy of PIA involves two classes of drugs: dopamine agonists and serotonin antagonists, as pars intermedia secretion is under tonic inhibitory control by dopaminergic drugs and serotonin antagonists [12, 52]. The dopamine agonists bromocriptine (up to 0.09 mg/kg BW, po, BID [7]) or pergolide mesylate (gradually increased up to 0.011 mg/kg BW, po, q24h [12]) can be used. The serotonin antagonist that has been used is cyproheptadine hydrochloride, at doses up to 0.26 mg/kg BW, po, q24h. Horses that do not respond to cyproheptadine often improve with pergolide [55, 75]. Pergolide must be given initially at a very low oral dose (0.001 mg/kg BW), which is increased every 3–4 days by 0.25–0.50 mg to a maximum of 0.011 mg/kg BW. Side effects include anorexia, colic, diarrhoea and depression [55]. One horse given 10 mg bromocriptine orally per day became anorexic [55], a side effect not seen in Utrecht cases. Both dopaminergic agonists can induce clinical improvement within several weeks (Figure 5) [7, 55].

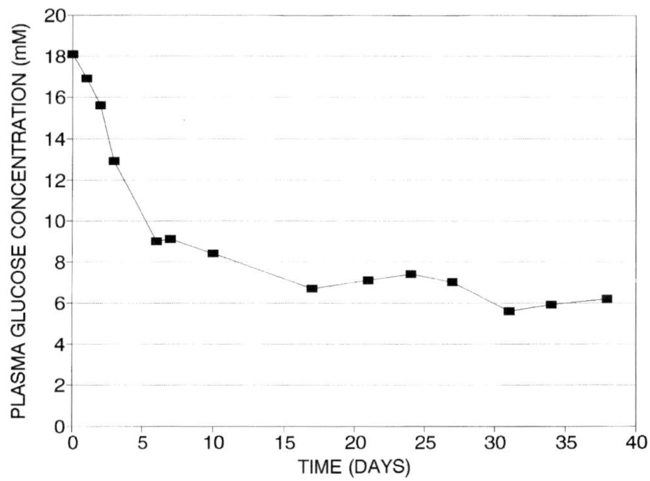

Figure 5. Plasma glucose concentration (mmol/L) during treatment with 0.025 mg of bromocriptine/kg BW orally bid in a 19-year-old pony gelding with hyperadrenocorticism.

The adrenocorticolytic agent, mitotane (op'DDD), is usually ineffective in horses with PIA [55, 75]. Bilateral adrenalectomy via bilateral transcostal approaches through the 18th rib is also not an option. Adrenalectomized horses can be maintained by administering up to 75 mg of desoxycorticosterone pivilate by intramuscular injection every 2–4 weeks and up to 50 mg of prednisolone orally once daily [18]. Development of antibodies against porcine as well as bovine insulin during the 6th treatment week has been reported [13], precluding long-term use of insulin for management of diabetes mellitus in horses.

Prognosis

The mean survival time (from discharge to the development of complications that required euthanasia) of seven horses without treatment was 162 days, with a range of 86–368 days. A mare was discharged and died 7 months later [8].

References

1. Pallaske G. Zur kasuistik seltnere Geschwülste bei den Haustieren. *Z Krebsforsch.* 1932; **36**, 342.
2. Eriksson K, Dyrendahl S & Grimfelt D. A case of hirsutism in connection with hypophyseal tumour in a horse. *Nord Vet Med.* 1956; **8**, 807–814.
3. Loeb WF, Capen CC & Johnson LE. Adenomas of the pars intermedia associated with hyperglycemia and glycosuria in two horses. *Cornell Vet.* 1966; **56**, 623–626.

4. Allen JR, Barbee DD & Crisman MV. Diagnosis of equine pituitary tumors by computed tomography – part 1. *Compend Contin Educ Pract Vet.* 1988; **10**, 1103–1106.
5. Baker JR & Ritchie HE. Diabetes mellitus in the horse: a case report and review of the literature. *Eq Vet J.* 1974; **6**, 7–11.
6. Auer DE, Wilson RG, Groenendijk S & Filippich LJ. Glucose metabolism in a pony mare with a tumour of the pituitary gland pars intermedia. *Aust Vet J.* 1987; **64**, 379–382.
7. Beck DJ. Effective long-term treatment of a suspected pituitary adenoma with bromocriptine mesylate in a pony. *Eq Vet Educ.* 1992; **4**, 119–122.
8. Field JR & Wolf C. Cushing's syndrome in a horse. *Eq Vet J.* 1988; **20**, 301–304.
9. Horvath CJ, Ames TR, Metz AL & Larson VL. Adrenocorticotropin-containing neoplastic cells in a pars intermedia adenoma in a horse. *J Am Vet Med Assoc.* 1988; **192**, 367–371.
10. Moore JN, Steiss J, Nicholson WE & Orth DN. A case of pituitary adrenocorticotropin-dependent Cushing's syndrome in the horse. *Endocrinology.* 1979; **104**, 576–582.
11. Moore BR, Abood SK & Hinchcliff KW. Hyperlipemia in 9 miniature horses and miniature donkeys. *J Vet Intern Med.* 1994; **8**, 376–381.
12. Orth DN, Holscher MA, Wilson MG, Nicholson WE, Plue RE & Mount CD. Equine Cushing's disease, plasma immunoreactive proopiolipomelanocortin peptide and cortisol levels basally and in response to diagnostic tests. *Endocrinology.* 1982; **110**, 1430–1441.
13. Staempfli HR, Eigenmann EJ & Clarke LM. Insulin treatment and development of anti-insulin antibodies in a horse with diabetes mellitus associated with a functional pituitary adenoma. *Can Vet J.* 1988; **29**, 934–936.
14. Holscher MA, Linnabary RL, Netsky MG & Owen HD. Adenoma of the pars intermedia and hirsutism in a pony. *Vet Med/Small Anim Clin.* 1978; **73**, 1197–1200.
15. Wilson MG, Nicholson WE, Holscher MA, Sherrell BJ, Mount CD & Orth DN. Proopiolipomelanocortin peptides in normal pituitary, pituitary tumor and plasma of normal and Cushing's horses. *Endocrinology.* 1982; **110**, 941–954.
16. Heinrichs M, Baumgärtner W & Capen CC. Immunocytochemical demonstration of proopiomelanocortin-derived peptides in pituitary adenomas of the pars intermedia in horses. *Vet Pathol.* 1990; **27**, 419–425.
17. Irvine CHG & Alexander SL. A novel technique for measuring hypothalamic and pituitary hormone secretion rates from collection of pituitary venous effluent in the normal horse. *J Endocrinol.* 1987; **113**, 183–192.
18. Slone DE, Vaughan JT, Garrett PD, Vaden MF & Purohit RC. Vascular anatomy and surgical technique for bilateral adrenalectomy in the equid. *Am J Vet Res.* 1980; **41**, 829–832.
19. Evans MJ, Kitson NE, Livesey JH & Donald RA. The effect of cortisol on the secretion of ACTH by anterior pituitary cells of the horse in culture. *J. Endocrinol.* 1993; **137**, 403–412.
20. Livesey JH, Donald RA, Irvine CHG, Redekopp C & Alexander SL. The effects of cortisol, vasopressin (AVP), and corticotropin-releasing factor administration on pulsatile adrenocorticotropin, alpha-melanocyte-stimulating hormone, and AVP secretion in the pituitary venous effluent of the horse. *Endocrinology.* 1988; **123**, 713–720.
21. Ng TB, Chung D & Li CH Isolation and properties of β-endorphin-(1–27), *N*-acetyl-β-endorphin, corticotropin, gamma-lipotropin and neurophysin from equine pituitary glands. *Int J Pept Prot Res.* 1981; **18**, 443–450.
22. Bottoms GD, Roesel OF, Rausch FD & Akins EL. Circadian variation in plasma cortisol and corticosterone in pigs and mares. *Am J Vet Res.* 1972; **33**, 785–790.
23. Kirkpatrick JF, Wiesner L, Baker CB & Angle M. Diurnal variation of plasma corticosteroids in the wild horse stallion. *Comp Biochem Physiol.* 1977; **57A**, 179–181.
24. Hoffsis GF, Murdick PW, Tharp VL & Ault K. Plasma concentrations of cortisol and corticosterone in the normal horse. *Am J Vet Res.* 1970; **31**, 1379–1387.
25. Irvine CHG & Alexander SL. Factors affecting the circadian rhythm in plasma cortisol concentrations in the horse. *Domest Anim Endocrinol.* 1994; **11**, 227–238.
26. James VHT, Horner MW, Moss MS & Rippon AE. Adrenocortical function in the horse. *J Endocrinol.* 1970; **48**, 319–335.

27. Kumar MSA, Liao TF & Chen CL. Diurnal variation in serum cortisol in ponies. *J Anim Sci.* 1976; **42**, 1360.
28. Larsson M, Edqvist LE, Ekman L & Persson S. Plasma cortisol in the horse, diurnal rhythm and effects of exogenous ACTH. *Acta Vet Scand.* 1979; **20**, 16–24.
29. Ralston JM, Stenhouse AM, Stenhouse NS, Buck GJ, Lucks SF, Reynoldson JA & Bolton JR. Cortisol concentrations in blood and urine of horses. *Austr Vet J.* 1988; **65**, 1–5.
30. Luna SPL & Taylor PM. Pituitary-adrenal activity and opioid release in ponies during thiopentone/halothane anaesthesia. *Res Vet Sci.* 1995; **58**, 35–41.
31. Messer NT, Johnson PJ, Refsal KR, Nachreiner RF, Ganjam VK & Krause GF. Effect of food deprivation on baseline iodothyronine and cortisol concentrations in healthy, adult horses. *Am J Vet Res.* 1995; **56**, 116–121.
32. Redekopp C, Irvine CHG, Donald RA, Livesey JH, Sadler W, Nicholls MG, Alexander SL & Evans MJ. Spontaneous and stimulated adrenocorticotropin and vasopressin pulsatile secretion in the pituitary venous effluent of the horse. *Endocrinology* 1986; **118**, 1410–1416.
33. Hoffsis GF & Murdick PW. The plasma concentrations of corticosteroids in normal and diseased horses. *J Am Vet Med Assoc.* 1970; **157**:1590–1594.
34. Seal US & Doe RP. Vertebrate distribution of corticosteroid-binding globulin and some endocrine effects on concentration. *Steroids.* 1965; **5**, 827.
35. Slone DE, Ganjam VK, Purohit RC & Ravis WR. Cortisol disappearance rate and pathophysiologic changes after bilateral adrenalectomy in equids. *Am J Vet Res.* 1983; **44**, 276–279.
36. Toutain PL & Brandon RA. Steroidal anti-inflammatory agents in the horse, pharmacokinetics and action on the adrenal gland. In, Ruckebusch Y, Toutain PL & Koritz GD. *Veterinary Pharmacology and Toxicology.* Boston: MTP Press Ltd 1983; 353–366.
37. MacHarg MA, Bottoms GD, Carter GK & Johnson MA. Effects of multiple intramuscular injections and doses of dexamethasone on plasma cortisol concentrations and adrenal responses to ACTH in horses. *Am J Vet Res.* 1985; **46**, 2285–2287.
38. Reilly L, Habecker P, Beech J, Johnston J, Sweeney C & Hamir A. Pituitary abscess and basilar empyema in 4 horses. *Eq Vet J.* 1994; **26**, 424–426.
39. Boujon CE, Bestetti GE, Meier HP, Straub R, Junker U & Rossi GL. Equine pituitary adenoma, a functional and morphological study. *J Comp Path.* 1993; **109**, 163–178.
40. Evans LH, Siegel ET & Hubben K. Clinico-pathologic conference. *J Am Vet Med Assoc.* 1968; **152**, 1778–1786.
41. Fix AS & Miller LD. Equine adrenocortical carcinoma with hypercalcemia. *Vet Pathol.* 1987; **24**, 190–192.
42. Kolk JH van der, Mars MH & Gaag I van der. Adrenocortical carcinoma in a 12-year-old mare. *Vet Rec.* 1994; **134**, 113–115.
43. Raker CW & Fegley H. Clinico-pathologic conference. *J Am Vet Med Assoc.* 1965; **147**, 848–860.
44. King JM. Pituitary tumor and mycotic pneumonia in a gelding. *Vet Med.* 1993; **88**, 836.
45. Kolk JH van der, Kalsbeek HC, Garderen E van, Wensing T & Breukink HJ. Equine pituitary neoplasia: a clinical report of 21 cases (1990–1992). *Vet Rec.* 1993; **133**, 594–597.
46. Millington WR, Dybdal NO, Dawson R Jr, Manzini C & Mueller GP. Equine Cushing's disease: differential regulation of β-endorphin processing in tumours of the intermediate pituitary. *Endocrinology.* 1988; **123**, 1598–1604.
47. Green EM & Hunt EL. Hypophyseal neoplasia in a pony. *Compend Contin Educ Pract Vet.* 1985; **7**, S249–S257.
48. King JM, Kavanaugh JF & Bentinck-Smith J. Diabetes mellitus with pituitary neoplasms in a horse and a dog. *Cornell Vet.* 1962; **52**, 133–145.
49. Orth DN & Nicholson WE. Bioactive and immunoreactive adrenocorticotropin in normal equine pituitary and in pituitary tumors of horses with Cushing's disease. *Endocrinology.* 1982; **111**, 559–563.
50. Naylor JM, Kronfeld DS & Acland H. Hyperlipemia in horses, effects of undernutrition and disease. *Am J Vet Res.* 1980; **41**, 899–905.

51. Eyre P, Elmes PJ & Strickland S. Corticosteroid-potentiated vascular responses of the equine digit, a possible pharmacologic basis for laminitis. *Am J Vet Res.* 1979; **40**, 135–138.
52. Dybdal NO, Hargreaves KM, Madigan JE, Gribble DH, Kennedy PC & Stabenfeldt GH. Diagnostic testing for pituitary pars intermedia dysfunction in horses. *J Am Vet Med Assoc.* 1994; **204**, 627–632.
53. Hillyer MH, Taylor FGR, Mair TS, Murphy D, Watson TDG & Love S. Diagnosis of hyperadrenocorticism in the horse. *Equine Vet Educ.* 1992; **4**, 131–134.
54. Kolk JH van der, Wensing T, Kalsbeek HC & Breukink HJ. Laboratory diagnosis of equine pituitary pars intermedia adenoma. *Domest Anim Endocrinol.* 1995; **12**, 35–39.
55. Beech J. Treatment of hypophysial adenomas. *Compend Contin Educ Pract Vet.* 1994; **16**, 921–923.
56. Sweeney CR, Stebbins KE, Schelling CG, Beech J & Schilling DA. Hypertrophic osteopathy in a pony with a pituitary adenoma. *J Am Vet Med Assoc* 1989; **195**, 103–105.
57. Chiba S, Okada K, Numakunai S & Ohshima K-I. A case of equine thyroid follicular carcinoma accompanied with adenohypophysial adenoma. *Jpn J Vet Sci.* 1987; **49**, 551–554.
58. Kolk JH van der. Relation between relative pituitary weight in horses with Cushing's disease and some plasma and clinical parameters. *Proceedings of 35th Congress of British Equine Veterinary Association.* 1996; 82–83.
59. Andreasen M, Olsen SN, Jensen AL & Basse A. Hypofysetumor hos hest. *Dansk Veterinaertidsskr.* 1994; **77**, 97–103.
60. Ellison RS & Jacobs RM. The isoelectric focusing properties of serum alkaline phosphatase in disease and following prednisolone and phenylbutazone administration in the horse. *Can J Vet Res.* 1990; **54**, 126–131.
61. Cohen ND & Carter GK. Steroid hepatopathy in a horse with glucocorticoid-induced hyperadrenocorticism. *J Am Vet Med Assoc.* 1992; **200**, 1682–1684.
62. Beech J & Garcia M. Hormonal response to thyrotropin-releasing hormone in healthy horses and in horses with pituitary adenoma. *Am J Vet Res.* 1985; **46**, 1941–1943.
63. Levy M, Blevins WE & Janovitz EB. Radiological diagnosis of pituitary adenoma in the horse. *Proceedings of the 3rd Congress of the World Equine Veterinary Association. Geneva, Switzerland.* 1993; 18.
64. Garcia MC & Beech J. Equine intravenous glucose tolerance test: glucose and insulin responses of healthy horses fed grain or hay and of horses with pituitary adenoma. *Am J Vet Res.* 1986; **47**, 570–572.
65. Kolk JH van der, Kalsbeek HC, Wensing T & Breukink HJ. Urinary concentration of corticoids in normal horses and horses with hyperadrenocorticism. *Res Vet Sci.* 1994; **56**, 126–128.
66. Eiler H, Oliver J & Goble D. Adrenal gland function in the horse: effect of dexamethasone on hydrocortisone secretion and blood cellularity and plasma electrolyte concentrations. *Am J Vet Res.* 1979; **40**, 727–729.
67. Sojka JE, Johnson MA & Bottoms GD. The effect of starting time on dexamethasone suppression test results in horses. *Domest Anim Endocrinol.* 1993; **10**, 1–5.
68. Alm CC, Sullivan JJ & First NL. Induction of premature parturition by parenteral administration of dexamethasone in the mare. *J Am Vet Med Assoc.* 1974; **165**, 721–722.
69. Eiler H, Oliver J & Goble D. Combined dexamethasone-suppression cosyntropin-(synthetic ACTH) stimulation test in the horse: a new approach to testing of adrenal gland function. *Am J Vet Res.* 1980; **41**, 430–434.
70. Thompson JC, Ellison R, Gillet R & Badcoe L. Problems in the diagnosis of pituitary adenoma (Cushing's syndrome). *NZ Vet J.* 1995; **43**, 79–82.
71. Johansson B & Segall T. Meningiom – en ovanlig tumörform hos häst. *Svensk Vet Tidning.* 1994; **46**, 123–126.
72. Dowling PM, Williams MA & Clark TP. Adrenal insufficiency associated with long-term anabolic steroid administration in a horse. *J Am Vet Med Assoc.* 1993; **203**, 1166–1169.
73. Kolk JH van der, Wensing T, Kalsbeek HC & Breukink HJ. Lipid metabolism in horses with hyperadrenocorticism. *J Am Vet Med Assoc.* 1995; **206**, 1010–1012.

74. Freestone JF, Wolfsheimer KJ, Ford RB, Church G & Bessin R. Triglyceride, insulin, and cortisol responses of ponies to fasting and dexamethasone administration. *J Vet Int Med.* 1991; **5**, 15–22.
75. Love S. Equine Cushing's disease. *Br Vet J.* 1993; **149**, 139–153.

4

Disorders of Adrenal Gland Function

Jill Beech

Key Points

- Primary adrenal gland dysfunction is uncommonly diagnosed in horses.
- Primary adrenal insufficiency has been reported in premature foals, whose survival is at risk owing to the requirements of cortisol for the final development.
- Secondary adrenal insufficiency may be associated with administration of glucocorticoids or anabolic steroids.
- Neoplasms of the adrenal cortex and medulla have been recorded at necropsy, but do not appear to have been associated with endocrine dysfunction.
- Clinical signs of adrenal insufficiency in adult horses include poor performance, depression, lethargy, long or dull haircoat, dermatitis, and weight loss.
- Adrenal insufficiency is best diagnosed by measurement of baseline plasma cortisol concentrations and response to adrenocorticotrophic hormone. An interval of up to 14 days from last administration of steroids may be necessary prior to endocrinological testing.
- Treatment for adrenal insufficiency should encompass rest, minimizing stress and discontinuing steroids. Glucocorticoid replacement therapy may be required in some cases.

Introduction

Primary adrenal gland dysfunction is relatively uncommonly diagnosed in horses. Adrenal cortical hyperplasia secondary to pituitary pars intermedia adenoma is more common and has been referred to as Equine Cushing's or Cushingoid syndrome (see Chapter 3). Signs of hyperadrenocorticism can be induced by glucocorticoid therapy. Primary adrenocortical tumours and pheochromocytomas are both rare [1–12] and often not diagnosed antemortem. Adrenal insufficiency, likewise, is unusual and to the author's knowledge there are no data from a sizable equine patient group.

Adrenal Insufficiency

Primary adrenal insufficiency in the horse has been reported in premature foals [13, 14] and experimentally in bilaterally adrenalectomized animals [15]. In addition to hypoglycaemia and undetectable cortisol, hyponatraemia, hyperkalaemia, and haemoconcentration owing to lack of mineralocorticoid production can occur in the latter [15]. Premature foals with evidence of incomplete development, poor cardiovascular stability and abnormal cerebral function had low plasma cortisol concentrations and were diagnosed as having hypoadrenocorticism [13, 14]. However, plasma cortisol values can be highly variable just prior to parturition and higher values correspond to older gestational age [16]. Premature foals failed to show the same amount of increase in plasma cortisol or responsiveness to exogenous adrenocorticotrophic hormone (ACTH) following birth and their ACTH levels appeared more variable compared with those of term foals [13]. Premature foals born prior to the normal late periparturient increase in plasma cortisol would appear to have hypoadrenocorticism and be at risk for survival owing to lack of cortisol required for final development [16].

Suspected cases of secondary adrenal insufficiency in the horse have been presumed to be associated with glucocorticoid administration [17, 18], and chronic anabolic steroid administration followed by abrupt cessation was implicated in one horse [19]. Exogenous glucocorticoid administration results in suppression of endogenous ACTH production, resulting in decreased synthesis and secretion of cortisol. Long-term suppression of ACTH may result in atrophy of the zona reticulata and fasciculata of the adrenal cortex. As mineralocorticoid secretion is spared, sodium and potassium balance is often normal [20]. Clinical signs are not specific and have included dullness or lethargy, weight loss and a dull haircoat with no signs of infectious disease or primary dysfunction of another organ system. In one horse, laminitis, muscle wasting and a long haircoat were reported [19]. Because of relatively limited endocrinologic testing it is possible that horses with secondary adrenal insufficiency remain undiagnosed.

In a group of 10 horses with suspected hypoadrenocorticism based on baseline low cortisol concentrations and signs (Beech and Reimer, unpublished data), seven had poor racing performance and six were noted to be unusually quiet, depressed, or lethargic. A dull haircoat and/or dermatitis was noted in six, and

Table 1. **Clinical features of adrenal insufficiency**

Primary adrenal insufficiency
- premature foals with incompleted development and poor cardiovascular stability

Secondary adrenal insufficiency	Blood biochemistry in experimental adrenal insufficiency
• dullness, lethargy	• hypoglycaemia
• weight loss	• hyponatraemia
• dull haircoat	• hyperkalaemia
• poor racing performance	• haemoconcentration
	• undetectable cortisol

seven were underweight. No evidence of significant cardiovascular, pulmonary, or musculoskeletal disease was found on physical examination. Laboratory data (white blood cell count, packed cell volume, total protein, and fibrinogen in all 10 horses and serum electrolytes in five) were normal. None showed signs of hypoglycaemia.

Plasma cortisol concentrations were below the laboratory's normal range (35–70 ng/mL) in all horses, with a mean of 14.4 ng/mL (range 3.09–24.0 ng/mL). An ACTH response test was performed in six horses and a combined dexamethasone-suppression/ACTH stimulation test was performed in two. Although there was a two to almost fivefold increase in cortisol after ACTH administration, except in one horse in each test group the peak values were low and did not rise above 70 ng/mL. The cortisol concentration six hours after ACTH administration in one horse had decreased below the low baseline level. A history of previous systemic or intra-articular corticosteroid administration prior to one month before testing was later admitted in three horses, and three had a history of anabolic steroid administration.

All horses were subsequently rested and all corticosteroids and anabolic steroids were discontinued. In addition, one was treated with oral prednisolone at a dosage of 0.1 mg/kg BW, every other day for 10 days. Cortisol concentrations were normal in five horses re-evaluated 1–3 months later and response to ACTH was 1.7 to 2.9 times the baseline value with peak levels greater than 70 ng/ml. All five horses were reported to have improved in attitude and appearance 1–6 months later. The one horse treated with ACTH continued to deteriorate and cortisol concentrations fell below baseline. The latter increased seven fold following ACTH but peak was still below normal range; he was euthanased but post mortem revealed no changes in the adrenal or pituitary glands.

In one horse with hypoadrenocorticism suspected to be associated with discontinuing chronic anabolic steroid administration, the baseline plasma cortisol concentration was normal and had normal negative response to dexamethasone but showed no rise following ACTH stimulation [19]. The horse's endogenous plasma ACTH concentration was normal. Following glucocorticoid treatment (prednisolone, 0.5 mg/kg BW, po, q48h) the horse appeared clinically normal within 2 months and an ACTH response test after 9 months was normal. Prednisolone was then slowly withdrawn and the horse remained clinically normal. In another horse administered excessive glucocorticoids, baseline cortisol was undetectable and there was evidence of incomplete adrenocortical suppression based on a low peak response to ACTH [21].

In most cases of suspected adrenal insufficiency, exogenous steroid administration is documented or suspected, and when testing adrenal gland function, the effects of both systemic and intra-articular steroids must be considered. Transient suppression of cortisol concentrations has been reported following intramuscular administration of dexamethasone [22, 23] and triamcinolone [25]. Intramuscular administration of prednisolone acetate has been shown to suppress basal plasma hydrocortisone concentrations for up to 21 days [22]. A dose of dexamethasone as low as 5–10 μg/kg BW IM reportedly can suppress the pituitary adrenal axis [26]. By 4 days following administration of dexamethasone (0.044 and 0.088 mg/kg BW IM) plasma cortisol concentrations had returned to normal, and ACTH responses were normal 8 days following the last of six dexamethasone injections administered at these dosages every five days [23]. In another study, cortisol concentrations did not return to baseline for 7 days after dexamethasone (0.044 mg/kg BW IM) or for 14 days following triamcinolone (0.044 mg/kg BW IM) [24]. Plasma cortisol (hydrocortisone) concentrations were suppressed for three days following intra-articular administration of methylprednisolone acetate but ACTH response tests were normal [27]. Following intravenous prednisolone sodium succinate plasma hydrocortisone concentrations returned to normal after 24 hours [22]. After intra-articular triamcinolone (6 mg in three joints), serum cortisol concentration decreased within hours, reaching the lowest level by 12 hours; it began to rise on day 3 and by day 5 following injection it had returned to baseline [25].

Short term anabolic steroid therapy (1.1 mg/kg BW boldenone undecylenate IM or 0.55 mg/kg BW stanozolol IM, on days 1 and 8 prior to testing on day 12) had no effect on cortisol concentrations nor adrenal gland responsiveness to ACTH [28]. The effect of very protracted use has not been documented. Administration of ACTH also may affect results [29, 30]. Following the ACTH induced peak, cortisol concentrations were reported to fall below baseline and were out of phase with the diurnal pattern for approximately 24 hours [30]. Unless the exact dosage and drug are known, to allow one to determine the appropriate interval, the author usually suggests a 10–14 day interval prior to endocrinologic testing. If triamcinolone is likely to have been used and the dosage is unknown, the interval should probably be at least 14 days.

Diagnosis of Adrenal Insufficiency

As clinical signs of adrenal insufficiency are nonspecific, diagnosis depends on endocrinological testing (Table 2). A history of frequent steroid administration is supportive of the diagnosis of adrenal insufficiency. Resting cortisol levels may be normal or subnormal in individuals with adrenal gland insufficiency. Single samples are usually not adequate because of variability in basal cortisol concentrations.

Ultradian rhythms in both cortisol and ACTH have been reported in both adult horses (pregnant and nonpregnant) and equine foetuses [16, 31]. In one study, pulsatile release occurred in most (but not all) horses between 11 and 17 minutes [16] and in another study pulsatile release of ACTH occurred every 16–24 minutes [31]. Because peaks and troughs could be over 50% different from the mean value for the entire sampling series, obtaining a single plasma sample for basal ACTH or cortisol concentrations could misrepresent an animal's pituitary–adrenal status [16]. Because of this, obtaining samples every

***Table 2.* Endocrinological testing for adrenal gland function**

Test	*Normal Response*	*Reference*
ACTH Stimulation		
100 U Cosyntropin IV baseline and 2 hour samples	80% increase above baseline cortisol in 2 hours with peak exceeding normal baseline range	29
200 IU Corticotropin gel IM baseline and 1 and 4 hour samples	100% increase in cortisol by 1 hour, persisting at least 4 hours	29
1 U ACTH gel/kg IM baseline and 2 hour sample	2- to 3-fold increase in cortisol by 2 through 12 hours	26
Dexamethasone Suppression		
40 μg/kg IM basal samples and at 12 or 16 and 20–24 hours	$>$ 80% decrease in cortisol by 8 through 24 hours	26, 33
	$<$ 1 μg/dl by 20–24 hours	26
Combined Dexamethasone-suppression Cosyntropin Stimulation		
baseline cortisol close to 9 a.m. 10 mg dexamethasone IM cortisol sample 3 hours later 100 IU cosyntropin IV Cortisol sample 2 hours later	nondetectable cortisol (RIA) at 3 hours 1.5–2.5-fold increase above baseline 2 hours post cosyntropin	29

5 minutes over a 20 minute duration so as to cover a time period longer than that of the normal oscillation was suggested [16]. This wide oscillation was not seen in unstressed horses studied by the author. Significant hourly fluctuations in cortisol have been reported [32, 29]. In some studies diurnal variation in plasma cortisol concentrations was reported. Cortisol levels were reported to be higher between 8 a.m. and 4 p.m., with lower values at 8 p.m., 12 a.m. and 4 a.m. [26] and another study reported peak values a 6 a.m. and lowest values at about 6 p.m. [30]. Another study in stabled regularly fed horses showed a small circadian rhythm with a peak at mid morning and a value approximately one half that in late afternoon or evening [32]. Other studies failed to show diurnal variation in horses sampled many times daily [33] or at 8 a.m. and 8 p.m. [34]. A study of mares at pasture showed neither baseline cortisol concentrations nor responses to metyrapone (an inhibitor of 11β-hydroxylase and thus conversion of 11-deoxycortisol to cortisol) were related to time of day [35].

In attempts to study the pituitary–adrenal axis, efforts have been made to stimulate ACTH release in the horse through exercise, induction of hypoglycaemia and administration of adrenalin. Pharmacological doses of adrenalin did not significantly raise cortisol levels and only after induction of severe hypoglycaemia was any significant increase in cortisol level observed [36]. Effect of exercise on cortisol levels has been variable and most likely was related to the stress of the exercise [36–38].

The most useful test for adrenal insufficiency is baseline cortisol concentrations and an ACTH stimulation test. A lack of response to ACTH may indicate primary or advanced secondary adrenal insufficiency. Horses may show a blunted response indicative of incomplete adrenocortical suppression. One should evaluate the difference in serum or plasma cortisol concentrations pre- and post-ACTH stimulation as well as the peak serum or plasma cortisol concentrations. Based on available data, prior to ACTH stimulation, several baseline samples should be obtained because of normal fluctuation in concentrations; a mean baseline can then be determined. Intravenous administration of 100 U ACTH doubled the plasma cortisol concentration in 2 hours in normal horses [29]. Alternatively, 1 U/kg BW of ACTH gel can be administered intramuscularly and blood samples taken before and after ACTH administration. Normal horses have a two- to three-fold increase in cortisol (Table 2) [26].

A normal response to ACTH does not exclude decreased ACTH reserve. In other species studied, not unexpectedly, ACTH levels are decreased in secondary adrenal insufficiency, and increased in primary adrenal insufficiency. Although equine ACTH can be assayed [16, 31, 39–42] the test is not readily available to many veterinarians. Its measurement would be helpful in diagnosing adrenal and pituitary–adrenal axis disorders.

Treatment and Management

To the author's knowledge, there are no published data on which to base definitive recommendations. Therapy for cases of adrenal insufficiency should include rest, minimizing stress, supportive care and discontinuing unnecessary medications including systemic and intra-articular corticosteroids, and anabolic steroids. Treatment of these cases with ACTH is controversial. Experimentally, ACTH has been shown to cause a rebound lowering of cortisol [30, 35]. Glucocorticoid replacement therapy [prednisone administered at small dosages (0.1–0.3 mg/kg BW)] should be considered in horses with adrenal insufficiency if they have extremely low plasma cortisol concentrations, show inappetence, debilitating disease, or are undergoing unavoidable stress.

Tumours of the Adrenal Gland

Both adrenocortical tumours and tumours of the medulla have been reported. In most reported cases the tumours have not caused signs of endocrine dysfunction.

Adrenocortical Neoplasia

Two horses with adrenocortical carcinomas and metastasis and one with an adrenocortical adenoma had clinical signs, including seizures, hindlimb and scrotal oedema, abdominal pain, lethargy and stiffness; two had weight loss and two polydipsia with a low urine specific gravity [2]. All three had hyponatraemia and one had hypoglycaemia; no endocrinological testing was performed.

In another report of an adrenocortical carcinoma, the major clinical signs were intermittent colic and weight loss; a large mass was palpated in the sub-lumbar region. Serum chloride and sodium were in the low end of normal range but potassium and calcium were normal, as was basal cortisol concentration [1]. There was no evidence that the tumour was functional in these cases.

Diagnosis of a tumour would appear to be based mainly on palpation per rectum and probably ultrasonographic examination. Percutaneous biopsy, using ultrasonographic guidance, could be considered. Laparoscopy via the flank could also be used. If plasma cortisol concentrations were consistently significantly elevated, one would suspect the tumour to be functional. Dexamethasone suppression testing could be used as one would not expect a tumour to be under normal pituitary feedback. However, horses with pituitary adenomas/hyperplasia also fail to show normal dexamethasone suppression and have a more rapid return to baseline concentrations. Although late in the day performance of dexamethasone suppression testing has been advised, so as to precede the normal diurnal increase in ACTH [26], in a small group of normal horses there was no significant difference in values between 9 a.m. or 9 p.m. initiated tests [34]. To the author's knowledge there are no documented cases of increased adrenal activity in horses except those with pituitary pars intermedia dysfunction and, therefore, ACTH or dexamethasone response test results are speculative. The usual tests employed to evaluate adrenal function are outlined in Table 2.

Adrenal Medulla Neoplasia

Well encapsulated phaeochromocytomas, usually unilateral and benign, have been reported in horses. There is one report of metastasis of a phechromocytoma with compression of the spinal cord in a 6-month-old foal [7]. With phaeochromocytoma one would expect signs attributable to increased production and release of catecholamines – sweating, tachypnoea and tachycardia, abdominal pain, muscle tremors, mydriasis, and less often diarrhea. Hypertension is a frequent sign in humans but to the author's knowledge has not been documented in equine cases. However, in horses phaeochromocytomas may be non-functional and be incidental findings at necropsy. In several cases, abdominal pain has been the major clinical sign. Retroperitoneal haemorrhage and/or haemoperitoneum secondary to ruptured phaeochromocytomas has been documented [5, 12].

Diagnosis has usually been at necropsy. The tumour is unlikely to be palpable per rectum except when large and involving the left kidney, and retroperitoneal haemorrhage and/or haematoma may or may not be palpable. One would expect blood pressure to be increased, possibly intermittently, but there are no data in horses to substantiate how frequently this occurs. Catecholamine assays are not usually available, although elevated concentrations combined with clinical signs would be highly suggestive. The usefulness of ultrasonography or other imaging modalities is unknown.

As most reports have been based on necropsy diagnoses and some of these horses were apparently asymptomatic, no definitive recommendations can be made. Surgical removal is performed in humans but to the author's knowledge has not been attempted in horses. There is no documented medical treatment in horses.

References

1. van der Kolk JH, Mars MH & van der Gaag I. Adrenocortical carcinoma in a 12-year-old mare. *Vet Rec.* 1994; **134**, 113–115.
2. Raker CW & Fegley H. Clinico-pathologic Conf. *J Am Vet Med Assoc.* 1965; **147**, 848.
3. Evans LH, Siegel ET & Hubben K. Clinico-pathologic Conference (Adrenal Neoplasm in a Horse). *J Am Vet Med Assoc.* 1968; **152**, 1778.
4. Fix AS & Miller LD. Equine adrenocortical carcinoma with hypercalcemia. *Vet Pathol.* 1987; **24**, 190.
5. Johnson PJ, Goetz TE, Foreman JH *et al.* Pheochromocytoma in two horses. *J Am Vet Med Assoc.* 1995; **206**(6), 837–841.
6. Gelberg H, Cockerell GL & Minor RR. A light and electron microscopic study of a normal adrenal medulla and pheochromocytoma from a horse. *Vet Pathol.* 1979; **16**, 395–404.
7. Froscher BG & Power HT. Malignant pheochromocytoma in a foal. *J Am Vet Med Assoc.* 1982; **181**, 494–496.
8. Evans LH, Stewart J & Dodd DC. Clinico-pathologic Conference. *J Am Vet Med Assoc.* 1971; **159**, 209–219.
9. Yovich JV, Horney FD & Hardee GE. Pheocromocytoma in the horse and measurement of norepinephrine levels in horses. *Can Vet J.* 1984; **25**, 21–25.
10. Buckingham JDE. Pheochromocytoma in a mare. *Can Vet J.* 1970; **11**, 205–208.
11. Duckett WM, Snyder JR, Harkema JR *et al.* Functional pheochromocytoma in a horse. *Comp Cont Educ Pract Vet.* 1987; **9**, 1118–1121.
12. Yovich JV & Ducharme NG. Ruptured pheochromocytoma in a mare with colic. *J Am Vet Med Assoc.* 1983; **183**, 462–464.
13. Silver M, Ousey JC, Dudan FE, *et al.* Studies on equine prematurity 2: postnatal adrenocortical activity in relation to plasma adrenocorticotrophic hormone and catecholamine levels in term and premature foals. *Equine Vet J.* 1984; **16**, 278–286.
14. Rossdale PD, Ousey JC & Silver M. Studies on equine prematurity 6: Guidelines for assessment of foal maturation. *Equine Vet J.* 1984; **16**, 300–302.
15. Slone DE, Ganjam VK, Purohit RC, *et al.* Cortisol (hydrocortisone) disappearance rate and pathophysiologic changes after bilateral adrenalectomy in equids. *Am J Vet Res.* 1983; **44**, 276–279.
16. Cudd TA, LeBlanc M, Silver M *et al.* Ontogeny and ultradian rhythms of adrenocorticotropin and cortisol in the late-gestation fetal horse *J Endocrinol.* 1995; **144**, 271–283.
17. Kirk MD. Field diagnosis and treatment of secondary adrenal insufficiency in the horse. *Vet Med Small Anim Clin.* 1974; **69**, 1383–1386.
18. O'Connor JT. The untoward effects of the corticosteroids in equine practice. *J Am Vet Med Assoc.* 1968; **153**, 1614–1617.
19. Dowling PM, Williams A & Clark TP. Adrenal insufficiency associated with long term anabolic steroid administration in a horse. *J Am Vet Med Assoc.* 1993; **204**, 1166–1169.
20. Feldman EC & Peterson ME. Hypoadrenocorticism. *Vet Clin North Am* (*Small Animal Pract*). 1984; **14**, 751–766.

21. Cohen ND & Carter GK. Steroid hepatopathy in a horse with glucocorticoid induced hyperadrenocorticism. *J Am Vet Med Assoc.* 1992; **200**, 1682–1684.
22. Toutain PL, Brandon RA, dePomyres H, *et al.* Dexamethasone and prednisolone in the horse, pharmacokinetics and action on the adrenal gland. *Am J Vet Res.* 1984; **45**, 1750–1756.
23. MacHarg MA, Bottoms GD, Carter GK, *et al.* Effects of multiple intramuscular injections and doses of dexamethasone on plasma cortisol concentrations and adrenal responses to ACTH in horses. *Am J Vet Res.* 1985; **46**, 2285–2287.
24. Slone DE, Purohit RC, Ganjam VK, *et al.* Sodium retention and cortisol (hydrocortisone) suppression caused by dexamethasone and triamcinolone in equids. *Am J Vet Res.* 1983; **44**, 280–283.
25. Chen CL, Sailor JA, Collier J *et al.* Synovial and serum levels of triamcinolone following intra-articular administration of triamcinolone acetonide in the horse. *J Vet Pharmacol Therap.* 1992; **15**, 240–246.
26. Dybdal NO, Hargreaves KM, Madigan JE *et al.* Diagnostic testing for pituitary pars intermedia dysfunction in horses. *J Am Vet Med Assoc.* 1994; **204**, 627–632.
27. Autefage A, Alvinerie M & Toutain PL. Synovial fluid and plasma kinetics of methylprednisolone and methylpredisolone acetate. *Equine Vet J.* 1986; **18**, 193–198.
28. Morris DP & Garcia MC. Effect of phenylbutazone and anabolic steroids on adrenal and thyroid glands functions tests in healthy horses. *Am J Vet Res.* 1985; **46**, 359–364.
29. Eiler H, Goble D & Oliver J. Adrenal gland function in the horse, effects of cosyntropin (synthetic) and corticotropin (natural) stimulation. *Am J Vet Res.* 1979; **40**, 724–726.
30. Larrson M, Edqvist LE, Ekman L, *et al.* Plasma cortisol in the horse, diurnal rhythm and effects of exogenous ACTH. *Acta Vet Scand.* 1979; **20**, 16–24.
31. Redekopp C, Irvine RA, Livesey JH *et al.* Spontaneous and stimulated adrenocorticotropin and vasopressin pulsatile secretion in the pituitary venous effuent of the horse. *Endocrinology.* 1986; **118**, 1410–1416.
32. Toutain PL *et al.* Diurnal and episodic variation of plasma hydrocortisone concentrations in horses. *Dom Animal Endocrinol.* 1988; **5**, 55–59.
33. Hoffsis GF, Murdick PW, Tharp VL *et al.* Plasma concentrations of cortisol and corticosteroids in normal horses. *Am J Vet Res.* 1970; **31**, 1379.
34. Sojka JE, Johnson MA & Bottoms GD. The effect of starting time on dexamethasone suppression test results in horses. *Dom Anim Endocrinol.* 1993; **10**(1), 1–5.
35. Alexander SL, Irvine CHG, Livesey JH *et al.* The acute effect of lowering plasma cortisol on the secretion of corticotropin-releasing hormone, arginine vasopressin, and adrenocorticotropin as revealed by intensive sampling of pituitary venous blood in the normal horse. *J Endocrinol.* 1993; **133**(2), 860–866.
36. James VHT, Horner MW, Moss MS *et al.* Adrenocortical function in the horse. *J Endocrinol.* 1970; **48**, 319–335.
37. Garcia MC & Beech J. Endocrinologic, hematologic, and heart rate changes in swimming horses. *Am J Vet Res.* 1986; **47**, 2004–2006.
38. Seren E, Tamanini C, Gaiani R, *et al.* The effect of submaximal exercise on blood lactate, creatine phosphokinase and cortisol (corticosterone) levels in the horse during training. *Archiv Vet Ital.* 1977; **28**, 65–712.
39. Ng TB Chung D & Li CH. Isolation and properties of *β*-endorphin-(1–27), Na-acetyl-*β*-endorphin, corticotropin, gamma-lipotropin and neurophysin from equine pituitary glands. *Int J Pept Prot Res.* 1981; **18**, 443–450.
40. Orth DN, Holscher MA, Wilson MG *et al.* Equine Cushing's disease: plasma immunoreactive pro-opiolipomelanocortin peptide and cortisol levels basally and in response to diagnostic tests. *Endocrinology.* 1982; **110**, 1430–1441.
41. van der Kolk JH, Kalsbeck HC & van Garderen E. Equine pituitary neoplasia, a clinical report of 21 cases (1990–1992). *Vet Record.* 1993; **133**, 594–597.
42. Couëtil L, Paradis MR, Knoll J. Plasma adrenocorticotropin concentration in healthy horses and in horses with clinical signs of hyperadrenocorticism. *J Vet Int Med.* 1996; **10**, 1–6.

5

Disorders of Thyroid Gland Function

Jill Beech

Key Points

- Hypothyroidism has been associated with the feeding of goitrogens and diets both deficient in iodine and containing excessive iodine. Dams fed such diets are often normal, but give birth to foals that are weak and dysmature, and suffer a number of orthopaedic problems.
- In older animals, hypothyroidism has been suggested as a cause of poor growth, infertility, prolonged gestation, agalactia, obesity, poor performance, muscle dysfunction and laminitis.
- Diagnosis of hypothyroidism is based upon measurement of plasma throxine and tri-iodothyronine concentrations, together with their response to exogenous thyroid stimulating or thyrotropin releasing hormones.
- Hypothyroidism should be treated with thyroxine, with correction of any dietary anomalies.
- Tumours of the thyroid gland are frequent, incidental findings and are not associated with thyroid dysfunction.
- There are no documented cases of equine hyperthyroidism.

Introduction

The thyroid secretes thyroxine (T_4) and small amounts of tri-iodothyronine (T_3); the majority of T_3 is formed in tissues from thyroxine. Circulating T_3 and T_4 are bound primarily to thyroxine binding globulin with smaller amounts bound to thyroxine-binding prealbumin and albumin. Less than 1% is in the free state. It is the free form that is active and there is hardly any metabolic function that is not affected by the thyroid hormones.

Although many horses are given exogenous thyroxine based on low plasma T_3 and/or T_4 levels, the incidence of thyroid disease in horses is probably not accurately known. Tumours of the thyroid gland are frequently incidental findings in older horses. These tumours may enlarge sufficiently to cause clinical problems and sometimes are locally invasive or metastasize; because thyroid function itself has been normal in reported cases, they will be mentioned only briefly. The author knows of no documented cases of hyperthyroidism in horses.

Hypothyroidism

Goitrogenic feeds have been associated with hypothyroidism. Mares fed iodine deficient diets have had foals born dead or weak and lacking hair [1, 2]. Mares fed excessive amounts of iodine, usually in the form of kelp or seaweed extracts, although appearing clinically normal themselves have had foals born weak with limb deformities, prognathism and goitres and there have been some foetal deaths. Idiopathic hypothyroidism has been reported in foals mainly in western Canada and sporadically elsewhere in North America; gestation is often prolonged with dystocia and premature lactation [1] but dams are otherwise normal. The foals are born weak and dysmature and nearly always have retarded ossification and crushing of the tarsal and carpal bones, forelimb contractures and ruptured common digital extensor tendons and prognathism. One foal also was hypothermic and had respiratory distress attributed to atelectasis and impaired surfactant production; it failed to show the expected rise in T_3 and T_4 following thyrotropin releasing hormone (TRH) administration, and at postmortem examination the thyroids were enlarged and colloid filled [3].

Hypothyroidism was documented by lack of response to thyroid stimulating hormone (TSH) in a foal that was lethargic, stunted, had an abnormal rough long haircoat, decreased rectal temperature, angular limb deformities and 'flabby' muscles. The foal was also anaemic, hypercholesterolaemic and lipaemic [4]. Some of these foal's signs were the same as those reported in young thyroidectomized horses.

Hypothyroidism has been suggested as a cause of poor growth, agalactia, muscle dysfunction, prolonged gestation, infertility, poor performance, obesity, 'cresty neck' and laminitis (Table 1) but data are lacking to substantiate these associations. Agalactic mares were reported to have reduced basal serum T_4

Table 1. **Clinical features of hypothyroidism**

Foals
- weakness
- prognathism
- limb deformities
- poor growth
- goitre

Other animals (N.B. many of these associations have not been substantiated or proven)
- reproductive dysfunction – infertility, prolonged gestation, agalactia
- poor performance
- obesity
- laminitis
- 'cresty neck'

values but response to TRH was the same as in normally lactating mares. The basal T_3 concentration was the same as that in the normal mares but the rise following TRH was greater [5]. Horses with chronic laminitis were reported to have normal T_4 concentrations. Mildly affected horses had higher T_3 levels, although the range of values was wide. Their responses to TSH were the same as in control horses. The authors suggested that increased T_3 levels might be a consequence and not a causative factor in laminitis [6]. Poor performance in six racehorses with muscle stiffness or weakness in five of the six, and lethargy and anaemia in one were attributed to hypothyroidism based on low resting T_4 and clinical improvement following iodinated casein supplementation [7]. As their T_4 response to TSH was normal, thyroid gland function itself would appear to have been normal, and decreased basal circulating T_4 levels possibly were caused by some other factor(s).

When young horses were thyroidectomized they developed lethargy, anaemia, leukopenia, decreased rectal temperature, coarse thickened facial features, a dull haircoat and limb oedema, and stopped growing. Feed consumption and weight gain were markedly decreased. Epiphyseal plate closure and incisor teeth eruption were delayed. Neither laminitis nor obesity was reported [8, 9]. The role of hypothyroidism in infertility in mares is unclear, especially as conception has been reported after thyroidectomy [10]. Thyroidectomized stallions had decreased libido, increased time to ejaculation and a decreased sperm concentration; however, the latter was offset by increased semen volume [10].

Diagnosis of Abnormal Thyroid Function

Diagnosis of hypothyroidism is based on T_3 and T_4 concentrations and response to TSH or TRH stimulation. Diagnosis of hypothyroidism should not be made solely on the basis of T_3 and/or T_4 levels because of the many factors that influence T_3 and T_4 concentrations and the fact that low values can exist in normal horses [11]. It is unclear whether there is diurnal variation in T_3 and T_4 concentrations. One study showed no significant difference between a.m./p.m. samples [11] but in another T_4 tended to be higher between 5 and 8 p.m. than at 8 a.m. [12]. Both T_3 and T_4 can be decreased by phenylbutazone (2 g IV, BID) [12]. In another paper a similar dose (4.4 mg/kg IV, q12h for 7 days) caused a decrease in T_4 (total and free) but not T_3 concentrations [11]. In foals, accurate measurement of T_3 and T_4 may be difficult because of the high concentration of strong affinity T_3 and T_4 binding proteins; use of kitsets without validation on equine (foal) plasma may give erroneous results [13]. Levels of T_4 are highest at birth, decline rapidly in the first 4–6 days and then steadily through day 28 [13, 14]. The T_3 rises for 24–48 hours after birth before plateauing for several days and then declining, parallel to T_4 [13]. The levels in foals are much higher than in other species or adult horses [13]. Interpretation of values in neonatal foals may not be possible because of the high variability; in 1-day-old foals baseline T_3 and T_4 concentrations were reported to have a wide range

(26.0–732.7 ng/dL and 4.4–25.1 μg/dL, respectively [15]. A seasonal or pasture effect has been suggested in brood-mares with baseline concentrations lower at certain times of the year (R Douglas, personal communication, 1995). However, in one study, plasma concentration of thyroxine was not significantly different between winter and summer or different stages of pregnancy vs non pregnancy. Lactating mares, however, had significantly lower levels of T_4 compared with nonlactating mares. Acute cold exposure caused a 63% increase in plasma T_4 [16]. Since greater than 99% of the circulating T_3 and T_4 is protein bound and it is the free form that is in equilibrium with intracellular levels and gives a better idea of tissue thyroid hormone status, it has been suggested that the measurement of free forms is more desirable. In normal horses, however, measuring free T_4 (by single-stage radio-immunoassay, RIA) provided no additional useful information over total T_4 measurement [11].

Because of the potential problems in interpreting baseline T_3 and T_4 concentrations, thyroid stimulating tests have been devised. Both TSH and TRH have been used (Table 2). Various protocols have been suggested for the TSH stimulation test. Five international units of TSH IM is adequate to evoke an increase in T3 and T4 in a healthy mature horse [12] and the same dose has been administered IV to foals and mature horses. A dose of 2.5 IU IV has also been reported to evoke a response [17]. Blood samples are obtained prior to TSH administration and at 2 and 4 or 6 hours later. In normal horses T_3 increased to more than twice baseline at 2 hours and T_4 doubled at 4 and 6 hours [12, 18]. In foals, T_3 shows the greater response to TSH with a peak increase between 1 and 3 hours. It is possible that the decline in circulating T_4 concentration that normally occurs during the first 24 hours of the foal's life obscured its response to TSH administration [11].

Table 2. Endocrinological testing of thyroid function

Test	*Normal Response*	*Reference*
TRH stimulation		
0.5 mg IV in ponies or 1.0 mg IV in horses with samples obtained prior to and at 2 and 4 hours after TRH	T_4 increases 1.5-fold by 2 hours and 2-fold by 4 hours T_3 increases approx. 3-fold by 2 hours	18
	Significant increase in T_4 by 2 hours with peak at 4–10 hours; peak in T_3 at 2 or 4 hours.	19
	T_3 and T_4 significantly increase by 1 hour with T_4 peaking at 4 hours	20
TSH stimulation		
5 IU IM with samples pre TSH and at 3 and 6 hours	T_3 significantly increases at 1–3 hours with < variation and peak at 3 hours T_4 increases significantly by 3 hours and is approx. 2 × baseline at 6 hours	12
5 IU IV with samples pre TSH and at 2–3 hours	T_4 increases 2 × baseline by 2–3 hours and peaks (2.4 × baseline) at 4 hours T_3 increases 2 × baseline by $\frac{1}{2}$–1 hour and peaks (5 × baseline) at 2 hours	24

At least in some areas, TSH is frequently difficult to acquire, and TRH has become more widely used for evaluating thyroid function. A dose of 0.5 mg in ponies or 1 mg in horses is administered intravenously. Plasma or serum samples are taken before and at 2 and 4 hours after injection of TRH; T_4 shows a significant rise by 2 hours and peaks between 4 and 10 hours and T_3 peaks at 2 or 4 hours [19]. Another study showed a significant rise in both T_3 and T_4 by 1 hour, although T_4 continued to rise, peaking at 4 hours [20]. Therefore, if one is able to take only two samples these should be at 0 (i.e. pre TRH administration) and 4 hours.

Treatment of Hypothyroidism

A dosage of 10 mg L-thyroxine po once daily is used for treatment of hypothyroidism, based on the report that this dose in adult horses (500 kg, estimated BW) can increase serum levels of T_3 and T_4, with the latter remaining elevated for 24 hours [19]. Clinical signs and plasma concentrations of T_3 and T_4 should be monitored and dosage adjusted if needed. One should eliminate potential goitrogens from the horse's environment.

Thyroid Gland Neoplasia

Adenomas, C cell tumours, carcinomas, and hyperplasia of thyroid glands have been reported in horses [21–23]. Adenomas are not uncommon in older horses. Clinical signs are usually referable to the size of the thyroid gland and/or tumour and, to the author's knowledge, no signs of hypo- or hyper-thyroidism have been seen in any of these cases. Gulping or gurgling was reported in two horses with C cell tumours and signs resolved following tumour removal [21]. In addition to physical examination, scintigraphy, and or ultrasonography can be useful diagnostically. Biopsy for histology should confirm the diagnosis.

References

1. Allen AL, Doige CE, Fretz PB *et al.* Congenital hypothyroidism, dysmaturity and musculoskeletal lesions in Western Canadian foals. *Proc AAEP.* 1993; **39**, 207–208.
2. McLaughlin BG & Doige CE. Congenital musculoskeletal lesions and hyperplastic goiter in foals. *Can Vet J.* 1981; **22**, 130–133.
3. Murray MJ. Hypothyroidism and respiratory insufficiency in a neonatal foal. *J Am Vet Med Assoc.* 1990; **197**, 1635–1638.
4. Vivrette SL, Reimers TJ & Krook L. Skeletal disease in a hypothyroid foal. *Cornell Vet.* 1984; **74**, 373–386.
5. Thompson FN, Caudle AB, Kemppainen RJ *et al.* Thyroidal and prolactin secretion in agalactic mares. *Theriogenology.* 1986; **25**(4), 575–580.

6. Hood DM, Hightower MS, Amoss MS Jr *et al.* Thyroid function in horses affected with laminitis. *The Southwestern Veterinarian.* 1987; **38**(2), 85–91.
7. Waldron-Mease E. Hypothyroidism and myopathy in racing thoroughbreds and standardbreds. *J Equine Med. Surg.* 1979; **3**, 124–128.
8. Lowe JE & Kallfelz FA. Thyroidectomy and the T-4 test to assess thyroid dysfunction in the horse and pony. *Proc AAEP.* 1980; **16**, 135–154.
9. Lowe JE, Baldwin BH, Foote RH *et al.* Equine hypothyroidism: The long-term effects of thyroidectomy on metabolism and growth of mares and stallions. *Cornell Vet.* 1974; **64**, 276–296.
10. Lowe JE, Baldwin BH, Foote RH *et al.* Semen characteristics in thyroidectomized stallions. *J Reprod Fertil Suppl.* 1975; **23**, 81–86.
11. Sojka JE, Johnson MA & Bottoms GD. Serum tri-iodothyronine, total thyroxine, and free thyroxine concentrations in horses. *Am J Vet Res.* 1993; **54**, 52–55.
12. Morris DD & Garcia M. Thyroid-stimulating hormone response test in healthy horses and effect of phenylbutazone on equine thyroid hormones. *Am J Vet Res.* 1983; **44**, 503–507.
13. Irvine CHG. Hypothyroidism in the foal. *Equine Vet J.* 1984; **16**, 302–306.
14. Murray MJ & Luba NK. Plasma gastrin and somatostatin, and serum thyroxine (T_4), tri-iodothyronine (T_3), reverse tri-iodothyronine (T_3) and cortisol concentrations in foals from birth to 28 days of age. *Equine Vet J.* 1993; **25**, 237–239.
15. Shaftoe S, Schick MP & Chen CL. Thyroid-stimulating hormone response tests in one-day-old foals. *Equine Vet Sci.* 1988; **8**, 310–312.
16. Katovich M, Evans JW & Sanchez O. Effects of season pregnancy and lactation on thyroxine turnover in the mare. *J Anim Sci.* 1974; **38**(4), 811–818.
17. Harris P, Marlin D & Gray J. Equine thyroid function tests: A preliminary investigation. *Br Vet J.* 1992; **148**, 71–80.
18. Lothrop CD & Nolan HL. Equine thyroid function assessment with the thyrotropin-releasing hormone response test. *Am J Vet Res.* 1986; **47**(4), 942–944.
19. Chen CL & Li WI. Effect of thyrotropin releasing hormone (TRH) on serum levels of thyroid hormones in Thoroughbred mares. *J Eq Vet Sci.* 1985; **6**, 58–61.
20. Beech J & Garcia MC. Hormonal response to thyrotropin releasing hormone in healthy horses and in horses with pituitary adenoma. *Am J Vet Res.* 1985; **46**, 1941–1943.
21. Lucke VM & Lane JG. C Cell tumours in the thyroid in the horse. *Equine Vet J.* 1984; **16**, 28–30.
22. Hillidge CJ, Sanecki RK & Theodorakis MC. Thyroid carcinoma in a horse. *J Am Vet Med Assoc.* 1982; **181**, 711–714.
23. Schotthauer CF. The incidence and types of diseases of the thyroid gland in adult horses. *J Am Vet Med Assoc.* 1931; **78**, 211–218.
24. Oliver JW & Held JP. Thyrotropin stimulation test – new perspective on value of monitoring tri-iodothyronine. *J Am Vet Med Assoc.* 1985; **187**(9), 931–934.

6

Equine Rhabdomyolysis Syndrome

Pat A. Harris

Keypoints

- Primarily affects the muscles of horses of apparently any age, breed or gender resulting in a partial or complete inability to move.
- Sufferers have an underlying predisposition to the condition which is then triggered by one or more factors, usually including exercise, resulting in the clinical signs.
- The underlying predisposition, as well as the triggering factors, may differ between groups of sufferers.
- Two sub-groups with distinct pathophysiological processes have been identified recently. One involves a disorder in muscle contractility or excitation–contraction coupling and the other involves a defect in carbohydrate storage and/or utilization, polysaccharide storage myopathy (PSSM).
- Diagnosis is usually based on clinical history and signs together with plasma muscle enzyme activities. PSSM is diagnosed from a muscle biopsy.
- Treatment depends on the clinical severity but aims to limit further muscle damage, decrease pain and anxiety plus restore fluid balance.
- Guaranteed preventative managemental and therapeutic regimens not currently available.
- High fibre, low hydrolysable carbohydrate, +/− fat supplemented diets may be beneficial in some cases. Decreasing 'stress' levels and maintaining daily exercise with pasture turnout are also recommended.

Introduction

This condition primarily affects the muscles of horses of apparently any age, breed or gender, resulting in a partial or complete inability to move. Over the years, a number of names have been used, most of which are descriptive in nature, i.e. Setfast, Azoturia, Tying-Up, Paralytic Myoglobinuria, Monday Morning Disease, Exertional Rhabdomyloysis. As it is unlikely that a single pathophysiological process can explain all manifestations of the condition and exertion *per se* is not always involved (although movement tends to be the final 'triggering' factor), the author prefers to refer to this condition as the equine rhabdomyolysis syndrome (ERS). Fairly recently, two specific causes of recurrent episodes of rhabdomyolysis have been identified in the United States and it is likely that others will be found in the future. One of these is believed to be a disorder of muscle contractility or excitation-contraction coupling and the other a disorder in carbohydrate storage and utilization (polysaccharide storage myopathy). In the future, therefore, as more information becomes available about the pathophysiological processes involved, in different sub-groups of sufferers, it will be preferable and beneficial to subdivide the syndrome.

Pathophysiology

A number of features, which need to be taken into consideration when discussing the pathophysiology of the equine rhabdomyolysis syndrome, are summarized in Table 1. Even within an individual sufferer, for example, one episode may differ considerably from another as to the time of year it occurs, the clinical severity, the duration and intensity of any preceding exercise and so on. The author currently believes that sufferers have an underlying predisposition to the condition which is then triggered by one or more factors resulting in the clinical signs as outlined in Table 2.

Progress in understanding this syndrome has been slow, partly due to the difficulties in identifying and obtaining sufficient numbers of sufferers with the same pathophysical process to study as well as the intermittent nature of this condition. Although the recent work from the United States is helping to clarify certain of the potential pathophysiological processes, there are still many more theories than facts available about this syndrome. A number of the more popular theories are outlined below.

Table 1. **Some of the interesting features of the equine rhabdomyolysis syndrome**

- Primarily affects Type II muscle fibres
- Often recurrent
- Intermittent – the interval between episodes can vary from days to months
- Variable clinical severity – even within an individual
- Can affect one individual within a group all on the same management feeding and exercise regimen
- Exercise is a very common triggering factor – the nature and type of the exercise which precedes an episode often varies between *and* within individuals
- Between episodes, many sufferers are able to 'perform' as required

Table 2. **Pathophysiology**

- It is unlikely that one theory can explain all manifestations of this syndrome
- The pathophysiological pathways that lead to the initiation of the process(es) which result in the clinical signs are likely to vary within groups of individuals, although there may be a common pathway leading to the actual muscle damage
- 'Triggering' and 'Predisposing' factors are likely to vary from one individual to another
- Optimal treatment/preventative regimens for one sufferer (or group of sufferers) may differ from those required for another
- Possible sequence of events:

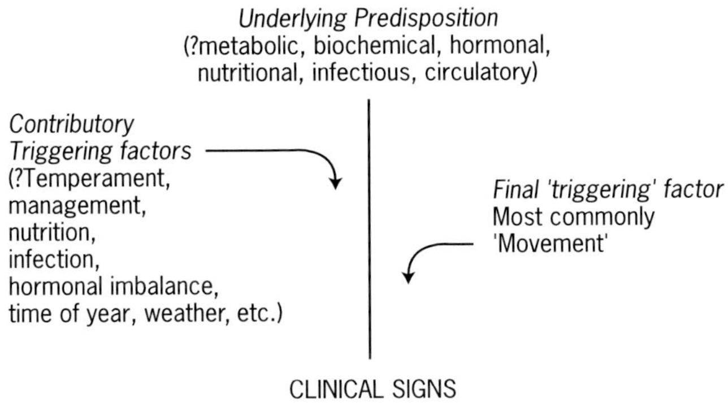

Carbohydrate Overloading

This has been one of the more popular and enduring theories. In the early 1900s, when oats were scarce and raw sugar was fed instead, an increase in metabolic diseases, especially 'Azoturia', was reported. Later studies reported that the condition could be induced by feeding horses 3 kg molasses per day and then exercising them after a rest period [1]. Since then, it has often been suggested that any factor which increases the rate of muscle glycogen deposition or utilization is likely to predispose to ERS, as would a decreased circulation to the muscle, because during exercise the glycogen would be metabolized anaerobically, resulting in the rapid production of lactic acid. This, in turn, would cause local tissue damage, vasospasm, decreased circulation and further reduction in lactic acid removal [2].

Recently, however, this theory has become less popular among research scientists. It has been shown, for example, that blood and muscle lactate concentrations during an episode of ERS tend to reflect the fitness of the animal and the nature of any preceding exercise [3, 4] rather than the syndrome itself. After race-like work, it has been shown that it takes several days to restore muscle glycogen content and therefore it seems unlikely that in such circumstances, glycogen overloading could occur after a single rest day. Studies in a number of countries, however, have found very high resting glycogen concentrations in the muscles of some recurrent sufferers, which it was suggested could be a marker for a subgroup with a certain pathophysiology [3, 4]. Interestingly, exercise was shown to result in muscle glycogen depletion in these affected animals to concentrations similar to those found in the control animals [4]. Resynthesis occurred rapidly so that within 24 hours, the initial high resulting values were established. The researchers did not, however, believe that intramuscular glycogen accumulation *per se* was a triggering factor for the syndrome or that a rapid rate of anaerobic glycolysis with excessive lactate accumulation was the cause of the muscle damage [4]. Studies at the single fibre level were not carried out.

Glycogen overloading in Man is associated with increased uptake of intracellular water, most likely owing to the increase in osmotic pressure. One possible effect of increased muscle fibre size would be a reduction in capillary perfusion owing to the increase in intramuscular pressure.

Polysaccharide Storage Myopathy (PSSM)

A subset of recurrent sufferers have been relatively recently found to have a glycogen storage disorder characterized by the accumulation of a non-bioavailable polysaccharide in up to 40% of their Type II muscle fibres; subsarcolemmal vacuoles and increased muscle glycogen concentrations [5, 6]. These acid mucopolysaccharide inclusions have been shown to consist of beta glycogen particles and filamentous material on electron microscopy. The muscle glycogen content can be up to four times that of normal horses.

The exact metabolic defect in glycolysis or glycogen synthesis has not been identified, although work is in progress. It has been postulated that the clinical signs occur because of the inability of glycolysis to generate ATP for mechanical work and maintenance of chemical gradients [7].

Whether this condition also occurs in Europe, and could explain at least some of the high muscle glycogens previously reported in European studies, is currently unknown. To date, in the USA, this disorder has been identified in Quarter Horses, Paints, Appaloosas, Draft and Draftcrosses, Warmbloods and a few Thoroughbreds.

A familial basis has been identified in Quarter Horse related breeds [8] and breeding trials are in progress in order to determine if this condition is inherited.

Other Potentially Genetically Determined Metabolic Abnormalities

A number of genetically determined conditions have been identified in man that produce signs similar to ERS including McArdle's Syndrome (lack of muscle phosphorylase) and Taru's Syndrome (lack of phosphofructokinase) in which muscle glycogen is not available for anaerobic metabolism. This leads to a characteristic lack of an increase in blood lactate concentration following ischaemic forearm exercise [9]. However, clinical signs tend to be present every time the sufferer exercises unlike the more intermittent nature of ERS and it is unlikely that a major abnormality of the carbohydrate glycolytic pathway is present in all ERS sufferers. One study of 22 affected horses could not find a predisposition to ERS based on an abnormal activity level of 20 intracellular enzymes, including phosphorylase, in muscle biopsy samples [10, 11]. However, it has been proposed that local areas of abnormality may occur. The analysis of whole muscle biopsies, which have a heterogeneous fibre composition, may be of little value owing to the possible marked variability in enzyme and intracellular buffering capacity of the different muscle fibre types.

Carnitine palmitoyltransferase is involved in the mitochondrial oxidation of long chain fatty acids and a deficiency in man results in very similar clinical signs to ERS, although it tends to occur more in males and to be precipitated by fasting prior to exercise. It also commonly involves the respiratory muscles [12]. A deficiency in this enzyme has been suggested to be a contributory factor to ERS [13] although these workers appeared to show that all horses, whether or not they were prone to ERS, had a low activity relative to man.

It is possible that other partial deficiencies or less severe enzyme abnormalities could be involved in certain subgroups of ERS sufferers. However, the techniques for detecting them would need to be validated for use in the horse and large numbers of sufferers screened in order to detect those (potentially small in number) with a particular abnormality.

Vitamin E/Selenium (Se) and Free Radical Induced Muscular Damage

The selenium-containing enzyme, glutathione peroxidase and vitamin E help to protect against free radical induced cellular damage [14].

Evidence for a role of vitamin E/Se deficiency in the pathophysiology of ERS has been based on anecdotal reports on the success of supplementation in preventing further episodes. These anecdotal findings have not been supported to date by scientific studies. Vitamin E/Se responsive myopathies of sheep and pigs have selective Type I fibre degeneration compared with the Type II fibre involvement in ERS [3, 15, 16]. However, little is known about the role of free radical induced muscular damage in ERS, delayed onset muscle soreness or even overexertion. It is possible that vitamin E may have a role in treating/preventing muscle damage owing to its free radical scavenging abilities.

Viral Aetiology

Muscle pain or myalgia is a commonly reported symptom in influenza and other viral illnesses in man. Anecdotal reports have been suggested that certain horses may be stiff and reluctant to work after an attack of the 'virus' and one study into an outbreak of muscle stiffness and poor performance in a flat racing stable of Thoroughbreds suggested prior equine herpesvirus-1 (EHV-1) infection [17]. Much more work into this area is needed. It may be, for example, that muscle can be directly affected by certain viruses resulting in an increased susceptibility to exercise induced damage. The author does tend to recommend that animals prone to ERS should have their work load and feed intake reduced until several days after all signs of infection have passed, if there is any suggestion of a viral infection being present where the horse is kept.

Malignant Hyperthermia

In this condition, which has been reported in man, pigs, dogs and cats, there is believed to be an abnormal release of calcium from the sacroplasmic reticulum (SR) in response to a triggering factor. The reaction may not occur immediately or on first exposure to the 'stressor' which most commonly is anaesthesia, but can be fighting for dominance, sudden changes in ambient temperature, exercise, excitement and other types of 'stress'. The primary metabolic defect seems to be in the ligand gated calcium channel of the SR rather than the Ca^{2+} sequestration mechanism and it tends to result in hyperthermia, metabolic and respiratory acidosis and muscle damage [18, 19].

The human diagnostic halothane–caffeine contracture test has been adapted and used in a small number of recurrent ERS sufferers [20]. Two out of the five animals evaluated gave contractures similar to those expected in humans with a susceptibility to malignant hyperthermia. Another study [21], found that the *in vitro* twitch characteristics of muscle samples from recurrent sufferers differed from a control group by having, in particular, prolonged relaxation times. It has been suggested that this could be a result of abnormal calcium fluxes [22].

Very recently, an abnormality in excitation–contraction coupling has been reported in Standardbred and Thoroughbred horses suffering from chronic intermittent rhabdomyolysis [7]. Studies have reportedly shown an altered relaxation of muscle following a contractile twitch, using intercostal muscle preparations, suggesting that abnormal intracellular calcium regulation is the cause of this type of ERS [7]. Elevated myoplasmic calcium concentrations have also been reported during acute episodes [7]. To what extent this pathophysiological process is responsible for chronic intermittent rhabdomyolysis episodes in horses throughout the world is currently unknown.

Phenytoin (diphenylhdantoin) has been shown to reduce the incidence of episodes in certain recurrent ERS sufferers and although its mechanism of action is not clear, it is thought to affect sarcolemmal and sacroplasmic reticulum, and thereby intracellular, calcium homeostasis [7, 21].

Dantrolene, which has been suggested to work by restabilizing the SR membrane [18] has been used to try and prevent episodes of malignant hyperthermia and to reverse anaesthetic-induced episodes. In the horse, it has been used both for ERS and generalized myositis associated with anaesthesia, but no controlled studies have been undertaken; the drug appears not to be very bioavailable in the horse, therapeutic doses are unknown and it is potentially hepatoxic [23]. Although it has been anecdotally reported to be of some benefit in some horses [7], further work is needed in this whole area.

Local Hypoxia/Mechanical Strain

The ERS histologically predominantly affects the larger Type II fibres [15, 16]. These fibres have a greater glycogen storage capacity and fewer capillaries supplying them than the slow twitch (Type I) fibres. The Type II fibres also tend, at least in man, to have a more delicate connective tissue structure which means that they are more likely to be damaged by eccentric exercise. It has been suggested that a local hypoxia could lead to increased lactic acid production in these highly glycolytic fibres. However, many episodes of ERS occur during the initial warm-up stages of exercise when, in theory, these fast twitch fibres are unlikely to have been recruited. More generalized hypoxia (as occurs with subacute/chronic aorto-iliac thrombosis) does not tend to result in sufficient muscle damage to increase peripheral plasma muscle enzyme activities (unless severe in nature).

A study of six horses, with a history of recurrent ERS, exercised sub-maximally on the treadmill found marked increases in plasma aspartate amino-transferase (AST), creatine kinase (CK) and myoglobin concentrations in three animals, one of which also appeared clinically 'stiff'. The post exercise muscle biopsies in these three animals showed randomly scattered swollen vacuolated Type IIA and IIB fibres on light microscopy (approximately 6%). On electron microscopy, irregular sacromeres, myofibrillar disruption, dilated sacroplasmic reticulum and enlarged rounded mitrochondria with degenerate cristae were found [16]. These workers suggested that the scattered pattern of fibre necrosis meant that the rhabdomyolysis was likely to have been specifically induced within particular motor units. They concluded that this implied a more specific aetiology than the commonly quoted theories of general hypoxia or general lactic acidosis.

Hormonal Disturbances

Reproductive

Samples collected from a group of Thoroughbreds over a 9-month period showed that the 2-year-old fillies had more marked fluctuations in CK and AST activities than the 3-year-old fillies and colts, although no correlation between the plasma muscle enzyme activities and the stage of the oestrous cycle was found [24]. Another study [25] confirmed that sex and/or age could have a significant effect on the occurrence of high CK and AST activities. Fillies being in general more likely to have elevated CK and AST activities than colts and 2-year-olds to have higher AST activities than 3-year-olds. A more recent study showed no correlation between plasma progesterone levels or oestradiol 17-β concentrations and CK and AST activities in a group of 2- and 3-year-old fillies in training when the whole group was evaluated. However, when those animals with high median AST activities (which can take weeks to return to base line activities even after a single insult) were excluded, a number of significant correlations were found (Serrantoni *et al.* unpublished data).

ERS has anecdotally been reported to occur more frequently around oestrus. In a preliminary study, the reproductive hormones, progesterone and oestradiol 17-β, were shown to have a possible influence on certain electrolyte 24-hour percentage fractional excretion (FE) values [26]. The extent of the hormonal influence upon electrolyte excretion appeared to vary considerably between individuals and the study suggested that there could be marked changes in individual electrolyte excretion during the reproductive cycle, despite a constant dietary intake. Such changes could have a profound effect on individual animals' electrolyte status, especially if an electrolyte deficient or imbalanced diet was being fed. This could be a contributory factor to ERS in certain individuals (see below), but further studies are needed to evaluate this.

Thyroid

Hypothyroidism in man is often accompanied by muscular involvement ranging from slight fatigue to overt muscle damage. It has been suggested that in the horse, poor racing performances and certain myopathies are related to some degree of hypothyroidism [27] and that oral thyroxine supplementation may improve performance or decrease the incidence of ERS. A few ERS sufferers have been shown to have an apparently lowered response to thyrotropin-releasing hormone which may reflect a decreased thyroid reserve [28]. However, too few cases have been investigated and, to date, there is insufficient scientifically based evidence to prove that thyroid dysfunction is involved in ERS.

Electrolyte imbalances

Electrolytes play an important role in neuromuscular function and electrolyte disturbances have been shown in other species to result in often pronounced muscular signs. Such signs tend to be either permanently present or consistently induced by a triggering factor such as exercise. It has therefore been suggested that electrolyte and thyroid hormone involvement in some cases of ERS may be associated with transient alterations in the ionic fluxes or concentrations across the muscle membranes.

There is some scientific support for electrolyte disturbances being involved in some cases, although the evidence is not conclusive. Over a number of years, the author has apparently been able either to reduce the frequency of episodes or to prevent further episodes in a number of recurrent sufferers by appropriate electrolyte supplementation. The supplementation was based on the results of the urinary FE test often, but not always, combined with appropriate managemental changes [29]. This regimen, as outlined in Figure 1, does not appear to be beneficial in all sufferers and in those where there is apparent success, this may be due to either an effect of the managemental and/or the dietary changes or the unpredictable nature of this syndrome. In a few cases, cessation of the recommended electrolyte supplementation has been known to result in the reoccurrence of episodes. The FE test, however, needs to be applied and interpreted with caution [30]. It must also be appreciated that different feeding practices within and between countries may mean that electrolyte supplementation based on the FE test may have more or less relevance. Horses in one study [31] in the United States with recurrent ERS had lower muscle potassium concentrations on a dry weight basis than the control group and although the ERS group tended to have lower %FE potassium values, the differences were not significant.

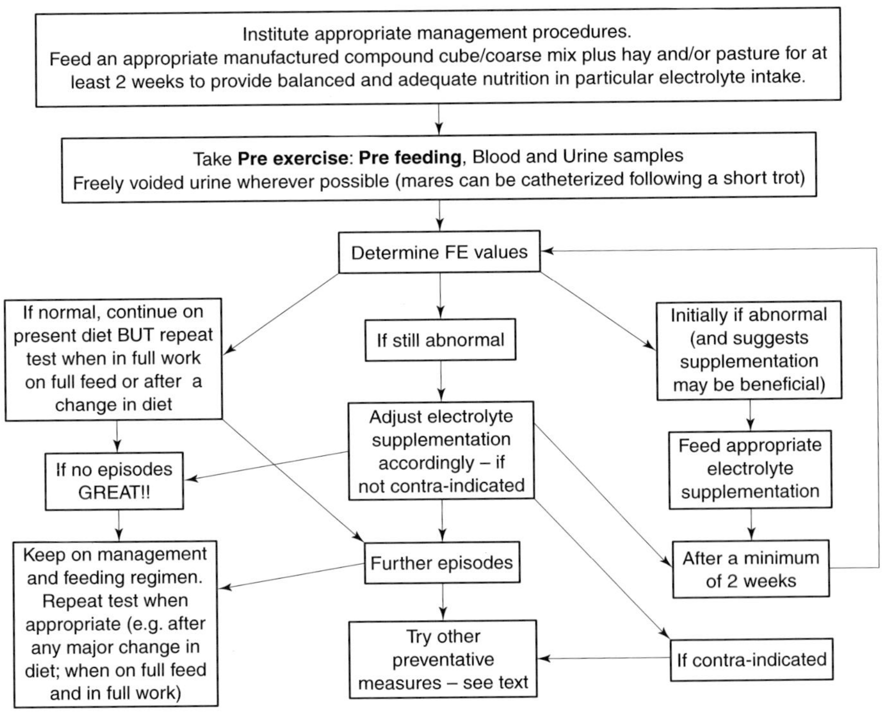

Figure 1. Protocol for fractional urinary electrolyte testing (based on Harris PA. Equine Rhabdomyolysis Syndrome. *Current Therapy in Equine Medicine,* 4, 1997)

Conclusion

It has been suggested that regardless of the initiating process, there is a common final pathway of muscle fibre degeneration [15]. However, much more work is needed to understand the pathophysiological processes involved in ERS so that the preventative and therapeutic regimens recommended can be more scientifically based and effective.

Epidemiology

Epidemiological studies of this syndrome are hampered, because at present, there is no simple and reliable method that will confirm that an individual is suffering, has suffered or will suffer from ERS (apart from PSSM). Any investigation tends, therefore, to base the inclusion of case material on a combination of appropriate clinical histories, clinical signs and laboratory data. Some epidemiological information for the UK is given in Table 3. A recent review from the United States suggested that about 5% of Thoroughbred racehorses develop recurrent exertional rhabdomyolysis during the racing season. Episodes most commonly occurred in the young fillies, especially 2-year-olds, of a nervous disposition. The PSSM sufferers, however, often have a calm and sedate manner. Typically, they suffer numerous episodes each year starting when they commence training. The milder cases however may only suffer one or two episodes a year [7, 8].

A familial predisposition has been suggested but not conclusively proved for ERS in general although a familial basis for the PSSM in Quarter Horse related

***Table 3.* Some epidemiological features of the equine rhabdomyolysis syndrome in the UK. Based on the results of a UK survey [33]**

• Time of Year
The highest apparent prevalence was between November and February, but this may no longer be correct with cases now occurring more consistently throughout the year. Possibility of an increased incidence with the availability of 'lush', hydrolysable carbohydrate rich, pastures.

• Breed
Most of the sufferers in the survey were Thoroughbred or Thoroughbred crosses, but a wide variety of breeds and types were represented. This breed prevalence may just reflect the higher competetive usage of these animals in the UK and the clientele of the laboratory concerned.

• Age
Can occur at any age, but seems to be more common in 2–15-year-olds which may just reflect that these tend to be the most active animals.

• Sex
Both sexes can be affected, but appears to be more common in the female, especially the young filly in training.

• Number
Around 2% of equine samples sent into the referral diagnostic laboratory used in this survey (excluding routine health checks from animals in training) came from apparent ERS sufferers.

breeds has been identified [8]. A much higher prevalence of the condition has been noted in offspring of one of two stallions bred and trained at the same farm [7]. Trials are underway to determine if PSSM is a heritable condition [7]. It has been reported that animals prone to raised plasma muscle enzyme activities differed significantly from a control population of Standardbreds when the homogeneity of a number of blood group systems was compared [32]. In a small survey carried out in the UK, 5% of owners reported that they were aware of a relative of their own horse that had also suffered from ERS [33]. This may perhaps be considered a high percentage as many horses in the UK are brought for non-racing purposes without any knowledge of their breeding. Prior corticosteroid administration has been suggested to be important by some [2] workers, but this has not been the finding of the author in the UK. This may reflect differences in the usage of corticosteroids between countries. Traditionally, this syndrome was most commonly seen in animals which were exercised after a period of rest without a reduction in feed intake (i.e. Monday Morning disease). This type of history is far less commonly reported today in the UK, with many episodes occurring in animals in regular exercise. A recent review [7] from the United States concluded that stress and a period of stall rest preceding exercise appeared to trigger recurrent exertional rhabdomyolysis in susceptible horses. Box stall rest for more than 12 hours per day appeared to increase the incidence of rhabdomolysis in PSSM sufferers.

Clinical Signs

In most cases, the clinical signs occur either during or after exercise (as the animal returns home or in the stable/field after exercise). A small number of cases, however, are reported when the animal is not in work or as it leaves the stable/field at the start of exercise. A few young Quarter Horses with PSSM have been found to develop moderate to severe rhabdomyolysis without any associated exercise.

The main clinical sign is some degree of muscular stiffness which can be very mild or result in a total inability to move. Recumbency can occur. Nowadays, only on rare occasions is the condition fatal. The hind limbs are most commonly affected, usually bilaterally. Forelimb involvement has been reported, but to the author's knowledge, confirmation of preferential Type II muscle fibre damage in such cases has not been reported.

Firm, swollen muscle groups may be present, especially in the more severely affected animals but this is not always the case. Palpation of the muscles may or may not be resented. Signs associated with pain and distress may be apparent to a variable extent, as shown in Table 4. It must be appreciated that temperament can be a very important factor affecting the apparent clinical severity in an individual. Abdominal disturbances can occur at the same time or following an episode of ERS. The incidence of myoglobinuria is difficult to determine as

***Table 4.* Equine rhabdomyolysis syndrome graded according to clinical severity (from Harris PA. In: *Practice*, vol. 11(1), 1989)**

Clinical signs	*Grade 1*	*Grade 2*	*Grade 3*	*Grade 4*	*Grade 5*
Mobility	Slight stiffness shortened stride	Reluctant to move	Unable to move	Unable to move, may become transiently recumbent	Rapidly becomes recumbent
Muscle	NAD	Often NAD	±Firm and swollen, resent palpation	Firm and swollen, may not resent palpation	Firm± wasting
Excessive sweating	–	±	+	++	++
Pulse and resp. rates elevated above expected levels	–	±	++	++	+++
Signs normally attributed to gastrointestinal (GIT) disturbance	–	±	+	++	+++
Discolored urine	–	±	+	++	+++
Comments	Easily confused with other conditions			?Palpation is actually felt by the horse	GIT stasis can occur. Shock may develop. Death may occur

Key: NAD = No abnormality detected
– = absent
± = sometimes present
+ = usually present
++ = prominent
++ = severe

many owners will not actually see their horse urinate. Table 4 is only a guide to the condition, but can be of value when discussing treatments. In the UK, the majority of episodes seem to be relatively mild, in which no signs are apparently seen other than some degree of stiffness with or without increased sweating. In one survey [33], 38% of cases were stiff but able to walk, 38% were able to walk with difficulty, 21.5% were unable to walk and 2.5% became recumbent. More detailed descriptions of typical clinical findings have already been reported [33, 34]. Rare clinical signs associated with PSSM are exercise intolerance, muscle atrophy, renal failure and respiratory distress [7].

Prognosis

Where the potential triggering factor(s) can be identified, such as exercising after a period of rest without a reduction of feed intake, provided that appropriate management safeguards are instigated, further episodes may not occur. The risk will be reduced further if the animal can be returned to work without a second episode. This is because, in the author's opinion, the period between an episode and the return to full work is the most crucial time, as there appears to be an increased risk of re-occurrence during this period. An individual that has suffered a number of episodes, especially when there appears to be no common set of triggering factors, is more likely to suffer another episode at some indeterminable point in the future.

In many cases, no apparent residual effects of the muscle damage that occurred during an episode are found once the animal has fully recovered. In some of the animals investigated in depth, electromyograph (EMG) and histological changes, similar to those found with other chronic myositic conditions, may be present, but this is not an invariable finding. In a few cases, slight muscular atrophy may be present initially, but in the majority of cases, even this may resolve in time.

Diagnosis

A number of conditions have been included in the differential diagnosis of the ERS [35] and are shown in Table 5. The likely differentials will vary to some extent according to the nature and the severity of the clinical signs [35].

Table 5. **Some of the differential diagnosis which have been suggested for the ERS in the literature (including [3, 21, 34, 37 and 38])**

- Over exertion*
- Pulled muscles*
- Delayed onset muscle stiffness
- Laminitis*
- Aorto-iliacthrombosis (see [39, 40])*
- Vitamin E/selenium responsive myodegeneration (see [41–43])*
- Atypical myoglobinuria (see [3, 44])*
- Post-exhaustion syndrome (see [45])
- 'Colic'
- 'Back' problems
- Proximal limb lameness
- Monensin poisoning (see [46])*
- Acorn poisoning (see [47])

'More unusual' conditions that have been included in the differential diagnosis of ERS

Anthrax
Castration sequelae
Tetanus
Pleuritis
Cystitis
Nephritis
Spinal cord disease

*Possibly the most common conditions to exclude.

Apart from the distinct group of PSSM sufferers at the moment, there is no practical test or group of tests that can confirm, in between episodes, that an individual has suffered from or will suffer again from the ERS. The diagnosis of a clinical episode of ERS involves confirmation that there has been skeletal muscle involvement and that it has occurred as a result of this syndrome. Owing to the relatively non-specific nature of the clinical signs associated with non-traumatic skeletal muscle disorders, the diagnosis is most commonly made on the basis of the clinical picture, often in association with laboratory investigations. Possible investigative techniques available include muscle histology, histochemistry, thermography, electromyography, scintigraphy and, most commonly in equine medicine, plasma/serum biochemical investigations. Although *muscle biopsies* can provide information, especially in generalized conditions, on the morphological, biochemical and physiological properties of the myofibrils examined, they currently are of limited general value in the diagnosis or monitoring of ERS. However, they can be of value in the diagnosis of specific subgroups such as the recently recognized polysaccharide storage myopathies [8]. Contraction–relaxation evaluations to identify those animals with a disorder of muscle contractility or excitation–contraction coupling are not routinely applicable as currently they involve the removal of intact intercostal muscle. *Thermography* and *scintigraphy* [36] may be of value in identifying muscular involvement, especially in 'poor performance' cases, but are of limited routine value in the field. The electromyographic changes seen in chronic myositis and certain ERS cases include fibrillation potentials and are of no routine value in the field.

Plasma muscle enzyme activities are most commonly used to confirm skeletal muscle involvement, assess severity and monitor recovery. An alteration in the plasma activity of an enzyme can occur through a variety of mechanisms, including cell necrosis, impaired removal or clearance of the enzyme and impaired or increased synthesis, but most commonly as a result of a change in the integrity (either transiently or permanently) of the membrane containing the enzyme. The most commonly used enzymes to monitor the muscular system are CK, AST and lactate dehydrogenase (LDH) (see Table 6). AST and CK activities are most commonly measured because the differences in the half-lives and times to peak activity following an insult can help to indicate whether muscular damage is active or resolving, as shown in Table 7. Difficulties, however, can arise when muscle activities alone are used to diagnose ERS (see Table 8). In PSSM the plasma muscle enzyme activities are often markedly elevated even after prolonged rest [7].

The use of exercise tests to determine susceptibility or otherwise to exercise induced muscular damage has often been recommended (see Tables 9 and 10). There are, however, no 'set rules' for AST/CK activities. Some horses seem, for example, to be able to race and win despite significantly elevated pre- (and often post-) exercise CK and AST activities. Although how much better they could perform if they did not have such increases is unknown [25]. PSSM sufferers

Table 6. Some details on the enzymes most commonly used for the monitoring of muscle disorders

Name	*Where found*	*Isoenzymes*	*What an increase can mean*	*Half life*	*Time to peak activity post single insult to muscle*	*Time taken for activity to return to normal post single insult*
CK (creatine kinase)	Mainly skeletal muscle myocardium and brain. Little exchange between CSF and plasma	At present, do not appear to be of confirmed diagnostic value	Increase in plasma activity suggests skeletal and/or cardiac damage. Large increases most likely reflect skeletal muscle damage. Inaccurate venepuncture technique can result in falsely elevated CK values	~ 2 hours	~ 4–12 hours	Days
AST (aspartate amino-transferase)	Most soft tissues, especially muscle and liver. Non-specific	cAST (originates from cytoplasm) mAST (from the mitochondria) of no apparent diagnostic significance, although high concentrations of mAST unlikely in plasma/serum unless severe muscle damage	Non-specific. Mild increases could reflect, for example, recovery from a previous muscle insult or some other soft tissue involvement. Large increases, especially if associated with increases in CK, reflect muscular involvement	~ 7–8 days	~ 24 hours	Weeks
LDH (lactate dehydro-genase)	Many tissues. Non-specific	5 isoenzymes LDH_{1-5} Locomotor muscles mainly LDH_5 (plus some LDH_4) training may increase proportion of LDH_{1-4} and decrease LDH_5, Heart mainly LDH_1 (plus LDH_2 and $_3$)	Isoenzyme profile may provide information as to which tissues are involved. Muscle damage tends to result in an increase mainly in LDH_5 (and LDH_4)	Unknown	~ 24 hours	Days

Table 7 Some guidelines on the interpretation of plasma CK and AST activities (u/L)

	1	*2*	*3*	*4*	*5*	*6*
AST	150–230	1500	6000	2000	220	330
CK	0–50	8500	3000	150	290	65

1 = Reference range for laboratory used
2 = Providing clinical signs are appropriate: acute episode of ERS
3 = Initial recovery from episodes of ERS providing history appropriate
4 = Later stages of recovery from muscular involvement
5 = Similar results may be found, for example, in a young racehorse 2 hours after its first gallop and most likely reflect some degree of over-exertion rather than 'subclinical' ERS
6 = Similar results could be found several weeks after an episode of ERS, but it should be noted that such AST activities could reflect previous injury to soft tissue other than muscle. The slight apparent increase in CK may not be clinically significant

Table 8. Difficulties in interpreting plasma CK and AST activities (from Harris PA [35])

- Level of activity may not correlate with severity of the clinical signs
  Possible explanations include:
  i. Temperament
  ii. Generalized but 'slight' muscular damage resulting in a low grade episode but high activities.
  iii. Localized limited muscular involvement, but more severe damage resulting in a high grade episode but lower activities
- High activities without clinical signs
  Possible explanations include:
  i. mild clinical signs of ERS missed
  ii. physiological variation, e.g. decreased clearance
  iii. increased sensitivity of the cell membrane to those processes that cause an alteration in permeability
- Clinical signs of ERS without raised AST/CK activities
  Possible explanations include:
  i. misdiagnosis
  ii. insufficient muscle damaged to cause a significant rise in activities, although sufficient damage to cause overt signs of myopathy and pain, possibility that damage to certain muscle groups may be more painful than others
  iii. a separate condition with a different pathophysiology that results in muscle spasm, but no cellular damage
- Differentiation from other myopathies that can also result in raised activities and similar clinical signs, especially over-exertion

often show significant increases in plasma CK activities (of more than 1000 u/L) post mild exercise (e.g. 15 minutes at the trot). Myoglobin may be present in the urine of ERS sufferers and although *per se* is not nephrotoxic, when combined with disturbances in fluid status, it can result in renal damage. Haemoglobinuria has also been reported in some cases, although this has not been the author's experience. Such haemoglobinuric cases, with or without myoglobinuria, may represent a sub-group of cases with a particular pathophysiology [3].

Table 9. Comments on the use of an exercise test for ERS cases

- In a healthy horse, the effect of exercise on CK and AST activities may depend on a number of factors, including:
  - i. the intensity of the exercise
  - ii. the duration of the exercise
  - iii. the nature of the exercise
  - iv. the fitness of the individual
  - v. the age of the individual
  - vi. the sex of the individual
  - vii. the diet of the individual
- Lunging an unfit animal for a set period of time may result in raised plasma muscle enzymes regardless of a susceptibility or otherwise to muscular damage. *May precipitate an episode of ERS.*
- Over-strenuous exercise may also result in raised plasma enzymes regardless of a susceptibility or otherwise to muscular damage.
- Exact nature of the ideal exercise test and the interpretation of the results is controversial.
- The author's recommendation is a submaximal individually tailor-made exercise test:
  - i. Blood sample pre-exercise
  - ii. Give the horse exercise that the owner/rider considers to be a fair workout with respect to the animal's recent exercise regimen. Should not be over-strenuous. Horse should have undertaken similar work in the recent past. Avoid lunging.
  - iii. Sample 2–6 hours post exercise ($\pm$ at 24 hours post exercise).
  - iv. Measure AST/CK activities

  Note that animals can have an apparently 'normal' response to such an exercise test and still suffer an episode of ERS the following day.
- Such a test can give an idea of whether there has been any muscular damage since a previous sample and whether any such damage occurred during this exercise test.

Table 10. Criteria for determining a 'normal' response to a submaximal individually tailor-made exercise test

1 Pre-exercise:
- i. CK activity < 100 u/L (laboratory resting refence range 0–50 u/L)
- ii. AST activity < 300 u/L (laboratory resting reference range 150–230 u/L)

Plus

2 Not more than a doubling of the resting CK activity at 2–6 hours post exercise

3 Return to close to baseline CK activities at 24 hours post exercise

4 Not more than a 50% increase in AST activities

Plus

5 No clinical signs of stiffness

(Needs to be interpreted with care)

Use in monitoring the return to work after an ERS episode

- Carry out after approximately 3 days of return to exercise
- If acceptable results obtained, continue to bring back into full work
- If unacceptable results obtained, check managemental procedures. Consider a further period of rest (but maintaining pasture or equivalent turnout wherever possible), and other preventative regimens including FE testing

Repeat after being in work around 7–10 days and then as and when required (such as 3 days after any significant change in work load).

continued

Table 10. *Continued*

Example plasma CK and AST activities u/L before and 2–6 hours following an exercise test (based on Harris PA In: *Current Therapy in Equine Medicine* 4, 1997)

	A	B	C	D	E
Pre-exercise CK	20	55	200	95	45
Post-exercise CK	25	300	600	1100	60
Pre-exercise AST	190	200	630	250	190
Post-exercise AST	195	230	800	1000	235
Clinical Signs	None	None	None	None	Stiff

A: 'Normal' exercise test results but a chronic intermittent ERS sufferer may have such values and suffer an episode the next day. *Advice:* if such values are found in an ERS sufferer, it could be acceptable to increase work-load.

B: Normal resting CK and AST activities, suggesting that there has been no muscular injury sufficient to raise peripheral muscle enzyme activities in the recent past. Increase in CK post exercise. *Advice:* if horse suffered from recurrent ERS and had not been given excessive exercise, its work-load should remain constant for a few more days and exercise rest should be repeated.

C: Raised AST and CK resting activities suggesting muscular injury in recent past. The increase with exercise suggests continued muscular involvement. *Advice:* decrease work-load, ideally stop exercise and turn out. Reassess dietary, managemental and therapeutic regimens.

D: Raised AST/CK activities although no apparent clinical signs seen. These may have been missed or very subtle. May reflect more widespread, but slight, muscular involvement, insufficient to cause obvious clinical signs, but there is an increased risk in a recurrent ERS sufferer that the individual will suffer a further episode if exercise is continued. *Advice:* as per C.

E: No marked increase in CK and AST – increases seen cannot be considered diagnostically significant. *Advice:* most likely it is not ERS which is causing the stiffness.

Treatment

The extent of any initial treatment will depend on the apparent clinical severity, the temperature of the animal and on the experience of the owner. A guidance for a suggested treatment schedule is given in Figure 2 and a few comments on the more common treatments suggested for ERS are given in Table 11. Unless over-exertion or some form of 'cramp' is the cause of the stiffness, an affected animal should be rested as soon as possible after signs first appear until all signs have clinically resolved. At this point, the animal should be turned out into a small paddock or school for a period of time before exercise recommences. Such managemental procedures will not prevent all cases from suffering a further episode, but they do appear to limit the number of animals that suffer a re-occurrence in this difficult post-episode phase.

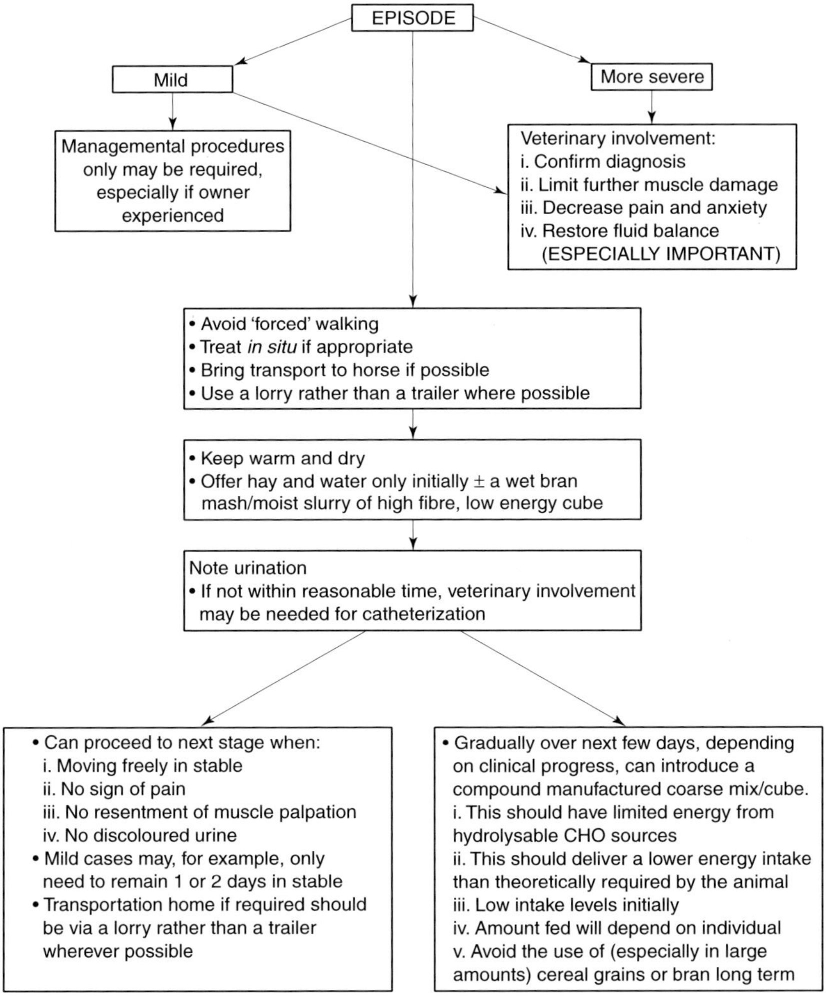

Figure 2. A suggested protocol for the management of an ERS case in the initial stages

Some workers recommend oral non-steroidal anti-inflammatory drugs (NSAIDs) for several days after the initial episode. The author tends to use, when required (usually only for the more severe cases), intravenous NSAIDs initially and then oral NSAIDs until the horse moves freely around the stable or a very small corral. NSAIDs are then stopped and, provided that the horse remains apparently pain-free, it is moved to a larger yard/small field for a period of time before exercise recommences. This may be several weeks in the more severe cases, but only a few days in the more mild.

***Table 11.* A few points about some of the more common treatments suggested for ERS (see also under Prevention)**

Fluids
MOST IMPORTANT TO MAINTAIN RENAL FUNCTION, ESPECIALLY IF MYOGLOBINURIA PRESENT
N.B. Especially in severe cases, it can be worth checking electrolyte and acid base status and treating accordingly
- Will be needed in the more severe cases, especially Grades 4 and 5 (see Table 4). Intravenous fluids may be combined with oral fluids in the more severe cases.
- Orally up to 5(–8) L every 30–60 minutes (provided no colic or ileus). Stop if any discomfort or gastric reflex occurs. Avoid hypertonic solutions.
- Use balanced IV solutions (some people have recommended that Glucose (5% dextrose saline) or 50% dextrose should be added to deliver between 50–100 g/hour).

It has been recommended to continue fluids until clear urine is produced.

Therapeutic agents
Sodium bicarbonate
- Not advisable to give sodium bicarbonate unless acid base status known – some suggest that should not be given unless plasma bicarbonate concentration is less than 15 mEq/L.
- Questionable efficacy post 'episode'.

Vitamin E/selenium
- May have some value in treatment due to their action against tissue damaging free radicals.
- Care with IV injections.
- Questionable efficacy.

Methocarbamol (robaxin)
- Supposedly acts to decrease pain by reducing muscle spasms.
- Animals can become ataxic and depressed.
- Questionable efficacy – several workers have reported it to be of little value.

Analgesics
- May not be required for Grade 1 severity cases.
- Care should be taken if ERS is likely to be complicated by other disease processes (the possibility 'of masking' signs).
- Care if renal compromise is likely as some may be potentially nephrotoxic.
- Some people recommend continued use post acute phase. This may be of value in the more severe cases, but not usually needed otherwise, see protocol outlined under management.
- Examples: phenylbutazone, flunixin meglumine, meclofenamic acid, butorphenol.

Sedatives/tranquilisers
- Phenothiazine derivatives may help peripheral circulation but care regarding possible hypotension if used when the circulation is compromised.
- Xylazine and detomidine are alternatives.

Corticosteroids
- May help to stabilize cellular membranes.
- May relax capillary sphincters and therefore improve tissue perfusion.
- Care regarding possible post-exercise laminitis, etc.
- May be more useful in the initial stages of the more severe cases (continued use not normally recommended).

Prevention

No single procedure or set of procedures are available that can guarantee no further episodes of ERS. Appropriate management and nutrition of susceptible animals may, however, help to reduce the likelihood or frequency of future episodes. Some of the recommended management procedures are shown in Figure 3. A few of the more commonly recommended 'preventative agents' are shown in Table 12.

Ready to proceed to next stage (see Fig. 2)

- Turn out into a small field/indoor school
  i. Avoid 'lush' pastures
  ii. Very occasionally, sedation may be required when initially turning out
  iii. Avoid getting 'cold'
  iv. Encourage 'gentle' movement in field
  N.B. In severe cases which occur at competitions this should occur before the horse is transported home.

↓

- Especially if a recurrent sufferer or has suffered a severe episode – monitor AST/CK activities
  i. Ideally, wait until both are within reference resting range before starting exercise or, following a severe episode at a competition, before transporting home
  iii. But, as a minimum – recommended that CK should be less than twice the upper limit of 'normal' for laboratory before exercise recommences.

↓

- When appropriate (could be after only 2–3 days in field for mild cases), start exercise
  i. Avoid lunging
  ii. Straight line work only
  iii. Slowly increase intensity and duration. Give plenty of warm-up
  iv. Provide regular exercise. Turn out if cannot exercise
  v. If misbehaves on own or in company, ride alone or with others as appropriate
  vi. Decrease work intensity and concentrate feed intake, if there is any suspicion of a respiratory viral infection being present on the premises where kept.

↓

Consider exercise testing (see Tables 9 & 10)

- Continue on as balanced a diet as possible
  i. Keep energy intake behind anticipated work load
  ii. Avoid high intakes of cereal grains
  iii. Consider fat supplementation of diet if additional energy required
  iv. Feed sufficient to maintain appropriate bodyweight and 'type' of ride
  v. Check that intake of trace elements and vitamins will be sufficient long term if feeding less than manufacturer's recommended intakes for a horse in a particular type of work. Additional sodium supplementation in particular may be required
- If the horse is given a day of rest the amount of concentrate feed should be halved from the evening before until the evening after the rest day
- If there is a longer period of rest it is worth decreasing the amount of feed further and/or changing to one with a lower energy level (see iv above)

↓

Consider checking FE values when been on 'balanced' diet for minimum of 2 weeks (see Fig. 1)

Figure 3. Later stages in the management of an ERS case – a suggested protocol

For those suffering from the recently recognized PSSM the recommended preventative measures include increasing the oxidative capacity of their skeletal muscle through gradual training and feeding a fat-supplemented diet (good quality grass hay, no grain or sweet feed, and a fat source plus an appropriate

Table 12. Comments on some of the more frequently recommended preventative agents.

Sodium bicarbonate
- Questionable relevance as most cases appear to have a metabolic alkalosis, but events at the single fibre level are presently unknown.
- Doses suggested of around 2–4 oz day (28–56 g) 3–6 hours before exercise.
- Efficacy unproven (possibility that any beneficial effect is due to the Na content).

Vitamin E and Se
- Unlikely to be deficient if on manufactured (compound) diets
- Questionable efficacy: effect, if any, may be due to role in preventing/limiting free radical induced muscular damage
- Oral Se recommended. Over-supplementation of Se can result in toxicity
- Higher levels of Vitamin E have been suggested to be advantageous in the performance animal, but unproven to date
- Supplementary doses recommended: 1.5–4.4 mg/kg BW.day of α-tocopherol acetate

Dimethylglycine (DMG)
- Results of studies controversial, most show no beneficial cardio-respiratory or metabolic effects
- Anecdotal success only: 1 mg/kg BW.day
- Efficacy unproven

Methyl sulfonyl methane (MSM)
- Suggested to be an oral natural anti-inflammatory alternative
- Anecdotally 5–15 g recommended
- Efficacy unproven

Thiamine
- Acts as a co-enzyme in the oxidative decarboxylation of pyruvate. Suggested that a deficiency could result in the accumulation of pyruvic and lactic acid in tissues as a result of a disturbance in carbohydrate metabolism
- Suggested levels: up to 500 mg/horse or 28 g/day brewer's yeast
- No scientific evidence as to efficacy

Acepromazine (ACP)
- 0.005–0.02 mg/kg approximately 30 minutes pre-exercise said by some to be of value, especially in nervous fillies
- No scientific evidence as to efficacy in preventing ERS

Phenytoin
- Care regarding clearance times/possible drug interactions/potential side effects
- A number of protocols have been recommended, but often have to be individually tailored
  - i. Initially 8–12 mg/kg BW, BID then check blood levels and maintain blood levels at 5–10 μg/mL, 4–6 hours post administration
  - ii. 8–12 mg/kg BW, BID for 3 days then 10 mg/kg BW, SID for a week then start training ($\pm$5–6 mg/kg BW, SID).

Thyroxine
- Suggested but unproven that some ERS sufferers have a decreased thyroid reserve (see [28])
- *But* optimal way of determining thyroid status in the horse is unknown at present
- Doses of around 5–10 mg L-thyroxine (500 kg horse) or 6–14 mg/kg BW iodinated casein have been recommended
- Potential negative effects of suddenly ceasing high-level supplementation have not been fully evaluated
- Efficacy unproven

Dantroline
- Pharmalogically effective dose not known for the horse
- Potentially hepatotoxic
- Effects on liver appear to be individually variable
- Advisable to monitor hepatic status
- A number of protocols available
  - i. 2–2.5 mg/kg BW in physiological saline given by stomach tube followed by 400–500 mg every 6–8 hours for more severe cases

continued

Table 12. *Continued*

ii. 2 mg/kg BW, po, SID initially for 3–5 days, then every 3rd day for up to a month
iii. Up to 1 g given with a small feed 1–2 hours before exercise for 3–5 days (more commonly used for animals in race training)
iv. 500 mg po, for 3–5 days, then 300 mg every 3rd day for a period of time: time will depend on circumstances and individual effect on the liver, prolonged treatment for more than 3 months is not, however, recommended

- Of little use in animals which suffer episodes very intermittently
- Efficacy unproven

Diazepam

- Used apparently at doses around 0.25 mg/kg BW, IV
- Efficacy unproven-care due to potential side effects

Electrolytes

- Electrolyte supplementation can be empirical, and usually involves Na and Ca supplementation, or preferably based on the results of a urinary electrolyte fractional electrolyte excretion test (FE) test
- FE test must be carried out appropriately and interpreted with care (see [30])
- Any apparent success could be an effect of associated management and/or dietary changes or the unpredictable nature of this syndrome
- *But*, the author has had the most success in helping to reduce episodes in recurrent sufferers using a combination of appropriate electrolyte supplementation based on the FE test and the managemental/dietary procedures shown in Figure 1

vitamin/mineral supplement) similar to that described in Figure 3. Daily riding as well as pasture turnout has also been recommended for this subgroup of sufferers [5, 7, 8]. For those suffering from the postulated contractility/excitation–contraction coupling disorder, standardized daily routines together with an environment that minimizes stress has been recommended [7]. Dietary advice is similar to that recommended in Figure 3. Low dose ACP administration, dantrolene and phenytoin have been suggested as possible therapeutic options to consider [7]. The avoidance of long slow work in some of these sufferers has been recommended, which is different from that recommended in Figure 3.

References

1. Carlstrom B. Uber die atiologie und pathogenese der kreuzlahme des pferdes (Haemoglobinaemia paralytica). *Scand Archiv.* 1933; **62**, 1–69.
2. Lindholm A, Johannson HE & Kjaersgaard P. Acute rhabdomyolysis (tying-up) in standardbred horses. A morphological and biochemical study. *Acta Vet Scand.* 1974; **15**, 325–335.
3. Harris PA. Aspects of the equine rhabdomyolysis syndrome. PhD thesis, Cambridge University, Cambridge, UK 1988.
4. Valberg S, Haggendal J & Lindholm A. Blood chemistry and skeletal muscle metabolic responses to exercise in horses with recurrent exertional rhabdomyolysis. *Equine Vet J.* 1993a; **25**(1), 17–22.
5. Valberg SJ, Cardinet GH III, Carlson GP & DiMauro S. Polysaccharide storage myopathy associated with recurrent exertional rhabdomyolysis in horses. *Neuromusc. Disord.* 1992; **2**(5, 6), 351–359.

6. Valberg SJ. Exertional rhabdomyolysis and polysaccharide storage myopathy in Quarter Horses. *41st A.A.E.P. Proc, Kentucky.* 1995; pp. 228–230.
7. Valberg S. Exertional rhabdomyolysis in the horse. *Proc. KER Equine Nutrition Conference, Kentucky*. 1997; 15–17.
8. Valberg SJ, Geyer CJ, Forum S & Cardinet III GH. Familial basis of polysaccharide storage myopathy and exertional rhabdomyolysis in Quarter Horses and related breeds. *Am J Vet Res.* 1996; **57**, 286–290.
9. Rennie MJ & Edwards RHT. Carbohydrate metabolism of skeletal muscle and its disorders. In, Randle PJ, Skeiner DF & Whelan WJ (eds) *Carbohydrate Metabolism and its Disorders*. London, Academic Press 1981; 75–99.
10. Van den Hoven R. Some histochemical and biochemical aspects of equine muscles, with special respect to equine exertional myopathy. Proefschrift Rijksuniversiteit, Utrecht 1987.
11. Van den Hoven R, Wensing T, Breukink HJ & Meijer AEFH. Enzyme histochemistry in exertional myopathy. In: Gillespie JR & Robinson NE (eds) *Equine Exercise Physiology*. Davis: ICEEP Publications 1987; 796–810.
12. Sadeh M & Gutman A. Carnitine palmitoyl transferase deficiency, A common cause of recurent myoglobinuria. *Israel J Med Sci.* 1990; **26**, 510–515.
13. Scholte HR, MHN, Ross JD, Van den Hoven R, Wensing T, Breuking HJ, Meijer AEFH & Van den Hoven E. Equine exertional rhabdomyolysis, activity of the mitochondrial respiratory chain and the carnitine system in skeletal muscle. *Equine Vet J.* 1991; **23**(2), 142–144.
14. Hitt ME. Oxygen-derived free radicals. *Comp Cont Educ Pract Vet.* 1988; **10**, 939–946.
15. McEwan SA & Hulland TJ. Histochemical and morphometric evaluation of skeletal muscle from horses with exertional rhabdomyolysis (tying-up). *Vet Pathol.* 1986; **23**, 400–410.
16. Valberg S, Jonsson L, Lindholm A & Holmgren N. Muscle histopathology and plasma aspartate aminotransferase, creatine kinase and myoglobin changes with exercise in horses with recurrent exertional rhabdomyolysis. *Equine Vet J.* 1993b; **25**(1), 11–16.
17. Harris PA. Outbreak of the equine rhabdomyolysis syndrome in a racing yard. *Vet Rec.* 1990; **127**, 468–470.
18. O'Brien PJ, Klip A, Britt BA & Kalow BI. Malignant hyperthermia susceptibility, Biochemical basis for pathogenesis and diagnosis. *Can J Vet Res.* 1990; **54**, 83–92.
19. Nelson TE. Malignant hyperthermia in dogs. *J Am Vet Med Assoc.* 1991; **198**, 989–994.
20. Hildebrand SV, Arpin D & Cardinet GH. Exertional rhabdomyolysis related to malignant hyperthermia using the halothane–caffeine contracture test. In: Gillespie JR & Robinson NE (eds). *Equine Exercise Physiology.* Davis: ICEEP Publications 1987; 786–795.
21. Beech J, Fletcher JE, Lizzo F & Johnston J. Effect of Phenytoin on the clinical signs and *in vitro* twitch characteristics in horses with chronic intermittent rhabdomyolysis and myotonia. *Am J Vet Res.* 1988; **49**, 2130–2133.
22. Hodgson DR. Exercise-associated myopathy, is calcium the culprit? *Equine Vet J.* 1993; **25**(1), 1–3.
23. Court MH, Engelkung LR, Dodman NH, Answer MS, Seeler DC & Clark M. Pharmokinetics of dantrolene sodium in horses. *J Vet Pharmacol Therap.* 1988; **10**, 218–226.
24. Frauenfelder HC, Rossdale PD, Ricketts SW & Allen WR. Changes in serum muscle enzyme levels associated with training schedules and stage of the oestrous cycle in Thoroughbred racehorses. *Equine Vet. J.* 1986; **18**, 371–374.
25. Harris PA, Snow DH, Greet TRC & Rossdale PD. Some factors influencing plasma AST/CK activities in thoroughbred racehorses. *Equine Vet. J.* 1990; **Suppl. 9**, 66–71.
26. Kinslow P, Harris P, Gray J & Allen WR. Influence of the oestrous cycle on electrolyte excretion in the mare. *Equine Vet. J.* 1995; **Suppl. 18**, 388–391.
27. Waldron-Mease E. Hypothyroidism and myopathy in racing thoroughbreds and standardbreds. *J Equine Med Surg.* 1979; **3**, 124–128.
28. Harris PA, Marlin DJ & Gray J. Equine thyroid function tests, A preliminary investigation. *Br. Vet. J.* 1991; **148**, 71–80.

29. Harris PA & Snow DH. Role of electrolyte imbalances in the pathophysiology of the equine rhabdomyolysis syndrome. In: Persson SGB, Lindholm A & Jeffcott LB (eds) *Equine Exercise Physiology 3*. Davis: ICEEP Publications 1991.
30. Harris PA & Gray J. The use of the urinary fractional electrolyte excretion test to assess electrolyte status in the horse. *Equine Vet Educ.* 1992; **4**(4), 162–166.
31. Beech J, Lindborg S & Braund KG. Potassium concentration in muscle, plasma and erythrocytes and urinary fractional excretion in normal horses and those with chronic intermittent exercise associated with rhabdomyolysis. *Res Vet Sci.* 1993; **55**, 43–51.
32. Lindholm A. Pathophysiology of exercise induced diseases of the musculoskeletal system of the equine athlete. In: Gillespie JR & Robinson NE (eds). *Equine Exercise Physiology* **711**, Davis: ICEEP Publications 1987.
33. Harris PA. The Equine Rhabdomyolysis Syndrome in the UK, Epidemiological and clinical descriptive information. *Br. Vet. J.* 1991; **147**, 373–384.
34. Arighi M, Baird JD & Hulland TJ. Equine exertional rhabdomyolysis. *Comp Cont Educ Pract Vet.* 1984; **6**, S726–S732.
35. Harris PA. Differential Diagnosis of the Equine Rhabdomyolysis Syndrome. In: Raw ME & Parkinson TJ (eds). *The Veterinary Annual.* Oxford, Blackwell Scientific Publications 1992; 175–191.
36. Morris E, Seeherman HJ & O'Callaghan MW. Scintigraphic identification of rhabdomyolysis in horses. *Proc AAEP.* 1991; **37**, 315–324.
37. McLean JG. Equine paralytic myoglobinuria ('Azoturia') a review. *Aust Vet J.* 1973; **49**, 41–43.
38. Freestone JF & Carlson GP. Muscle disorders in the horse: a retrospective study. *Equine Vet. J.* 1991; **23**(2), 86–90.
39. Maxie MG & Physick-Sheard PW. Aortic-iliac thrombosis in horses. *Vet Pathol.* 1985; **22**, 238–249.
40. Reef VB, Roby KAW, Richardson DW *et al.* Use of ultrasonography for the detection of aortic-iliac thrombosis in horses. *J Am Vet Med Assoc.* 1987; **190**, 286–288.
41. Hamir AN. White muscle disease in a foal. *Aust Vet J.* 1982; **59**, 57–58.
42. Dill SG & Rebhun WC. White muscle disease in foals. *Comp Cont Educ Pract Vet.* 1985; **7**, S627–S635.
43. Roneus B & Essen-Gustavsson B. Muscle fibre types and enzyme activities in healthy foals and foals affected by muscular dystrophy. *J. Am. Vet. Med. Assoc.* 1986; **33**, 1–12.
44. Whitwell KE, Harris PA & Farrington PG. An outbreak of a typical myoglobinuria. *Equine Vet. J.* 1988; **20**, 357–363.
45. Carlson GP. The exhausted horse syndrome. In: Robinson NE (ed) *Current Therapy in Equine Medicine.* Philadelphia: WB Saunders 1987; 482–485.
46. Amend JF, Mallon FM, Wren WB & Ramos AS. Equine monensin toxicosis. Some experimental clinicopatholgic observations. *Comp Cont Educ Pract Vet.* 1980; **2**, S173–S183.
47. Anderson GA, Mount ME, Vrins AA & Ziemer EL. Fatal acorn poisoning in a horse. Pathological findings and diagnostic considerations. *J Am Vet Med Assoc.* 1983; **182**, 1105–1110.

7

Hyperkalaemic Periodic Paralysis

Jonathon M Naylor

Key Points

- Hyperkalaemic periodic paralysis (HYPP) is caused by a point mutation in the gene that encodes the skeletal muscle sodium channel. The test for this mutation is commercially available.
- All affected horses are descendants of the Quarter Horse sire Impressive.
- The mutation is autosomal and dominant. It has been selected for at halter shows probably because it leads to a more muscular appearance. However, it impairs muscle working ability.
- Heterozygous, genotype H/N, horses account for about 0.4% of registered Quarter Horses. Most heterozygotes have relatively normal lives but occasional horses show clinical attacks of HYPP lasting from a few minutes to several hours.
- The most common signs are involuntary muscle fasciculation and increased respiratory rate. Prolapse of the third eyelid, stertor, involuntary recumbency and death may be observed. Serum potassium is usually elevated during attacks.
- Homozygotes are rare. They usually show clinical signs as foals. Respiratory stertor due to pharyngeal and laryngeal paralysis and muscle fasciculations are common signs. Dysphagia may occur. Serum potassium is often normal during attacks.

Introduction

Hyperkalaemic periodic paralysis is disease of horses descended from the Quarter Horse stallion Impressive [1, 2]. Impressive was born in 1969 and at an early age was recognized as having an outstanding conformation and good muscling. He had an excellent record in halter shows, which are judged mainly on conformation with the horse led from a halter. Although placed in race training he lacked stamina and was never raced. His first foals were born in 1973 and did extremely well in halter shows, by 1979 he was the leading sire of halter type Quarter Horses. In contrast, very few of his offspring performed well in racing events and at one stage some thought that his offspring were incapable of athletic performance [3]. It was not until 1985/86 that hyperkalaemic periodic paralysis was publicly recognized as a disease condition of Quarter Horses [4, 5]. The HYPP status of Impressive has not been officially reported.

By 1994 it was realized that HYPP affected horses were being inadvertently selected for by judges at American Quarter Horse halter shows. Unaffected offspring of the same sire had much less success in the show ring [6]. This is presumably because the gene that underlies HYPP gives a more pleasing phenotype – probably a more heavily muscled appearance. I assume that Impressive was either the first or one of the first horses to carry the mutation for HYPP and that one of the effects of the gene is to give horses a heavily muscled appearance. Selection for this pleasing phenotype underlies the success of his offspring in halter shows and the rapid dissemination of Impressive blood within the Quarter Horse breed; at the last count over 2% of registered Quarter Horses were descended from Impressive. Hyperkalaemic periodic paralysis is also found in related breeds such as American Paint Horses and Appaloosas and in cross breeds, but only in horses that can trace their ancestry to Impressive [1]. From the foregoing discussion it should be obvious that while HYPP causes signs of disease in some horses, its major effect is to alter the conformation of horses in a way that is pleasing to people.

Pathophysiology

Muscle cells are rich in potassium and low in sodium concentrations. The inside membrane has a negative potential difference with respect to the outside and is said to be polarized. Depolarization (less negative inside potential) produces muscle contraction when the threshold potential is reached. Membrane potential is the result of differences in ion concentration across the semipermeable cell membrane. It can be modified either by changing cellular ion concentrations (mainly controlled by Na/K ATPase) or by altering membrane ion permeability (by opening or closing ion channels). Depolarization can be produced by allowing increased entry of positively charged sodium ions, for example by opening sodium channels, or by slowing the exit of potassium ions, for example by raising serum potassium concentration.

Although HYPP is named for the characteristic increase in serum potassium that occurs during most attacks it is the result of a point mutation in the skeletal muscle sodium channel gene [7]. This changes one amino acid in one type of voltage dependent sodium channel (a number of different types of sodium channel exist) and allows the muscle to be more permeable to sodium. Normally, the sodium channel opens to allow rapid membrane depolarization in the initial phase of the action potential. Normal channels close once the membrane is depolarized but HYPP channels remain open. In consequence, the membrane potential is more depolarized, closer to threshold, and is more likely to contract spontaneously [8]. These changes are usually subclinical but increased muscle electrical activity can be documented by electromyography in almost all HYPP affected horses [9]. This activity is presumably associated with random muscle fibre contraction, which occurs on too small a scale to be grossly visible.

Hyperkalaemic periodic paralysis is a dominant genetic condition because the population of abnormal sodium channels affects membrane potential and thus influences all voltage dependent ion channels. Normal sodium channels are more likely to open and trigger a muscle contraction because resting membrane potential is closer to threshold. In severe attacks more complete depolarization inactivates normal sodium channels and the fibre can no longer contract.

Hyperkalaemia during clinical attacks is sometimes the result of excessive potassium ingestion. However, hyperkalaemia is more marked than that seen in normal horses given a similar dose of potassium. Hyperkalaemia is partly caused by increased muscular contraction since potassium is released from myocytes as potassium channels open to repolarize the membrane. Myocytes from HYPP affected horses have abnormally low potassium concentrations [10]. At the end of attacks potassium concentrations return to normal as a result of muscle paralysis, clearance of potassium by the kidneys or re-entry into muscle cells.

Random, spontaneous, fibre contraction would explain the apparent muscle hypertrophy in affected horses. It could also explain the need for greater muscular activity to maintain a given speed in affected horses, as random contractions would oppose voluntary action. At a given speed HYPP affected horses generate more lactate than their unaffected siblings [10].

Overt clinical attacks of HYPP are characterized by spontaneous contraction of large numbers of muscle fibres giving rise to grossly visible muscle fasciculations or muscle spasms. Known predisposing factors for attacks include cold and large oral doses of potassium chloride. Sodium channels of HYPP affected horses are unusually sensitive to cold and become more permeable in a cold environment making the muscle even more excitable [8]. Feeding potassium salts increases extracellular fluid potassium concentration and raises membrane potential closer to threshold because there is less diffusion pressure for potassium ions to leave the cell. Studies also show that elevated serum potassium favours additional repetitive openings of HYPP type sodium channels and further depolarization [11]. In humans, adrenocorticotrophic hormone may precipitate attacks [12]. Adrenaline stimulates the Na-K ATPase and produces slight membrane hyperpolarization [10], thus reducing the risk of attacks. It has also been recognized that there is individual variation in the sensitivity to attacks. This is related to differential rates of transcription of the normal and abnormal genes [13], but the factors responsible are not clearly defined.

Severe attacks of HYPP can include signs of weakness [14, 15]. Normal sodium channels initially open in response to membrane depolarization but close (become refractory) with further depolarization. If defective HYPP sodium channels produce sufficient membrane depolarization then the normal channels close and the muscle is refractory to contraction.

Clinical Syndromes

Subclinical Signs

Subclinical effects of HYPP can include a pleasing conformation. Hyperkalaemic periodic paralysis affected horses often appear heavily muscled, and HYPP positives horses are more likely to show well in halter classes than their non-affected siblings [16]. On the adverse side, HYPP affected horses have higher blood lactates at a given exercise intensity than non-affected horses of similar breeding and training, indicating decreased exercise tolerance (Figure 1).

Clinical Signs

Clinical signs occur irregularly and are only seen in some horses carrying the HYPP gene. Experimentally, however, attacks can be induced in almost all affected horses. Predisposing factors for disease attacks are not well defined but probably include long distance transportation [14, 15], young age [15], anaesthesia [14, 17, 18], and chilling. Most reports of attacks are in 2- to 3-year-old, well muscled, intact males being shown at halter [4]. Experimentally, males and females are equally susceptible [14], so the observed predilection for show males

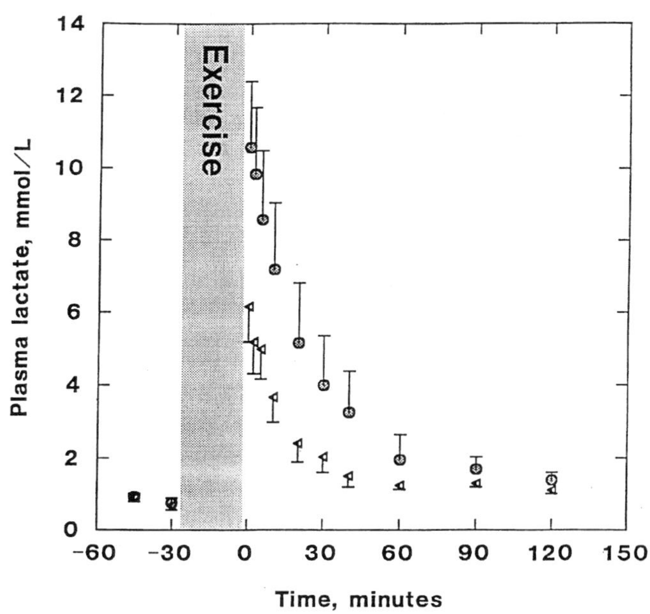

Figure 1. Plasma lactate concentrations, mean ±SE, in HYPP affected (◍) and unaffected horses (◁) before and after moderate excercise. Reproduced with permission from Steele DS, Naylor JM. Hyperkalemic periodic paralysis, plasma lactate and exercise tolerance. *J Equine Vet Sci* 1996; **16**, 327–323.

may be related to the high frequency with which these horses are observed or to other environmental factors such as diet or hormonal therapy.

Two forms of HYPP exist, heterozygous horses (H/N) usually have either no or infrequent clinical attacks lasting from a few minutes to several hours. Occasional horses suffere from repeated attacks. Although the disease is named a paralysis, the more common clinical signs are fine muscle fasciculations and an increase in respiratory rate (Table 1) [15]. There are many other causes for these signs so these findings are non-specific. Some horses sweat, show gross continuous muscle contractions, intermittent prolapse of the third eyelid, respiratory stertor, spasm of the facial or locomotory muscles, drooling of saliva, weakness or involuntary recumbency (Figure 2) [4, 14, 15]. The condition is usually non-painful but occasional horses will paw or roll as if they were uncomfortable. During attacks serum potassium is usually elevated but occasionally serum potassium is within the normal range [15, 19]. Hyperkalaemia can produce arrhythmias in HYPP affected horses [21] but there are no consistent changes in heart rate during attacks [15].

Homozygous horses (H/H) occur at a low frequency in the equine population. Limited experience suggests that these horses show a distinct syndrome with clinical signs within the first month of life. Owners report frequent, intermittent,

***Table 1.* Signs of HYPP arranged in order of likelihood of occurrence. Reproduced with permission of the author.**

Heterozygotes
Common:
- Increased respiratory rate
- Sweating
- Continuous muscle fasciculations*
- Weakness

Less Common:
- Prolapse of the third eyelid
- Respiratory stertor
- Recumbency
- Muscle spasm
- Pawing
- Rolling
- Arrhythmia
- Death

Homozygotes
- Respiratory stertor
- Increased respiratory rate
- Prolapse of the third eyelid
- Continuous muscle fasciculation*
- Weakness
- Sweating
- Cyanosis
- Drooling saliva
- Dysphagia
- Death

*Intermittent muscle fasciculation (lasting 1–3 seconds) is very common but is difficult to distinguish from that normally observed in response to flies or other irritants.

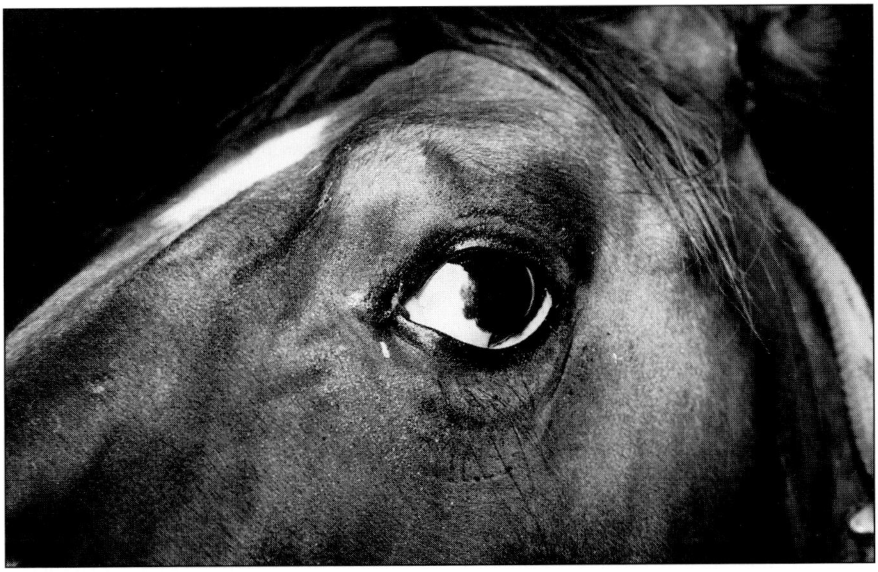

Figure 2. Prolapse of the third eyelid in a horse undergoing a clinical attack of hyperkalaemic periodic paralysis. The prolapse was intermittent. Reproduced with permission from Naylor JM. *Canadian Veterinary Journal.* 1994; **35**, 279–285.

attacks of respiratory stertor, occasional dyspnea and, rarely, drooling or dysphagia. Endoscopy during attacks reveals laryngeal and pharyngeal paralysis. In some horses the guttural pouch orifices remain open during attacks. Signs seem to diminish as the horse ages. Our homozygous stallion had severe signs as a foal but now shows clinical signs only when stressed. He is incapable of successfully breeding mares because he either falls off prior to ejaculation or contaminates the ejaculate with urine. In homozygotes clinical signs often occur without concurrent hyperkalaemia.

Clinical signs associated with anaesthesia have been reported as attacks of muscle fasciculation, hyperthermia (up to 40°C), and tachycardia in a young horse [20] that was probably homozygous for HYPP. Attacks with classical signs of HYPP have been reported during recovery from anaesthesia and probably occur in horses of either genotype [14, 17, 18].

Because attacks of HYPP are often brief, signs may be missed, particularly when horses are kept at pasture. However, abrasions and wounds may be incurred as a result of ataxia or recumbency during attacks and HYPP affected horses have more problems with these types of condition [15].

Differential Diagnoses

Initially, many clinical attacks of HYPP were confused with colic, probably because muscle fasciculation, sweating and recumbency can be seen in both conditions. HYPP may also be confused with rhabdomyolysis because of sweating, fasciculation and stiffness. Some attacks of HYPP follow exercise but many are unrelated to work. If the horse is being transported, early signs of HYPP may be missed and the recumbency phase looks like accidental recumbency during transportation (trailer wrecks). In addition, stiffness and prolapse of the third eyelid mimic tetanus; however, signs in HYPP are usually short lived.

Diagnosis

Diagnosis of attacks of HYPP disease is made on the basis of clinical signs, the intermittent nature of the attacks and an elevated serum potassium concentration during the attacks. It is important that blood is drawn while the horse is symptomatic and that serum or plasma is rapidly separated from the blood – ideally within an hour of collection. Potassium leaks out of erythrocytes and will spuriously elevate serum potassium concentrations if the blood is stored for long periods or if the cells haemolyse during collection or storage. If in doubt a second sample can be collected from a normal horse as a control and the two samples can be handled identically. The presence of clinical signs and hyperkalaemia indicates a clinical attack of HYPP. Occasionally, HYPP attacks are accompanied by normokalaemia so a single normal potassium concentration does not rule out HYPP [15, 19]. This is particularly the case in homozygotes where the combination of clinical signs, onset as a foal and an H/H genotype are sufficient to make a clinical diagnosis.

The presence of the gene that codes for HYPP can be determined using commercially available gene probe testing services (Table 2). A sample of tissue, usually blood, is collected. For consistent results it is important to get the sample to the laboratory rapidly and samples are usually pre-cooled, packed in styrofoam and sent to the laboratory by courier. I try to avoid collecting samples late in the week so that the samples do not get held up over the weekend. At the laboratory DNA is separated, amplified by the polymerase chain reaction and

***Table 2.* Laboratories performing HYPP gene probe testing**

Veterinary Genetics Laboratory,
University of California,
Davis, 95616–8737

If outside of USA contact the laboratory first to get USDA permit number for importation of blood (Fax 916 752 0414).

Dr Doug Nickel
Room 2234
Health Science Center
3330 Hospital Drive
Calgary T2N 4N1

Send whole EDTA treated (purple top) blood by courier. It is best to collect and send the samples on the same day, at the beginning of the week. To avoid fraud check that the blood is drawn from a horse matching the description on the registration papers and include the registered name of the horse with the sample.

the presence of normal and HYPP alleles of the skeletal muscle sodium channel gene detected. Results are reported as the N/N (no susceptibility to HYPP), N/H (heterozygotes, common, susceptible to HYPP disease), or H/H (homozygous affected, rare, very susceptible to HYPP disease) genotypes. A positive gene test result does not mean that the horse will necessarily show signs of HYPP, almost all H/N horses are capable of showing signs but the appropriate environmental factors needed to trigger attacks may not be present.

Other tests that have been used to determine HYPP susceptibility are the potassium chloride challenge test and electromyography. Potassium chloride challenge testing involves administering sequential doses of potassium chloride and observing for clinical signs of HYPP. It is time consuming and carries a slight risk of inducing death from a severe HYPP attack [15]. For these reasons it is only used experimentally. Electromyography is a safe and quick. Horses are usually deeply sedated and needle electromyography is performed using either unipolar or bipolar needles. Characteristic features of HYPP are prolonged insertional activity, spontaneous activity, and some mixture of myotonic discharges, high frequency complex repetitive discharges or trains of doublets (Figure 3) [9, 14]. These findings are not specific for HYPP but so far HYPP is the only reported cause of these findings in horses descended from Impressive. Characteristic electromyographic changes are present between attacks in about 80–90% of H/N horses. Gene probe testing is used in preference to routine diagnostic purposes because of its greater reliability.

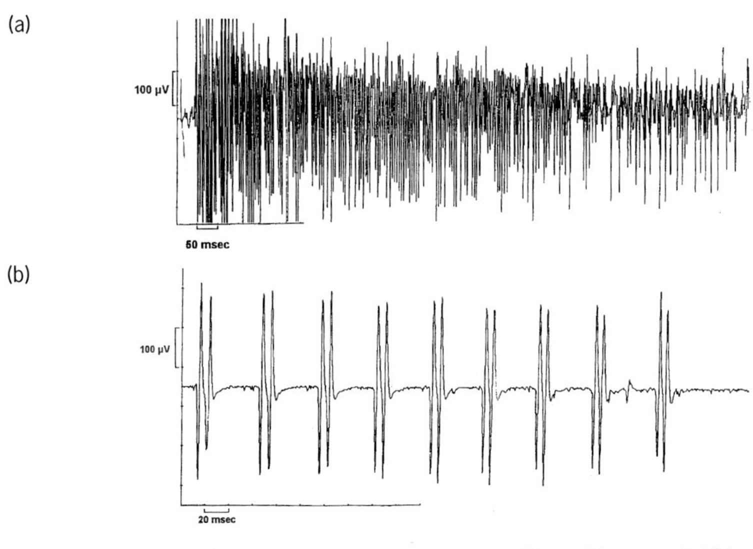

Figure 3. Electromyographic features of HYPP affected horses. (a) Myotonic discharges recorded in a HYPP affected horse while it was clinically normal; (b) trains of doublets recorded in a HYPP affected horse while it was clinically normal. Reproduced with permission from Naylor JM. *Canadian Veterinary Journal.* 1994; **35**, 279–285.

Treatment

Treatment of attacks centres on rapidly restoring serum potassium concentrations to normal by administering potassium free fluids to dilute out the hyperkalaemia and speed renal potassium excretion together with dextrose (5% dextrose, 2 ml to 6 ml/kg BW) and sodium bicarbonate (1 to 2 mmol/kg BW) to encourage potassium to re-enter the cells. I use a cocktail consisting of 2 L of isotonic, 0.9%, saline, 2 L of isotonic, 1.3% sodium bicarbonate and 250 mL of 50% dextrose. This can be run in rapidly intravenously over a period of 30–60 minutes. In horses over 300 kg the entire treatment can be repeated over an additional 60 minute period if clinical signs do not abate.

Calcium gluconate (0.2 mL/kg BW of 23% calcium gluconate) has been used intravenously to abort attacks. This treatment does not affect serum potassium concentrations. However, calcium antagonizes the effects of hyperkalaemia on the heart [22, 23], possibly by activating calcium dependent potassium channels which help repolarize the cell membrane. Although treatment can be successful, I have ceased to use it following the loss of one horse during therapy. In humans, beta-adrenergics are sometimes used to treat hyperkalaemia. They stimulate the Na/K ATPase which pumps potassium into cells. Slow intravenous infusion of isoproterenol has been tried in one horse but had to be discontinued because of tachycardia and premature ventricular contractions [18], making this a poor choice for routine use.

Prevention

Prevention of further attacks involves environmental and dietary modification as a first step and chronic medication with potassium wasting diuretics if these fail. If a horse is suffering from repeated HYPP attacks potential predisposing factors should be evaluated. A high potassium diet, long distance transportation, chilling and 'stress' are all thought to be potential predisposing factors. High potassium feeds include early cutting, lush, alfalfa (about 2.6% potassium, dry matter basis) and grass (about 2–3% potassium) hays, molasses (6% potassium), and soybean meal (about 2.2%). Potential lower potassium substitutes include later cutting, poorer quality hays (1–2% potassium). Sugar beet pulp is a palatable roughage with a particularly low potassium content (about 0.2%) but it is also low in phosphorus (0.1%) and vitamin A. For adult horses it should be fed with grain, some high quality grass hay, and balanced with phosphorus and possibly vitamin A supplements as required. Grains are low in potassium (oats about 0.4%) but bran is higher (1.4%) [24]. A commercial complete pelleted, low potassium, feed is marketed for HYPP affected horses (*Montana Pride Feeds*, Dillon, Montana). Some owners add sodium bicarbonate (15–30 g once or twice a day) to the grain portion of the feed as a prophylactic treatment.

Medication involves the continuous administration of potassium wasting diuretics. Acetazolamide at 2–4.4 mg/kg BW, po, BID is most commonly used

[4, 25, 26]. Hydroclorthiazides has been used at doses of 0.5 to 1 mg/kg BW, po, BID. Although it has fewer side effects than acetazolamide in humans [27, 28], it is not widely used in veterinary medicine to treat HYPP. With careful monitoring, diuretic dosages can often be gradually decreased until the lowest dose that prevents attacks is found. Another treatment that reduces the incidence of signs following experimental potassium chloride challenge, but not the severity of hyperkalaemia, is phenytoin [26, 29]. Because high doses of phenytoin can induce weakness and it appears not to protect the heart against hyperkalaemia [26], I do not routinely recommend it as a treatment for HYPP.

Genetics and Selection

Hyperkalaemic periodic paralysis likely originated as a point mutation in the germ cells that gave rise to Impressive, and all affected horses can trace their ancestry to this sire (Figure 4). The mutation has rapidly disseminated within the American Quarter Horse breed and has also penetrated related breeds as a result of selective breeding. One point of selection is at halter shows where HYPP

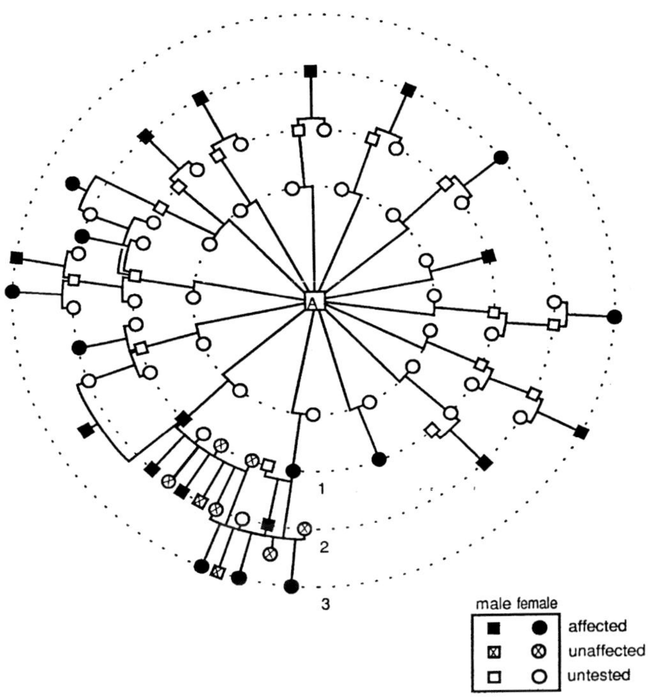

Figure 4. Interrelationship of HYPP affected horses. Note that where testing over several generations was possible, every affected horse has an affected parent. Reproduced with permission from Naylor JM. *Canadian Veterinary Journal.* 1994; **35**, 279–285.

affected phenotypes are preferred [6]. Some breeding farms also have an unusually high percentage of affected brood mares [30]. The exact number of affected horses is unknown but in 1989, 20 years after Impressive's birth, 2% of all American Quarter Horses could trace their ancestry to him and about 0.4% were affected [32].

HYPP is inherited in an autosomal dominant fashion [2, 7, 31]. This means that every affected horse has at least one affected parent, thus a positive gene test (H/N or H/H) on a horse indicates that at least one parent is also affected. If an affected (H/N genotype) horse is mated to an unaffected horse (N/N) then approximately half the offspring will be HYPP affected and half unaffected. Matings of two affected individuals (H/N) will result in unaffected (N/N), affected (H/N), and severely affected (H/H) offspring in a 1:2:1 ratio (Figure 5). With the advent of gene testing, control is relatively easy since horses descended from Impressive can be readily screened for the condition and need not be used in breeding programmes. If both parents are known to be HYPP negative (N/N) then the foals do not have to be routinely tested since genetic transmission is impossible. Similarly, there is little point in routinely testing horses that are not decended from Impressive because the condition has not been recorded outside this line. However, an extended pedigree is often needed to be sure of ancestry back to 1969 and occasional misrecording of breeding records is possible. Although not using affected horses for breeding makes veterinary sense, some in the industry are less convinced of this need, partly because clinical attacks of HYPP are rare in heterozygotes, partly because positive horses can do very well at shows, and partly because of the money invested in some positive horses. On the other hand homozygotes are severely affected and exercise ability is impaired in heterozygotes.

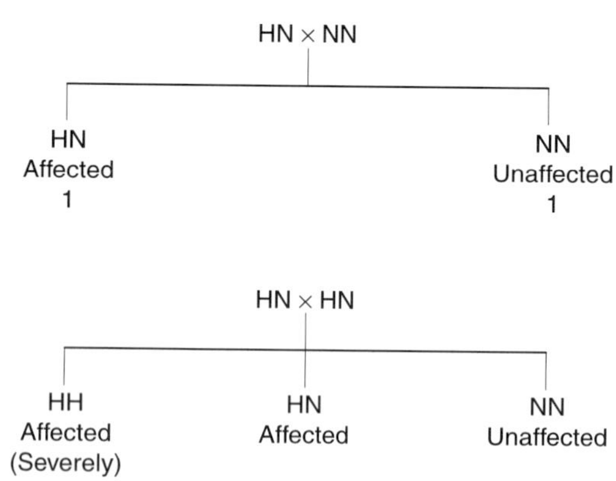

Figure 5. Predicted ratios of affected and unaffected offspring for the common matings of HYPP affected and normal parents. Reproduced with permission of the author.

Conclusions

Hyperkalaemic periodic paralysis in heterozygotes has a reasonably distinct clinical syndrome of muscle fasciculation and muscle spasm with an elevated respiratory rate and occasional respiratory stertor. Serum potassium concentrations are usually elevated during attacks. In homozygotes, the signs are more severe and are characterized by intermittent respiratory stertor and muscle fasciculations from an early age and serum potassium is often normal during attacks. In addition, sweating, drooling, prolapse of the third eyelid, weakness and collapse may be seen in either syndrome. Owners may confuse HYPP with colic, rhabdomyolysis, or accidental recumbency. Veterinarians need to be particularly cognizant of the disease when performing prepurchase examinations: affected horses are likely to appear normal but the presence of HYPP gene can have major implications for breeding and insurance. Affected horses are also less likely to perform well under conditions of strenuous exercise. HYPP should also be considered as part of the preanaesthetic work up as there are several reports of positive horses having difficulties during anaesthesia.

References

1. Naylor JM, Robinson JA & Bertone J. Familial incidence of equine hyperkalemic periodic paralysis in Quarter Horses. *J Am Vet Med Assoc.* 1992; **200**, 340–343.
2. Naylor JM. Equine Hyperkalemic periodic paralysis – review and implications. *Can Vet J.* 1994; **35**, 279–285.
3. Chamberlain R. Impressive. *Am Quarter Horse Assoc J.* December 1985; 146–151.
4. Cox JH. An episodic weakness in four horses associated with intermittent serum hyperkalaemia and the similarity of the disease to hyperkalemic periodic paresis in man. *Proc Am Assoc Equine Practitioners.* 1986; **31**, 383–391.
5. Steiss JE & Naylor JM. Episodic muscle tremors in a quarter horse: Resemblance to hyperkalemic periodic paresis. *Can Vet J.* 1986; **27**, 332–335.
6. Naylor JM. Selection of Quarter Horses affected with hyperkalemic periodic paralysis by show judges. *J Am Vet Med Assoc.* 1994; **204**, 926–928.
7. Rudolph JA, Spier SJ, Byrns G, *et al.* Periodic paralysis in Quarter Horses, a sodium channel mutation disseminated by selective breeding. *Nat Genet.* 1992; **2**, 144–147.
8. Pickar JG, Spier SJ, Snyder JR & Carlsen RC. Altered ionic permeability in skeletal muscle from horses with hyperkalemic periodic paralysis. *Am J Physiol.* 1991; **260**, 926–C933.
9. Robinson JA, Naylor JM & Crichlow EC. Use of electromyography for the diagnosis of equine hyperkalemic periodic paresis. *Can J Vet Res.* 1990; **54**, 495–500.
10. Steele DS, Naylor JM. Hyperkalaemic periodic paralysis, plasma lactate and exercise tolerance. *J Equine Vet Sci.* 1996; **16**, 321–323.
11. Cannon SC, Brown RH Jr & Corey DP. A sodium channel defect in hyperkalemic periodic paralysis, potassium-induced failure in inactivation. *Neuron.* 1991; **6**, 619–26.
12. Riggs JE. Review. Periodic Paralysis. *Clin Neuropharmacol.* 1989; **12**, 249–257.
13. Zhou J, Spier SJ, Beech J & Hoffman EP. Pathophysiology of sodium channelopathies: correlation of normal/mutant mRNA ratios with clinical phenotype in dominantly inherited periodic paralysis. *Hum Mol Genet.* 1994; **3**, 1599–1603.

14. Spier SJ, Carlson GP, Holliday TA & Cardinet III GH. Hyperkalemic periodic paralysis in horses. *J Am Vet Med Assoc.* 1990; **197**, 1009–1017.
15. Naylor JM, Jones V & Berry S-L. Clinical syndrome and diagnosis of hyperkalemic periodic paralysis in Quarter Horses. *Equine Vet J.* 1993; **25**, 227–232.
16. Naylor JM. Selection of Quarter Horses affected with hyperkalemic periodic paralysis by show judges. *J Am Vet Med Assoc.* 1994; **204**, 926–928.
17. Traub-Dargatz JL, Ingram JT, Stashak TS & Kiper ML. Repiratory stridor associated with polymyopathy suspected to be hyperkalemic periodic paralysis in four Quarter Horse foals. *J Am Vet Med Assoc.* 1992; **201**, 85–89.
18. Robertson SA, Green SL, Carter SW *et al.* Postanesthetic recumbency associated with hyperkalemic periodic paralysis in a Quarter Horse. *J Am Vet Med Assoc.* 1992; **201**, 1209–1212.
19. Stewart RH, Bertone JJ, Yvorchuk-St Jean K & Reed SM. Possible normokalemic variant of hyperkalemic periodic paralysis in two horses. *J Am Vet Med Assoc.* 1993; **203**, 421–424.
20. Cornick JL, Seahorn TL & Hartsfield SM. Hyperthermia during isoflurane anaesthesia in a horse with suspected hyperkalemic periodic paralysis. *Equine Vet J.* 1994; **26**, 511–514.
21. Castex A-M & Bertone JJ. ECG of the Month. *J Am Vet Med Assoc.* 1989; **194**, 654–655.
22. Bisogno JL, Langley A & Von Dreele MM. Effect of calcium to reverse the electrocardiographic effects of hyperkalemia in the isolated rat heart: A prospective, dose–response study. *Crit Care Med.* 1994; **22**, 697–704.
23. Leitch SP & Paterson DJ. Role of Ca^{2+} in protecting the heart from hyperkalemia and acidosis in the rabbit: implications for exercise. *J Appl Physiol.* 1994; **77**, 2391–2399.
24. Naylor JM. The major minerals (macrominerals). In: Naylor JM & Ralston SL (eds). *Large Animal Clinical Nutrition.* St Louis: Mosby Year Book, 1991.
25. Cox JH, De Bowes RM & Boyer JE Jr. Response of Normal and Acetazolamide Treated Horses To Oral Potassium Chloride Challenge. *Proc Sixth Annu Vet Med Forum, Am Coll.* 1988; **6**, 728.
26. Beech J & Lindborg S. Prophylactic efficacy of phenytoin, acetazolamide and hydroclorthiazide in horses with hyperkalemic periodic paralysis. *Res Vet Sci.* 1995; **59**, 95–101.
27. Gamstorp I, Hauge M, Helweg-Larsen HF & Mjones H. Adynamia episodica hereditaria. A disease clinically resembling familiar periodic paralysis but characterized by increasing serum potassium during the paralytic attacks. *Am J Med.* 1957; **23**, 385–390.
28. Lewis ED, Griggs RC & Moxley RT. Regulation of plasma potassium in hyperkalemic periodic paresis. *Neurology.* 1986; **29**, 1131–1137.
29. Beech J, Fletcher JE, Tripolitis L & Lindborg S. Effect of phenytoin in two myotonic horses with hyperkalemic periodic paralysis. *Muscle Nerve.* 1992; **15**, 932–936.
30. Naylor JM, Robinson JA, Crichlow EC & Steiss JE. Inheritance of myotonic discharges in American Quarter Horses and the relationship to hyperkalemic periodic paralysis. *Can J Vet Res.* 1992; **56**, 62–66.
31. Spier SJ, Carlson GP, Harrold D *et al.* Genetic study of hyperkalemic periodic paralysis in horses. *J Am Vet Med Assoc.* 1993; **202**, 933–937.

8

Metabolic Manifestations of Hepatobiliary Disease in Horses

Thomas J Divers

Key Points

- Hepatobiliary disease may arise from a variety of pathological mechanisms, but clinical signs generally only become apparent when greater than 70% of liver function is lost.
- Hepatoencephalopathy is frequently observed and is the most pronounced and troublesome clinical entity. Neurological signs are attributable to excessive ammonia, gamma-amino butyric-acid and other neurotransmitters, and may be complicated by hypoglycemia.
- Other clinical manifestations may include icterus, bilirubinuria or hemoglobinuria, polyuria, bleeding abnormalities, signs of sepsis, polypnea, photosensitivity, colic, weight loss, edema, ascites and diarrhea.
- Diagnosis is based upon elevations in serum activities of gamma-glutamyl transferase and sorbitol dehydrogenase together with measures of hepatobiliary function, namely serum concentrations of conjugated and total bilirubin and bile acids.
- Microscopic examination of the liver is often necessary to obtain a pathological description of the disease, provide evidence of causative factors, identify an infectious agent, and help determine prognosis.
- The treatment of liver failure is largely supportive and should include specific therapies for hepatoencephalopathy, fluid therapy, nutritional management, and antibiotics.

Anatomy and Pathophysiology of Liver Disease and Failure – A Brief Summary

Anatomically the liver can be divided into hexagonal lobules with rows of hepatocytes oriented around the central vein. At the periphery of the lobules are portal triads, each composed of a portal vein, hepatic artery and bile duct.

The liver receives nutrients and oxygen from both the portal vein and the hepatic artery, while it is drained by the hepatic vein and lymphatics. The central lobular area (around the central vein) is the most distant point from the portal vein and hepatic artery and is most susceptible to ischemic changes. Located within the vascular framework of the liver are the reticuloendothelial cells which help to protect against portal movement of endotoxin and/or bacteria. The predominant functional cell in the liver is the hepatocyte. Hepatocytes are responsible for hepatic carbohydrate and fat metabolism, synthesis of many proteins (e.g. albumin, clotting factors), catabolism of some proteins (e.g. immunoglobulin A, insulin) and metabolism of other nitrogenous materials (e.g. ammonia and aromatic amino acids). The hepatocyte is also important for metabolism of many drugs, mostly via the hepatocyte's cytochrome p450 enzymes. The fact that the liver serves as a clearance organ for many drugs and toxins makes it particularly susceptible to hepatic disease from some of the products. The hepatocyte is also the cell responsible for the uptake and conjunction of bilirubin and other organic anions (e.g. free fatty acids and bile acids). In addition, it serves as a storage site for many vitamins and minerals [1].

Anatomically aligned with the rows of hepatocytes are the bile ducts, which serve as an excretory pathway for bile products, including bile acids, conjugated bilirubin and many drugs. Most diseases of the liver affect both structural units, hepatocytes and bile ducts, although damage to one may be more pronounced than to the other. For example, Theiler's disease, which is believed to be a viral hepatitis, has a predominant effect on hepatocellular function and this is reflected by the clinical signs (e.g. frequent occurrence of hepatoencephalopathy) and laboratory findings (e.g. marked increases in the serum activity of hepatocellular enzymes and blood ammonia concentration). In contrast, ascending bacterial cholangiohepatitis has the most pronounced effect on biliary function, causing significant differences in laboratory findings (e.g. more marked elevations in biliary enzyme activity in the serum of the patient and greater elevations in conjugated bilirubin) and clinical signs (e.g. severe icterus but without neurologic signs in most cases) [2]. Hepatic disease may initially occur from a variety of pathological mechanisms including hepatocellular inflammation, necrosis, degeneration, infiltration (fat, amyloid neoplasia), atrophy and abnormal mitosis or from biliary inflammation, hyperplasia and obstruction. The general reaction to these mechanisms of liver injury is either regeneration and/or fibrosis [1]. Bile duct hyperplasia from a variety of insults is unusually common in the horse.

Fortunately, the liver has a very large functional reserve and 70% or more of liver function must be lost before signs of hepatic failure occur, offering a chance for regeneration in many cases. Diseases affecting less than 70% of the liver function may cause clinical signs but not of liver failure. Those hepatic diseases that produce clinical abnormalities without liver failure are most often hepatic neoplasm or abscessation.

Clinical Signs of Hepatic Failure

Clinical signs of hepatic failure occur only when the liver is severely diseased or dysfunctional such that it cannot sufficiently perform its normal functions. This generally equates to at least 70% loss of mass and/or function. The clinical signs of liver failure in the horse are often quite variable depending upon the primary site of structural and/or functional damage (Table 1). Neurologic signs are frequently observed with hepatic failure and are referred to as *hepatoencephalopathy*. Neurological signs are the most pronounced and clinically troublesome signs in most cases of equine hepatic failure. These signs may vary from depression to bizarre maniacal behaviour (Table 2). Apparent blindness, ataxia, head pressing (Figure 1), propulsive circling and frequent yawning are common clinical findings. The pathophysiological mechanism of these signs is undoubtedly complex but is mostly due to abnormal hepatic protein metabolism [3]. For example, the failing liver may be unable to sufficiently convert colonic-derived ammonia to urea via urea cycle enzymes located in the hepatocyte. The effect of excessive ammonia on the central nervous system (CNS) may include one or more of the following: enhancement of neurotransmitters, interference with normal neurotransmission, structural changes in the blood–brain barrier, changes in cerebral blood flow and/or interference with biochemical or electrophysiological pathways in the brain. Cerebral edema with development of Alzheimer type II cells are characteristics of high CNS ammonia. Alzheimer type II cells may arise from hepatic failure, primary hyperammoninemia or severe uraemia. Additionally, there may be decreased hepatic extraction of gut-synthesized gamma-aminobutyric acid (GABA) which may also serve as a potent inhibitory

Table 1. Clinical manifestations of hepatobiliary disease

- Hepatoencephalopathy
- Icterus
- Orange (bilirubinuria) or red (haemoglubinuria) discoloration of urine, polyuria
- Prolonged bleeding: spontaneous or associated with self trauma and nasogastric intubation
- Signs of sepsis: red-purple mucus membranes, tachycardia, scleral injection, pyrexia
- Photosensitivity
- Colic
- Weight loss
- Oedema, ascites and diarrhoea

Table 2. Common clinical signs of hepatoencepatholopathy

- Depression
- Apparent blindness
- Ataxia
- Head pressing
- Propulsive circling
- Frequent yawning
- Maniacal behaviour
- Polypnea

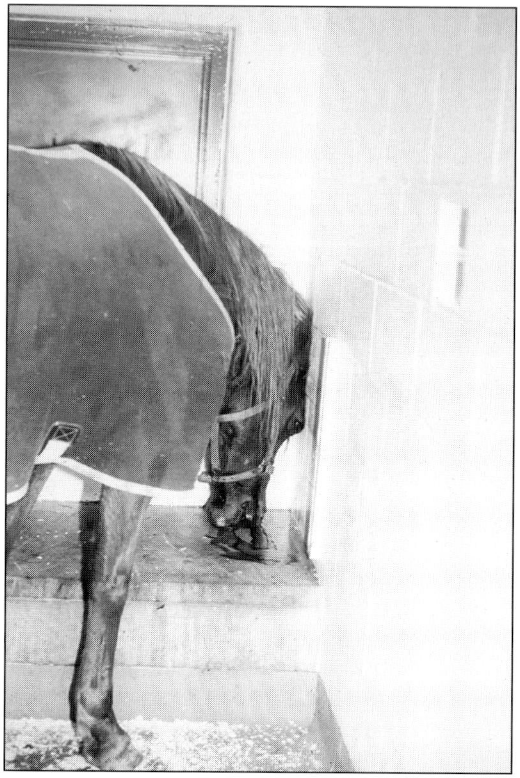

Figure 1. Head pressing is one of the signs of equine hepatic failure.

neurotransmittor. The movement of GABA into the CNS may be aided by an increased aromatic to branched-chain amino acids ratio in the plasma and by increased concentrations of plasma bile acids. Increased amounts of aromatic amino acids, which are normally metabolized by the liver, may serve as false neurotransmittors. Frequently in foals with hepatic failure, yet rarely in adult horses, the CNS sign of severe depression may be attributable to hypoglycemia caused by inadequate hepatic gluconeogenesis. Foals with porto-systemic shunts, toxic hepatopathy, or Tyzzer's disease often have profound hypoglycemia [4–6]. In foals with Tyzzer's disease the hypoglycemia is undoubtedly a result of both hepatic failure and toxemia. Additionally, increased plasma insulin has been reported in other species with liver failure as a result of the inability of the liver to degrade the insulin [1].

Icterus in the horse may be a result of hemolytic disease, liver dysfunction, or anorexia without liver disease or hemolysis. Bilirubinaemia caused by haemolytic disease is almost totally a result of an increase in unconjugated bilirubin, although in more protracted cases (e.g. neonatal isoerythrolysis) the conjugated bilirubin may progressively increase with time. Hyperbilirubinaemia in fasted or anorexic horses without liver disease or haemolysis appears to be related to decreased uptake of organic anions, including bilirubin. There is a strong positive correlation between the concentration of free fatty acids (FFA) and the unconjugated bilirubin concentration in the serum of fasted horses [7]. This suggests that an increase in FFA concentration may influence bilirubin metabolism as a result of competition for binding to hepatic intracellular transport proteins. The unconjugated bilirubin concentration in the serum of horses with icterus associated with anorexia is usually $< 120\ \mu$mol/L although some cases may be as high as $188\ \mu$mol/L. Bile acids are generally slightly increased with icterus associated with anorexia and are generally in the 10–22 μm/L range. Exogenous organic anions (e.g. sulfobromophthalein) have decreased hepatic clearance, although there is little if any indication for their diagnostic use in the horse.

Hyperbilirubinaemia and clinical icterus without haemolysis, liver disease or anorexia in healthy horses does exist. Serum bilirubin concentrations in a very few healthy horses may fluctuate from 85 to 205 μmol/L, with $> 90\%$ of the bilibrubin being of the unconjugated form. It seems most likely that in these healthy but jaundiced horses, there is a deficiency in hepatic conjugating mechanisms, possibly an incomplete deficiency of bilirubin-uridine diphosphate glucuronyl transferase (UDP-GT) activity [8]. Serum bile acids are normal (10.0 μm/L) in affected horses. Clinical icterus may not be noted until horses are young adults, which is similar to the histories of human patients with Gilbert's syndrome and Crigler–Najjar type II syndromes, which are both associated with decreased activity of UDP-GT.

Horses with hepatic failure generally have increases in both conjugated and unconjugated bilirubin, with the increase in unconjugated being the most pronounced in all diseases except biliary obstruction. The unconjugated portion becomes elevated because of lost hepatocellular function, with reduced uptake and conjugation of the bilirubin. The conjugated bilirubin level increases because of leakage of some conjugated bilirubin from the diseased liver back into the plasma. If there is an obstructive process, the increase in the conjugated portion of the bilirubin may equal or exceed the unconjugated portion.

Orange discoloration of the urine occurs in many cases of equine hepatic failure and is mostly a result of the increase in conjugated bilirubin, which is freely filtered by the glomerulus. Horses with biliary obstruction would therefore have the most pronounced orange discoloration of the urine. Normal horse urine can vary greatly in colour, so urine dipstick examination for bilirubinuria should be performed in order to help confirm the diagnosis of hepatic failure. False positive reactions to urine dipstick examination for bilirubinuria do occur but are not common. A relatively insensitive field test for bilirubinuria is to shake the urine in a test tube; if a green discolouration of the urine foam is noted this is indicative of bilirubinuria [9]. Foals with severe bilirubinaemia caused by neonatal isoerythyrolysis may develop orange (bilirubinuria) urine following two or more days of haemoglobinuria. This is most likely a result of bile stasis and increased plasma conjugated bilirubin rather than unconjugated bilirubin exceeding a renal threshold (a renal threshold for unconjugated bilirubin in horses is unknown).

Intravascular haemolysis and red discolouration of the urine may be seen on occasion, associated with equine hepatic failure. This most frequently occurs with acute hepatic necrosis (Theiler's disease) and is often but, not always, a terminal event. The cause of the haemolysis may be a microangiopathic haemolytic anemia caused by the physical damage to the red cells as they pass through the necrotic liver or fibrin within small capillaries (disseminated intravascular coagulation, DIC). Increased urine production (polyuria) may be observed in a few horses with chronic hepatic disease and failure. This may be a result of a chronic decrease in hepatic urea production, with decreased urea concentration in the renal interstitium causing a diminished concentration gradient with a blunted reaction to antidiuretic hormone and polyuria. The diminished ability to concentrate the urine may help explain the persistent erythrocytosis and elevated plasma protein observed in many horses with acute onset hepatic failure. There are likely other coexisting mechanisms that may be more significant in explaining these abnormalities. These include splenic contraction and increased globulin production.

Clinical bleeding abnormalities are not commonly observed in horses with liver failure. When bleeding occurs, it is generally prolonged bleeding associated with hepatoencephalopathy and self-inflicted physical trauma. Excessive haemorrhage associated with stomach tubing may also occur, so this procedure should be performed with caution in horses with liver failure since any blood swallowed will worsen the hyperammonaemia and neurologic signs. Spontaneous hemorrhage may occur in a few cases of equine hepatic failure, especially those caused by chronic obstruction of the bile duct [10]. Haemorrhage in horses with liver failure is generally a result of failure in both the extrinsic and intrinsic pathways of coagulation causing prolongation of both prothrombin and partial thromboplastin times. These occur because of decreased hepatic production of clotting factors. Factor VII has the shortest half-life so prothrombin time would be expected to be prolonged prior to prolongation of partial thromboplastin time (PTT) with liver failure. In some horses with liver failure, the PTT may sometimes be prolonged beyond the normal range prior to the prothrombin time (PT) being prolonged. The reason for this is unknown. Disseminated intravascular coagulation may be present in some horses with acute severe liver failure. The cause of this is often multifactorial and may include decreased hepatic production of antithrombin III, plasminogen and high molecular weight proteins that inhibit excessive coagulation. Additionally, overwhelming hepatic tissue damage and/or increased circulating endotoxin may stimulate release of soluble proteins that affect coagulation. Fibrin degradation products (FDPs) are often abnormally high in horses with liver failure since the liver is the organ responsible for clearance of circulating FDPs. An increase in FDPs, PT and PTT would be expected in horses with liver failure and these findings should not be over interpreted as being diagnostic for DIC. If a liver biopsy is required, this can generally be performed safely despite the prolongation in PT and PTT since platelet counts generally remain normal in horses with liver failure.

Signs of sepsis (e.g. brick red to purple mucus membranes, tachycardia, scleral injection, fever, etc.) can be seen in horses with liver failure regardless of the cause. These signs are virtually always present with acute bacterial infections of the liver (e.g. Tyzzer's disease) but are mostly absent with chronic bacterial cholangiohepatitis. With non-bacterial causes of liver failure, the signs of sepsis are likely to be a result of loss of hepatic reticuloendothelial cell function and inability to clear gut-derived organisms or toxins (e.g. endotoxin). Tachycardia and red mucus membranes may also be a result of increased circulating catecholamines which may also help explain the often persistent erythrocytosis observed in many horses with acute onset hepatic failure. This erythrocytosis may persist for several days despite large volume fluid therapy. Polypnea can be pronounced in some horses with acute hepatic failure. Polypnea may be neurogenic in origin (associated with the hepatoencephalopathy) or it may occur as compensation for severe metabolic acidosis, which is frequently present with acute hepatic failure. Metabolic acidosis is a variable finding in horses with liver failure and must be determined by blood gas and/or electrolyte measurements. If metabolic acidosis is present with acute liver failure, it is usually the result of hypovolaemia and increased lactic acid production. Laryngeal paresis and upper airway obstruction has been reported in ponies with pyrrolizidine alkaloid poisoning [11]. The pathophysiological mechanism for this is unknown.

Photosensitivity is a common finding in horses with liver failure and white markings that are exposed to sunlight (Figure 2). Photosensitivity occurs because of the decreased hepatic metabolism of the gut-derived breakdown product of chlorophyll, phylloerythrin. If phyloerythrin is increased in non-pigmented skin exposed to ultraviolet light, an oxidative cascade causing inflammation and skin sloughing may result. Photosensitization may be seen with either acute or chronic hepatic failure but is most common with subacute to chronic diseases. It may be especially pronounced with some plant poisonings (e.g. alsike clover). In some cases of plant poisoning and/or chronic hepatic disease (e.g. pyrrolizidine alkaloids) photosensitivity may be the first clinical sign noted. Although it is most common on white areas of the muzzle or legs, the eyes, conjunctiva or vaginal mucus membranes may be affected. A more generalized dermatitis with production of large amounts of scales and crust may also be noted with chronic liver disease in horses. The cause of this in the horse is not proven but it may be a nutritional dermatosis caused by decreased circulating bile acids, diminished bile acids secretion into the intestinal lumen and diminished absorption of the fat-soluble vitamins.

Colic may occur in horses with either cholangiohepatitis/cholelithiasis, other obstructions of the common bile duct, acute hepatic necrosis, abdominal trauma with fracture of the liver or torsion of a lobe of the liver. Colic is a clinical finding in most cases of cholelithiasis-induced liver failure and many cases of

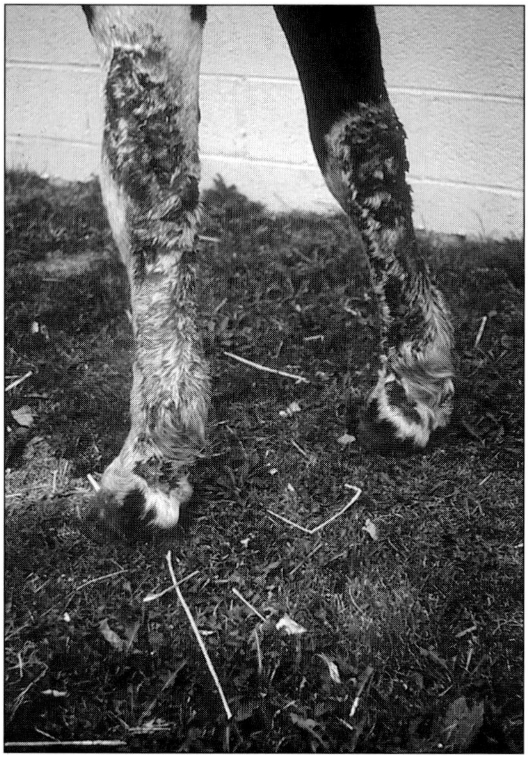

Figure 2. Photosensitivity exhibited on white markings of a horse with liver failure. (Photograph: RH Whitlock)

cholangiohepatitis. The pain is believed to be caused by hepatomegaly and acute stretching of the hepatic capsule. Most, if not all, cases of cholelithiasis in the horse are believed to be a result of a preceding bacterial cholangiohepatitis, rather than vice versa [12]. The high incidence of this disease in the horse compared with other domestic animals may be a result of the absence of a gall bladder in the equine and the proximity of intestinal bacteria to the biliary system. Offending organisms are mostly enteric Gram-negative organisms. A relatively common cause of colic and pronounced icterus (with hepatic disease and hyperbilirubinemia greater than that seen with anorexia alone) is 180 degree volvulus of the right colon [13]. In this condition the displaced colon may chronically stretch the mesentery surrounding the common bile duct, resulting in a lengthening of the bile duct by several inches, causing compression of its lumen.

Weight loss may be observed in horses with chronic liver disease and failure, and may be explained by a diminished appetite and/or decreased hepatic gluconeogenesis, fat metabolism and protein metabolism. In some cases of chronic liver disease (e.g. pyrrolizidine alkaloid toxicosis), the weight loss may precede other signs of liver failure such as photosensitivity, icterus or neurological signs. In many cases of chronic liver disease leading to hepatic failure, there may be no weight loss preceding the onset of fulminant signs of hepatic failure. In horses with liver disease caused by suppurative processes or neoplasia (e.g. hepatocellular carcinoma or cholangiocarcinoma), the weight loss is expected as a result of release of infection or tumor-induced cytokines and the loss in weight may be sustained without laboratory or clinical evidence of liver failure.

Edema, ascites and diarrhea are three relatively common findings with liver failure in other species that are rarely observed in horses. One explanation for the absence of hypoalbuminemia and edema in horses may be related to the long half-life of albumin in the horse in comparison with most other species [14]. Increased amounts of peritoneal fluid may be observed at post mortem in some horses that die of liver failure but ascites can rarely be appreciated in the live horse unless it is pronounced. If a peritoneal tap is performed in horses with liver failure, there may be an increase in peritoneal fluid protein caused by movement of high protein fluid across the vessel wall into the peritoneum. This hepatic sinusoidal leakage of high protein fluid is believed to be caused by the hepatic fibrosis and/or collapse of the hepatic parenchyma around the sinusoids resulting in an increase in hydrostatic pressure [1]. Diarrhoea occurs in other species in association with liver failure and is thought to be caused by decreased secretion of bile acids into the intestine, which does not permit normal emulsification of dietary fat, resulting in an osmotic diarrhoea [1]. The absence of diarrhoea in most horses with liver failure may be a reflection of the relatively low fat diet typically fed to horses.

Diagnosis of Hepatic Disease and Failure

The diagnosis of hepatic disease is based upon elevations in serum activity of hepatic-derived enzymes, increased plasma or serum bile acid concentration and microscopic examination of the liver [15–17]. The enzymes of the greatest predictive value for hepatic disease in the horse are gamma-glutamyl transferase (GGT) and sorbitol dehydrogenase (SDH) [15]. Although GGT is found in high concentrations in the equine pancreas and kidney, diseases of these organs rarely, if ever, cause elevations in GGT activity in the serum. The serum activity of GGT is greatest with diseases that predominantly affect the biliary tract: GGT has a relatively long half-life and remains elevated for several days after a hepatic insult has subsided. It may even increase for 2–3 days despite obvious clinical recovery in some hepatic diseases (e.g. Theiler's disease). This increase in enzyme activity in the face of clinical improvement is most likely a result of biliary hyperplasia, which is relatively non-specific and is commonly seen following a variety of different hepatic insults in a horse. There is no evidence that GGT is induced by drug therapy (e.g. corticosteroids) in the horse, as has been shown in some other species. Sorbitol dehydrogenase is both highly sensitive and specific for

Table 3. **Blood tests for the diagnosis of liver disease and failure. The diagnosis can usually be established using the primary tests listed below. The secondary tests may be of some value in the diagnosis and monitoring of therapy.**

	Primary Tests	*Secondary Tests*
Hepatocellular damage	Gamma-glutamyl transferase Sorbitol dehydrogenase	Aspartate amino transferase Glutamic dehydrogenase Isoenzyme 5 of lactate dehydrogenase
Hepatic function	Conjugated bilirubin Bile acids	Ammonia Prothrombin time Haemogram Leucogram Plasma proteins Blood gases

hepatocellular damage. In fact, it is so sensitive that SDH activity in the serum is frequently increased with any episode of endotoxemia and/or ischemia affecting horses. Increases in SDH, therefore, should not be over interpreted: SDH has a very short half-life and for that reason can be measured serially to more accurately predict prognosis in acute hepatic necrosis. Although it is not hepatic specific, the measurement of aspartate aminotransferase (AST) can be helpful in determining the presence of hepatocellular disease. Measurement of enzyme activity cannot accurately predict dysfunction, but AST values can give a crude index of the degree of hepatocellular damage in some equine hepatic diseases (e.g. Theiler's disease). If SDH measurements are not available in a practice area, measurement of other hepatocellular enzymes (e.g. AST, glutamic dehydrogenase (GD), isoenzyme 5 of lactate dehydrogenase (LDH-5)) may be needed in order to more accurately predict the type of disease processes occurring.

Hepatic failure is best determined by clinical signs and performing laboratory tests that estimate hepatic function. Most function tests do not become abnormal until 70% or more of hepatic function is lost. This generally corresponds to the onset of clinical signs of hepatic failure in horses. The function test that most often corresponds to hepatic failure is an abnormal elevation in plasma-conjugated bilirubin. Elevations in blood ammonia usually indicate severe compromise of hepatic function, but are not sensitive for hepatic failure and is not specific, since primary hyperammononaemia does occur in horses [13]. Prothrombin times are often prolonged with hepatic failure and urea nitrogen and fibrinogen are often abnormally low, but they are not highly sensitive or specific for hepatic failure. Drug excretion tests may be used to determine hepatic function (e.g. sulfobromophthalein) but these would rarely be expected to provide additional valuable information.

The most valuable battery of tests for evaluating hepatic disease and failure in the horse is a combination of serum enzyme activity (AST, GGT, SDH), conjugated and total bilirubin concentration, along with the measurement of serum total bile acid concentration. Bile acids become elevated in the serum prior to conjugated bilirubin in the progression of equine hepatic disease and are highly sensitive for hepatic failure in the horse. Serum bile acids are greater than 20 μmol/L in virtually all horses with significant hepatic dysfunction regardless of whether signs of hepatic failure are present and irrespective of whether the disease is acute or chronic. A single sample is all that is required since there is little diurnal variation in the serum bile acid concentration of the horse [18]. The measurement of serum or plasma bile acids would also detect hepatic dysfunction without disease (e.g. portosystemic shunt) [4].

Microscopic examination of the liver can be used to obtain a pathological description of the disease in the liver, identify an infectious agent, provide evidence suggesting causative factors and help in determining prognosis. A liver biopsy can be performed on either the right or left side of the horse, ideally after the liver is identified by ultrasound examination [19]. The ultrasound exam using a 5 mHz sector scanner is not only invaluable in identifying the location of the liver but also the size of the liver, evidence of biliary obstruction, presence of choleliths, traumatic tears, tumors or abscesses and severity of fatty infiltration and fibrosis. Microscopic examination of the liver is often unrewarding in determining the cause of the liver disease if periportal inflammation/fibrosis is the predominant finding. The periportal area is a common site for either toxic injury or ascending infection and in many cases it is not possible to differentiate the two causes by microscopic examination alone. Culture of the liver should always be performed when septic cholangitis is a consideration. Liver biopsy is relatively safe, even with hepatic failure and prolonged clotting times, but it should be recommended only when it is deemed likely to provide important diagnostic information that might be helpful in the treatment of the case or in providing a more accurate prognosis. In horses with chronic biliary obstruction and prior evidence of bleeding tendencies, fresh or frozen plasma may be given prior to the biopsy. The dosage is variable but 4–10 ml/kg BW would be an estimated recommended dose. Vitamin K_1 administration would not be useful with hepatocellular necrosis but may be useful if the primary disorder is biliary obstruction. If vitamin K_1 (0.025–2.5 mg/kg BW) is used for this purpose, it must be administrered intramuscularly or subcutaneously at least 6 hours prior to performing the biopsy.

Other laboratory tests that may be of some value in the diagnosis or treatment of liver diseases in the horse include: haemogram, leucogram, plasma proteins, blood ammonia, blood and gas determinations. Specific tests for toxicological purposes (liver concentration of iron, aflatoxins, etc.) should be performed when indicated [20]. Serum iron may be elevated in a variety of liver diseases. The haemogram often reveals an erythrocytosis that may be relatively unresponsive

Table 4. **Some guidelines for percutaneous liver biopsy**

- Perform on left or right side, ideally after identification of liver by ultrasound
- Culture the biopsy specimen where septic cholangitis is suspected
- Pretreat animals with chronic biliary obstruction and evidence of bleeding tendencies using fresh or frozen plasma and vitamin K_1

to fluid therapy. An absolute erythrocytosis, with packed cell volume (PCV) persistently greater than 60% has been reported with hepatocellular carcinoma [21]. Hepatocellular carcinomas most frequently occur in yearlings or young adult horses. The cause of the elevated haematocrit in horses with hepatocellular carcinoma is thought to be increased hepatic production of erythropoietin. If the hepatic disorder is a supportive cholangitis, the PCV may be low as a result of anaemia of chronic disease. The leucogram may reveal toxic appearance of neutrophils (vacuoles within the neutrophils), a left shift, and variable total neutrophil count with acute hepatic necrosis regardless of the etiology. A neutrophilia without immature neutrophils is expected with most cases of suppurative cholangitis.

Plasma protein concentration is increased in most horses with hepatic failure regardless of the cause. The increase in plasma protein may be associated with increased immunological response to intestinal-derived antigens resulting from diminished Kupffer cell function or increased immune reaction to damaged hepatic cell membranes, and/or decreased hepatic catabolism of immunoglubulins. Increased plasma protein concentration is expected in horses with bacterial cholangiohepatitis because of an increase in plasma fibrinogen and increased serum globulins in response to the infectious/inflammatory disease. Additionally, plasma volume contraction is often present in horses with liver failure prior to fluid treatment and would cause increases in both plasma protein and PCV.

Blood ammonia concentration is quite variable in horses with hepatic failure. Even with encephalopathy it may be within the normal range ($<100\ \mu$mol/L). With both hepatic disease and failure and in the primary hyperammononaemia syndrome, pronounced neurological signs are expected if the blood ammonia is greater than 140 μmol/L [13]. In foals with portosystemic shunts, pronounced neurologic signs may not occur unless the blood ammonia is of greater magnitude [4]. Congenital portosystemic shunts should be suspected in foals less than 4 months of age that have waxing and waning signs of encephalopathy, normal serum activity of liver enzymes, abnormally high plasma concentrations of bile acids and elevated blood ammonia. Primary hyperammononaemia occurs in some horses with intestinal colic and/or diarrhea and should be considered if encephalopathic signs are present, in addition to the intestinal signs [13]. In Morgan weanlings and yearlings, a hyperammononaemia condition exists that is most likely associated with an inherited abnormality in ammonia metabolism and causes progressive liver disease [22]. In order for ammonia measurements to be accurate, they should be performed on heparinized blood samples with the separated plasma being immediately cooled and measured or frozen after collection and separation.

Horses greater than 7 years of age with severe hepatic lipidosis should be appropriately tested for a pituitary adenoma. Peritoneal fluid evaluation is rarely helpful in the evaluation of equine hepatic failure, unless hepatic lobe torsion or traumatic injury to the liver is suspected, in which case bile crystals may be seen on microscopic examination of the fluid.

Treatment

The treatment of liver failure is largely supportive and should include: specific treatment for hepatic encephalopathy, fluid therapy, nutritional management and antibiotics [2, 17, 23]. If the horse is maniacal and cannot be safely handled, some chemical restraint will be necessary to prevent injury to the horse and the attending veterinarian. Small doses of xylazine (0.2–0.4 mg/kg BW) are usually sufficient in controlling the maniacal behaviour and will allow placement of an intravenous catheter. However, all sedatives should be avoided unless absolutely necessary and diazepam should not be given as this may worsen the hepatic encephalopathy.

Intravenously administered fluids are generally needed in most cases of hepatic failure for replacement of volume deficits, to improve organ perfusion, correct electrolyte and glucose abnormalities and to dilute circulating endogenous toxins. The preferred fluid in most cases is a polyionic fluid that has similar composition to plasma. Five grams of dextrose and 20–40 mEq of potassium chloride should be added to each litre. Additional dextrose can be added if the patient is confirmed to be hypoglycaemic or routinely in foals with hepatic failure. The potassium status of each patient should be monitored carefully since hypokalaemia may worsen the hepatic encephalopathy by increasing renal absorption of ammonia. Bicarbonate-containing fluids should be used with caution and only when blood pH is less than 7.1, and when polyionic fluids have not improved the blood pH. Too rapid infusion of bicarbonate may enhance transfer of ammonia into the CNS.

Moderate to low protein/high carbohydrate diets should be fed to horses with acute onset hepatic failure. This would ideally be a highly palatable 10–12%

Table 5. **Therapeutic objectives for horses with hepatobiliary diseases**

Objective	*Treatment*
Control maniacal behavior	Xylazine, 0.2–0.4 mg/kg BW
Restore circulatory volume, glucose and electrolytes, and dilute endotoxin	Intravenous polyionic fluids, with 5 g dextrose and 20–40 mEq potassium chloride per litre Use bicarbonate *only* when blood pH<7.1 and unresponsive to polyionic fluids
Reduce hepatic encephalopathy	Moderate to low protein diet, with high carbohydrate content and branch chain amino acids Oral neomycin, 10 mg/kg BW QID for 2 days Metronidazole, 7.5 mg/kg BW BID for 2 days
Treat septic cholangitis	Trimethoprim-sulfa (TMP/S) Ceftiofur or enrofloxacin where the organism is not sensitive to TMP/S or TMP/S is not effective
Obstructing cholelith	Surgery
Control chronic active hepatitis	Prednisolone, 0.4–1.0 mg/kg BW daily reducing to 0.4 mg/kg BW every other day

protein concentration mixed with sorghum and/or cracked corn to increase the branched-chain to aromatic amino acid ratio [24]. A commercial paste containing branched-chain amino acids is now available. Small amounts of this concentrate (top dressed with molasses) should be fed several times daily. Feeding small amounts of a high carbohydrate/moderate to low protein feed several times daily (as opposed to twice daily feedings of larger amounts) may prevent surges in plasma glucose, insulin release, and enteric ammonia production. A summer cut grass hay or oat hay should be fed. Alfalfa hay and lush spring grass should be avoided as these are often too high in protein. Summer and fall grazing would be ideal but exposure to sunlight must be avoided to prevent photosensitization. With chronic hepatic disease and failure, a slightly higher protein diet might be indicated.

Neomycin (10 mg/kg BW) should be given orally with molasses four times daily for 2 days in horses with acute hepatocellular necrosis or severe hepatic cirrhosis, to decrease enteric production of ammonia. If hepatic encephalopathy is severe and blood ammonia concentration is extremely high, metronidazole (7.5 mg/kg BW) can be administered in addition, two times daily for 2 days. Treatment to decrease enteric ammonia production is rarely needed in horses with cholangitis. Fulminant hepatic encephalopathy that does not respond to oral antibiotics and fluid therapy can be treated with the benzodiazepine receptor antagonist, flumazinil (0.02 mg/kg BW IV given slowly) but the expense is great and the efficacy is questionable.

Systemic antibiotic therapy is indicated for horses with septic supprative cholangitis. The therapy should be based upon the culture and sensitivity of the organisms(s) that can be cultured from the liver biopsy. When the offending organisms is sensitive to trimethoprim-sulfa (TMP/S), it is the preferred treatment. If the culture and sensitivity or the clinical response suggest that TMP/S is not effective, ceftiofur or enrofloxacin would be the next choices. Empirical treatment is often required because the success of identifying organisms from the liver biopsy is generally less than 50%. A successful response should include normal temperature and improved clinical appearance within 7 days of beginning antibiotic treatment and a decline in the serum GGT within 2–3 weeks. If a large obstructing stone is seen on the sonogram or is suspected based upon history, clinical and laboratory findings, surgery would be indicated. Dimethyl sulfoxide (DMSO) given intravenously may have some efficacy in dissolving calcium bilirubinate stones.

Chronic active hepatitis, not believed to be associated with bacterial infection, can be treated with 0.4–1.0 mg/kg BW prednisolone orally daily. If there is clinical improvement within 2 weeks, the dose can be reduced to a maintenance dose (0.4 mg/kg BW every other day). Ursodiol has not been proven to be safe or effective in the equine. If fibrosis is progressive and/or moderately severe, colchicine (0.03 mg/kg BW) can be given orally once daily but the efficacy of this is unknown. Treatment for hepatic lipidosis caused by a pituitary adenoma should include: cyproheptadine or pergolide (see chapter 3).

References

1. Crawford JM. The Liver and the Biliary Tract. In: Cotram RS, Kumar V, and Robbins SL (eds). *Pathologic Basis of Disease* 5th ed. Philadelphia: WB Saunders 1994; 831–896.
2. Divers TJ. Liver Disease and Failure in Horses. *Proc Am Assoc Eq Pract.* 1982; 213–223.
3. Madison JE. Hepatic encephalopathy – current concepts of the pathogenesis. *J Vet Int Med.* 1992; **6**, 341–353.
4. Fortier LA, Fubinin SL, Flanders JA & Divers TJ. Guidelines for the diagnosis and surgical correction of equine and bovine portosystemic shunts. *Vet Surg.* 1993; 379.
5. Divers TJ, Warner A, Vaala ME *et al.* Toxic hepatic failure in newborn foals. *J Am Vet Med Assoc.* 1983; **183**(12), 1407–1413.
6. Humber KA, Sweeney RW, Saik JE *et al.* Clinicopathologic findings in two foals with *Bacillus piliformis. J Am Vet Med Assoc.* 1988; **193**, 1425.
7. Naylor JN, Kronfeld DS & Johnson K. Fasting hyperbilirubinemia and its relationship to free fatty acids and triglycerides in the horse. *Proc Soc Exp Biol Med.* 1980; **165**, 86–90.
8. Divers TJ, Schappel KA, Sweeney RW & Tennant BC. Persistent hyperbilirubinemia in a healthy Thoroughbred horse. *Cornell Vet.* 1993; **83**, 237–242.
9. Cornelius CE. *Liver Function in Clinical Biochemisrty of Domestic Animals*, 4th ed. JJ Kaneko (ed). New York, Academic Press Inc. 1989; 373.
10. Tulleners EP, Becht JL, Richardson DW & Divers TJ. Choledocholithotripsy in a mare. *J Am Vet Med Assoc.* 1985; **186**(12), 1317–1319.
11. Pearson EG. Liver failure attributable to pyrrolizidine alkaloid toxicosis and associated with inspiratory dyspnea in ponies. *J Am Vet Med Assoc.* 1991; **198**, 1651–1654.
12. Johnson JK, Divers TJ, Reef BV & Acland H. Cholelithiasis in horses, Ten cases (1982–1986). *J Am Vet Med Assoc.* 1989; **194**(3), 405–409.
13. Divers TJ. Diagnosis of hepatic disease and dysfunction in the horse. *Proc 10th Annu Meet, Am Col Vet Int Med.* 1992; 430–432.
14. Parraga ME, Carlson GP & Thurmond M. Serum protein concentrations in horses with severe liver disease, A retrospective study and review of the literature. *J Vet Int Med.* 1994; **9**, 154–161.
15. Divers TJ. Biochemical diagnosis of hepatic diseased and dysfunction in the horse. *Eq Pract.* 1993; **15**(1), 15–17.
16. West HJ. Evaluation of total plasma bile acid concentrations for the diagnosis of hepatobiliary disease in horses. *Res Vet Sci.* 1989; **45**, 264–270.
17. Carlson GP. Icterus in the horse. In: Anderson NB (ed.) *Veterinary Gastroenterology.* Philadelphia: Lea & Febiger 1992; 688–702.
18. Kngelking LR & Gronwall R. Effects of fasting on hepatic bile acid clearance. *Proc Soc Exp Biol Med.* 1979; **161**, 123–127.
19. Rantanen NW. Diseases of the Liver. In: Rantanen NW (ed). Diagnostic Ultrasound. *Vet Cl N Am.* 1986; **2**(1), 105–115.
20. Pearson EG, Hedstrom OR & Poppenga RH. Hepatic cirrhosis and hemochromatosis in three horses. *J Am Vet Med Assoc.* 1994; **204**, 1053–1056.
21. Roby KAW, Beech J, Bloom JC & Black M. Hepatocellular carcinoma associated with erythocytosis and hypoglycemia in a yearling filly. *J Am Vet Med Assoc.* 1990; **196**(3), 465–467.
22. Divers TJ, Tennant BC, Murray MJ *et al.* Unusual cases of liver disease in Morgan foals. *Gastroent Viewpoint.* 1994; **2**, 6.
23. Divers TJ. Treatment of Hepatic Failure. In: BP Smith, (ed) *Large Animal Internal Medicine*, 2nd edn. St. Louis: Mosby Publishing Co. 1996.
24. Ralston SL. Clinical Nutrition of Adult Horses. In: HF Hintz (ed.) *Vet Clin N.A.–Eq Pract.* Philadelphia: WB Saunders 1990; **6**(2), 349.

9

Equine Renal Disease

Celia M Marr

Key Points

- Renal disease is an uncommon but important clinical problem in horses.
- Clinical signs of renal disease are often non-specific and, without a high index of suspicion, renal dysfunction can be overlooked because it usually accompanies other diseases such as enterocolitis or sepsis.
- Acute renal disease is most likely to be caused by nephrotoxins or haemodynamically mediated acute renal tubular necrosis in adult horses.
- Renal tubular necrosis due to asphyxia, neonatal septicaemia and, less commonly, leptospirosis and renal dysplasia are differential diagnosis for renal disease in foals.
- Acute renal tubular necrosis causes loss of urine concentrating ability and azotaemia.
- Measurement of serum creatinine concentration and urinary specific gravity is the simplest, and most important means of identifying renal dysfunction.
- Ultrasonography can provide valuable information on the size and architecture of the kidneys.
- Treatment of acute renal failure must be instituted early and aggressively if the disease is to be reversed.
- Many forms of acute renal failure can be treated successfully with intravenous fluids and diuretics, coupled with careful monitoring.
- Immunologically mediated glomerulonephritis is the most common cause of chronic renal failure.
- Chronic renal disease frequently leads to hypercalcaemia and hypophosphataemia and tends to carry a poor prognosis.
- Nephrolithiasis and interstitial nephrosis may be increasing in prevalence.
- Lack of response to therapy, ultrasonographic evidence of decreased renal size and severe fibrosis identified by renal biopsy are poor prognostic indicators.

Prevalence of Renal Disease

Primary renal disease is a fairly uncommon but, over the last fifteen years, an increasingly well documented clinical entity in horse [1–3]. Renal diseases can affect one or more of the four basic morphological components of the kidney:

glomeruli, tubules, interstitium and blood vessels. The clinical presentation is dependent on the location of the specific lesion was well as its nature and progression [4]. Currently, there is no specific information on the prevalence of the various forms of renal disease. Both renal papillary necrosis [5] and glomerulonephritis [6] have been found at post-mortem examination in horses showing no clinical signs of renal dysfunction. Acute tubular necrosis associated with haemodynamic or nephrotoxic causes appears to be the most common form of acute renal failure in horses [7, 8]. In these horses renal dysfunction can be complicated by pre-renal factors [1, 9]. Leptospirosis and hyperlipaemia are less common causes of acute renal failure [10–12].

Glomerulonephritis is a commonly diagnosed cause of chronic renal failure in horses [13, 14]. Immune mechanisms underlie most cases of glomerular disease in human beings [4] and in horses [15, 16]. There appears to be an association between group C streptococcal antigens and immune-complex glomerulonephritis in horses [16]. Less common causes of chronic renal failure include interstitial nephritis [17], pyelonephritis and oxalate nephropathy [1, 17–19]. Primary renal neoplasia is rarely described [20–24] and nephrocalcinosis secondary to hypercalcaemia of malignancy occurs occasionally [25, 26]. Nephrolithiasis with chronic renal failure has been reported with increasing frequency over the last two decades [27–32].

Congenital renal diseases such as renal agenesis also appear to be very uncommon in horses [33]. Congenital renal dysplasia and hypoplasia involve all of the nephron and can present both acutely and as chronic renal failure in foals and yearlings [34–38]. Polycystic renal disease presents as chronic renal failure during adult life and is probably a developmental defect [39–41]. Hydronephrosis has been reported in association with ectopic ureters [42], renal dysplasia [37], and nephrolithiasis [43].

Diagnosis of Renal Disease

Clinical Presentation

Horses with renal disease can be anuric, oliguric or polyuric. However, this can be difficult to document without the use of a urine collection device [44]. Measurement of water intake may reveal polydipsia. The major differential diagnosis for polydipsia and polyuria in the horse are pituitary adenoma, renal disease, liver disease, pseudohyperparathyroidism, diabetes insipidus and psychogenic water or salt consumption. Clinical signs of nephrotic syndrome are related to hypoalbuminaemia secondary to the loss of albumin through the glomerulus, and are characterized by marked ventral oedema. However, not all horses with glomerulonephritis present with the classic signs of nephrosis. In many cases of renal disease the clinical signs are non-specific ones such as weight loss, abdominal pain, anorexia and depression. Infrequently, buccal mucosal ulcers are seen with uraemia but these are more frequently seen in horses with pituitary adenoma. Enlargement of the left kidney, masses associated with the kidney, and dilation of the ureters may be detected on rectal examination.

Haematuria occurs with various renal diseases such as interstitial fibrosis, renal papillary necrosis [45], haemolytic uraemic-like syndrome [46], leptospirosis [47], nephrolithiasis [48], renal adenocarcinoma [20, 21] and renal pelvic adenoma [22], as well with haemorrhage arising from other areas of the urinary tract. Endoscopic examination of the urethra, bladder and ureters can be extremely valuable in demonstrating the level at which the blood is entering the urine (Figure 1). Samples of urine from each kidney can be obtained by ureteral catherization under cystoscopic guidance [49].

Clinical Pathology

The kidney has a central role in the excretion of the waste products of metabolism, and the maintenance of fluid, electrolyte and acid–base balance. Glomerular filtration is influenced by a balance between intravascular pressure in the afferent and efferent renal arterioles and plasma oncotic pressure. Glomerular filtration rate is controlled within strict limits by the renin–angiotensin mechanism. Normal horses produce 14.7–25.1 mL/kg BW of urine

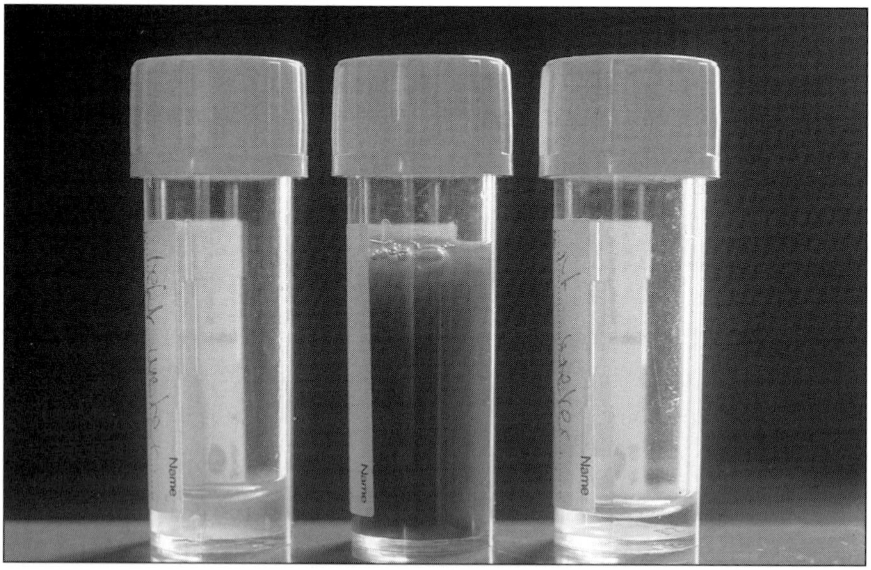

Figure 1. Urine samples taken from the bladder (centre) and both ureters (left and right) by endoscopically guided ureteral catheterization in a 7-year-old Thoroughbred gelding presenting with haematuria caused by a bladder calculi. Demonstration that the urine leaving the ureters was clear confirmed that the blood entered the urine in the bladder and not the kidneys.

per day with a urine specific gravity of 1.020–1.050. [50]. Equine urine contains large amounts of calcium carbonate crystals and mucus; therefore it is frequently cloudy and turbid [51]. Neonatal foals urinate frequently and have dilute urine, with the urine specific gravity typically in the range of 1.001–1.004 [52, 53].

Azotaemia

Serum creatinine concentration is a more reliable indicator of glomerular function than blood urea nitrogen since, having entered the filtrate, creatinine is not reabsorbed, while some urea is reabsorbed in the distal tubule as part of the concentrating mechanism and urea is influenced by non-renal factors such as diet and anabolic processes [51, 54]. Increased serum creatinine, azotaemia, arises due to prerenal, renal and post-renal disorders. Acute renal failure is characterized by increased serum concentrations of urea and creatinine coupled with loss of concentrating ability and isothenuria (urine specific gravity of less than 1.020). Seventy-five per cent or more of the functional capacity of the kidney must be permanently or temporarily lost to stimulate the development of azotaemia [1]. However, normal serum creatinine concentration does not preclude primary renal disease since it indicates only that 25% or more of normal glomerular filtration is occurring [51]. Normal or mildly increased serum creatinine concentrations can be observed in horses with chronic renal failure. Prerenal azotaemia implies structurally normal kidneys that cannot function normally because of decreased perfusion. Horses with cardiac disease or haemorrhagic, hypovolaemic, septic or endotoxic shock can develop prerenal azotaemia [1, 9]. With prerenal azotaemia, the urine is concentrated, and the azotaemia usually resolves following restoration of the circulating volume. Therefore, the response to the administration of intravenous fluids can help to differentiate intrinsic renal failure from prerenal azotaemia [52]. In some azotaemic horses, both renal and prerenal factors are present. Post-renal azotaemia develops in horses and foals with disruption of the urinary tract [52, 53].

Large increases in serum concentration of creatinine and moderate increases in blood urea nitrogen concentration have been observed in foals in the first day of life, with no evidence of renal disease [55]. This resolves within 24–48 hours, provided that the foals are well hydrated, and the finding reflects the dam's serum creatinine concentration and placental excetory function rather than the foal's renal function [52].

Urinalysis

Urinalysis is a simple but extremely important step in the investigation of renal disease [51]. Urine can be collected as a voided sample or by catheterization. Voided samples are suitable for most analyses but cannot be used for bacteriological culture where a sample must be collected aseptically by urethral catherterization to avoid contamination. If sedation for catheterization is necessary, alpha$_2$-adreno-ceptor agonists should be avoided because these drugs cause glycosuria and diuresis [56, 57].

The reference range for urine specific gravity in adult horses is 1.020–1.050 [51]. Isothenuria (urine specific 1.008–1.017) indicates renal dysfunction while hyposthenuria (urine specific gravity of less than 1.007) suggests that there is interference with the action of antidiuretic hormone, for example diabetes insipidus and pituitary adenoma [51]. Water deprivation tests can help to differentiate renal from non-renal causes of dilute urine. A normal horse will show an increase in urine specific gravity to greater than 1.038 after 24 hours of water deprivation and/or a decrease in body weight of 5% [58, 59]. Azotaemic horses should not be subjected to water deprivation.

Adult horses have alkaline pH while foals tend to have acidic urine [60]. An alkaline pH can invalidate the dipstick test for proteinuria. Protein should be analysed by alternative, chemical tests such as the sulfosalicylic acid or Coomassie brilliant blue methods [51]. Proteinuria can be caused by glomerular disease, or inflammation or haemorrhage. Glycosuria occurs most commonly with pituitary adenoma where the development of hyperglycaemia exceeds the renal tubular threshold for reabsorption of glucose. Glycosuria without hyperglycaemia occurs with renal proximal tubular cell dysfunction.

The occult blood test measures haem pigments, haemoglobin and myoglobin. Positive reactions are seen with haematuria, haemolytic disease and with myoglobinuria associated with myopathies. These processes can be differentiated readily since following centrifugation, in haematuria, intact red blood cells will be sedimented to the bottom of the sample, leaving a clear supernatant. With haemolysis, both the urine and the serum will be altered in colour whereas with myglobinuria, the urine is discoloured while the serum has a normal colour [51]. Examination of the urine sediment is easily performed since no staining is required. Following centrifugation, a drop of sediment is examined under a cover slip for the presence of casts, crystals and cells. Equine urine normally contains large amounts of calcium carbonate crystals. More than 10 red or white blood cells per high power field indicates haemorrhage or inflammation, respectively. Casts are moulds of protein and cells that have formed within the tubules. Casts of renal tubular cells are frequently seen with acute tubular necrosis from nephrotoxic or haemodynamic causes [51]. White blood cell casts suggest pyelonephritis [19].

Gamma glutamyl transferase (GGT) is found in the renal tubular cells as well as in the pancreas and liver [61, 62]. In horses with renal tubular damage, the urine concentrations of GGT increase and determination of the urine GGT to creatinine ratio can be a useful means of early diagnosis of renal disease [63]. However, clinical experience suggests that large increases in urinary GGT can be present with minor, subclinical renal pathology therefore the results should be interpreted with caution.

Serum Electrolytes

Hypochloraemia is the most consistent finding in polyuric renal failure while hyponatraemia and metabolic acidosis are seen slightly less frequently [7, 9, 63]. Severe hyperkalaemia is fairly uncommon in acute renal failure [51] and, particularly in foals, is more often observed with post-renal failure [64]. The horse is unusual in that serum calcium concentrations are often increased and serum phosphate concentrations are often decreased, particularly in chronic renal failure [13, 65, 66]. In acute haemodynamically mediated renal failure, hypocalcaemia and hypophosphataemia, the pattern typical in renal failure in small animals has been observed [7]. The pathophysiological mechanisms that lead to hypercalcaemia and hypophosphataemia in renal failure are not clear. The equine kidney has a unique role in calcium homoeostatis and loss of its regulation of excretion may be important [65]. Increase in the parathyroid hormone *C*-terminal, which is excreted through the kidney have been documented in acute renal failure. However, this is not the physiologically active portion of parathyroid hormone and the significance of this finding is uncertain [63]. The major differential diagnoses for hypercalcaemia and hypophosphataemia in the horse include hypercalcaemia of malignancy [26] and vitamin D toxicosis [67].

Distinguishing between Prerenal and Renal Azotaemia: Serum and Urine Osmolality, Creatinine, Urea and Electrolyte Ratios

The osmolality and concentration of creatinine and urea in the urine reflect both filtration and concentrating functions of the nephron, thereby indirectly assessing glomerular and tubular function. In prerenal azotaemia, tubular concentrating function is intact, therefore the urine to serum creatinine and urea ratios are increased (greater than 50:1 and 15:1, respectively). In renal azotaemia, with the loss of concentrating ability, these ratios fall (less than 37:1 and 15:1, respectively). The urine osmolality and the ratio of urine to plasma osmolality are also maintained (greater than 400 mOsm/kg of water and 1.5, respectively), [68].

The urinary clearance of electrolytes is the rate at which substance is removed from plasma or serum into the urine. To determine this it is necessary to collect urine formed over at least 6, and ideally 24 hours [69]. The fractional excretion (FE) of electrolytes is determined by the expression of the given electrolyte clearance as a ratio of creatinine clearance:

$$\mathrm{FE} = \frac{\mathrm{Ux}}{\mathrm{Sx}} \times \frac{\mathrm{Scr}}{\mathrm{Ucr}} \times 100$$

where Ux = urine concentration of electrolyte x; Sx = serum concentration of electrolyte x; Scr = serum concentration of creatinine; Ucr = urine concentration of creatinine.

The advantage of determining fractional clearances is that the test can be performed on urine and serum on one occasion, without prolonged and technically difficult urine collection [70]. However, there is diurnal variation [69], feeding can influence the results [71] and, in mares, the results can vary with the stage of the oestrous cycle [72]. Individual laboratories may provide specific recommendations on sample collection protocols for their reference range and, ideally, samples should be obtained from horses prior to exercise or feeding (Harris PA, personal communication). The fractional clearance of sodium can help to differentiate prerenal from renal azotaemia. Horses with renal dysfunction have sodium clearance ratios of greater than 0.50 [68]. Fractional excretions of potassium, calcium and magnesium are used to assess whole body electrolyte status and identify dietary deficiencies [73].

Assessing Effective Renal Plasma and Glomerular Filtration Rate

The classical method for assessing glomerular filtration rate is by inulin clearance. Inulin is freely filtered and is not reabsorbed to any significant extent. Consequently, the urinary and plasma concentrations of inulin are equal and the rate at which plasma is cleared after administration of inulin is equal to the glomerular filtration rate. Para-aminohippuric acid (PAH) is also filtered freely but any PAH that remains in the plasma after leaving the glomeruli is excreted from the peritubular capillaries into the tubules. Therefore, only around one-tenth of the PAH remains in the plasma after it has cleared the kidney and the PAH clearance can be used to estimate the effective renal plasma flow. Normal values for single injection and infusion inulin and clearances in adult horses and foals have been obtained [74, 75].

Alternative methods of estimation of glomerular filtration rate in horses include endogenous creatinine clearance [54, 75, 76] and sodium sulfanilate clearance [77, 78]. Clearance of the blood of radio-labelled diethylenetriamine-pentaacetic acid can also be used to estimate glomerular filtration rate and has the advantage that no urine samples are required [79]. These various techniques are most useful for physiological and pharmacological studies and are rarely used in clinical practice. The benefit of monitoring the reciprocal of serum creatinine concentration and sodium sulfanilate clearance half-time in determining the prognosis in one horse with polycystic renal disease has been demonstrated [40]. Estimation of glomerular filtration rate can occasionally be useful to identify renal dysfunction in horses with mild or no azotaemia [78].

Diagnostic Ultrasonography

Ultrasonography is an excellent means of assessing renal size and internal architecture. The right kidney lies immediately deep to the body wall, ventral to the subvertebral musculature, from the fifteenth to the seventeenth intercostal space [22, 43]. Cranial to the right kidney lies the liver and ventral to the right kidney lies the caecum and duodenum. Sector or microconvex transducers facilitate examination of this area between the ribs and, depending on the size of the horse, frequencies from 3.5 to 6.5 MHz are used. The left kidney is more variable in its position. It lies medial to the spleen in the left sublumbar fossa and sixteenth and seventeenth intervostal space [80]. Transducers at 3.5 MHz are usually used in adult horses because a deeper imagining field is needed [43, 81].

The cortex, medulla, calyces, renal pelvis and renal blood vessesl are visualized ultrasonographically. The kidneys should be less echogenic than the spleen and liver and it should be easy to distinguish the cortex from the medulla. The cortex is normally more echogenic than the medulla and fat in the renal pelvis produces very bright echoes [22, 43, 80]. It can be difficult to measure the kidneys precisely but in most adult horses they are 13–15 cm long [80].

The ultrasonographic features of a variety of equine renal conditions have now been documented. In acute tubular necrosis, the kidneys can be enlarged, with an increase in the echogenicity of the cortex [43, 82]. Perirenal oedema is frequently observed as an anechoic band around the kidneys in both haemodynamic and nephtotoxic acute renal failure [43, 82–84]. In cortical necrosis, there can be loss of the distinct corticomedullary junction, renal enlargement and areas of increased echogenicity in the cortex (Figure 2). However, in some cases of acute renal failure the ultrasonographic features may be subtle or

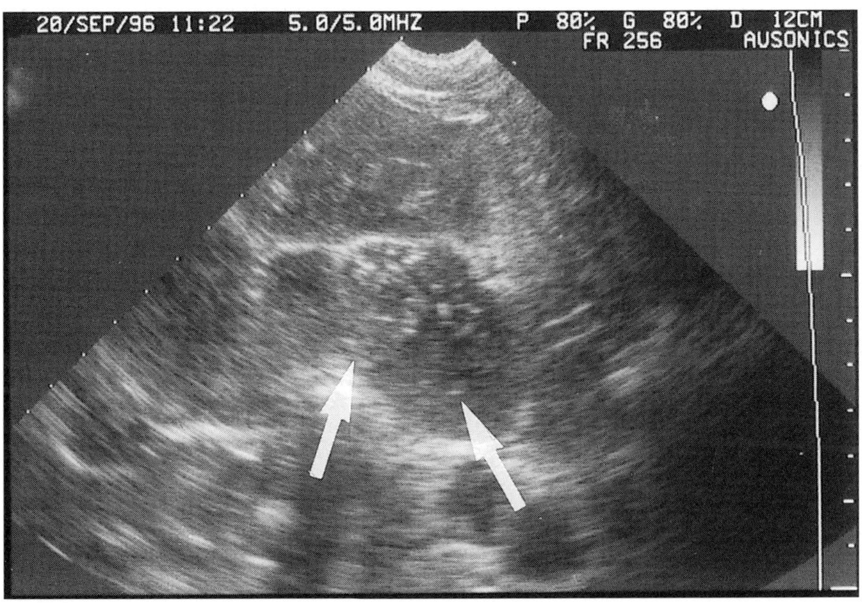

Figure 2. An ultrasonogram of the right kidney from a 3-month-old foal with bilateral renal cortical necrosis and staphylococcal cellulitis. The kidney is larger than expected, there is loss of the corticomedullary junction and there are numerous pin-point foci of increased echogenicity (arrows) throughout the cortex.

inapparent. In one horse with acute renal failure secondary to myositis no ultrasonographic abnormality was detected [85]. In an adult horse with leptospirosis the kidneys were enlarged but had normal internal architecture [10] and a weanling with leptospirosis had normal ultrasonographic findings in the early stages of the disease [11]. Likewise, in renal dysplasia, no specific ultrasonographic abnormalities have been recognized [38].

Chronic renal disease frequently results in a decrease in the renal dimensions, the kidneys may be nodular in shape, and there may be an increase in echogenicity with loss of the distinct corticomedullary junction. Assessment of the size of the kidney can be helpful in distinguishing acute from chronic disease, although not all horses with irreversible renal fibrosis have small kidneys [82, 85].

Ultrasonography is particularly valuable in the diagnosis of focal renal lesions. Fluid-filled lesions such as abscesses can be differentiated from solid masses [43]. Abscesses and haematomas are well differentiated from the surrounding renal parenchyma and usually have a uniform, hypoechoic appearance [85]. The ultrasonographic features of ureteropelvic polyps and associated hydronephrosis [37], polycystic renal disease [40] and isolated cystic lesions [82] have been reported. Cystic lesions usually contain anechoic fluid with associated acoustic enhancement [82]. Renal pelvic adenoma and renal adenocarcinoma are localized masses that may have a hypoechoic or mixed echogenicity [22, 85]. Renal lymphosarcoma can produce multiple masses of mixed echogenicity [82].

Renal calculi are usually strongly echogenic and produce strong acoustic shadows [29–31, 43, 44]. Care should be taken not to confuse these with fat in the renal pelvis. The sensitivity of the ultrasonography in the diagnosis of nephrolithiasis has not been studied specifically but in one study four out of eight cases were accurately diagnosed ultasonographically [32]. In horses with renal calculi, ultrasonography may provide information that is otherwise unattainable, such as the demonstration of the calculi, obstruction of the proximal portion of the ureter or renal pelvis, dilation of the renal calyces, size of the right kidney and the character of the renal parenchyma [30].

Renal Biopsy

Renal biopsy is most valuable in horses with chronic renal disease in which an assessment of the histological structure of the kidney is necessary to attempt to determine if irreversible changes are present to provide an accurate prognosis. Ideally, renal biopsy should be performed under ultrasonographic guidance since this will minimize the risk of penetration of blood vessels or adjacent intestine [85]. An ultrasonographic unit with a biopsy guide function allows more accurate placement of the biopsy instrument. The biopsy needle is secured through a plate attached to the ultrasound transducer and markers on the screen indicate the path of the needle. Biopsy needles with a spring-loaded or mechanical firing system are easiest to use because with manual sampling instruments there can be more movement of the apparatus as the sample is taken. The preferred site for biopsy of the right kidney is through the seventeenth intercostal space, in the lateral border of the kidney. This is around 15 cm away from the hilus and both poles of the kidney in a medium-sized horse (Figure 3). The kidney is imaged transversely and the needle is inserted

(a)

(b)

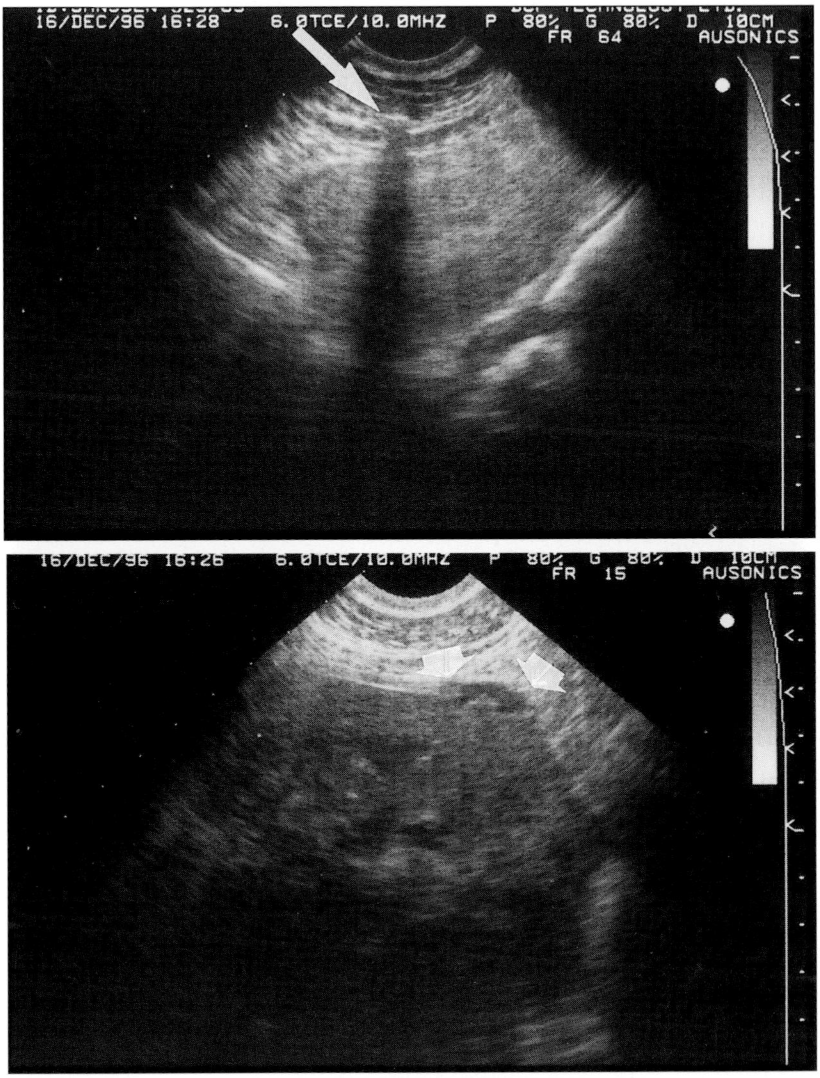

Figure 3. (a) An ultrasonogram of the lateral border of right kidney obtained from the right seventeenth intercostal space from a horse during ultrasound guided renal biopsy. The biopsy instrument (arrow) produces a strong acoustic shadow and can be seen adjacent to the renal capsule. (b) An ultrasonogram from the same horse a few minutes after the biopsy was completed. An anechoic area (arrows) representing sub-capsular haemorrhage is present.

approximately perpendicular to the body wall [86]. Transient haematuria may be observed following biopsy. On both ultrasonographic (Figure 3) and post-mortem examination subcapsular haemorrhage can be seen following renal biopsy but no major complications have been reported to date [86]. The left kidney is more difficult to biopsy, unless it can be pushed against the body wall by rectal examination by an assistant. It may be necessary to penetrate the spleen to reach the left kidney [86]. However, where ultrasonography is not available, biopsy of the left kidney with rectal immobilization may be preferable to blind biopsy of the right kidney [86].

Differentiation of Acute from Chronic Renal Failure

Horses that develop overt clinical signs of renal failure can have acute disease or this may represent an acute presentation of a chronic problem. The differentiation of these processes can be difficult. The clinical history may provide some useful clues; for example, insidious onset of clinical sign suggests chronic disease, and known exposure to nephrotoxins or concurrent predisposing factors such as endotoxaemia are suggestive of acute tubular necrosis. Hypercalcaemia can be present in acute renal failure but it is a more consistent finding in chronic renal failure. Ultrasonographic assessment of renal size may help to differentiate acute from chronic processes. Ultimately, until a specific diagnosis of the cause of the renal disease is reached, it may not be possible to differentiate acute and chronic processes. Equally, most types of acute renal dysfunction can progress to chronic renal failure.

Causes of Acute Renal Failure

Toxic nephropathies

Aminoglycoside toxicity

Aminoglycosides are taken up by the proximal tubular cells by endocytosis following binding to phospholipid receptors. They enter the lysosomes where they interfere with the activity of various enzymes and induce tubular necrosis. Obstruction of the tubules by necrotic debris and structural changes in the filtration barrier decrease glomerular filtration. Neomycin is more nephrotoxic than gentomycin and amikacin [87]. The combined use of gentomycin and ceftiofur has been shown in preliminary studies to induce higher concentrations of urinary GGT than gentomycin alone, although none of the horses developed clinical signs of nephrotoxicity (Livesey, personal communication).

Horses with systemic infection or dehydration and young foals are most at risk of developing aminoglycoside toxicity [88–90]. Ideally, every 3–4 days, the dosage and frequency of administration of gentomycin should be modified by measurement of peak (1 hour post administration) and trough serum concentrations of the drug to achieve target maximal concentration and minimal concentrations of

10 μg/mL and 1 μg/mL, respectively. In one study, nine of 12 horses with sepsis, that were considered to be at risk for developing gentomycin toxicity, required adjustement of dosing [89]. In another study of 35 horses with sepsis required dosage adjustment and one horse developed clinical signs of nephrotoxicosis on day 14 of treatment despite appropriate gentomycin concentrations 4 days previously [90]. In foals, a dose of 3 mg/kg BW, q12h has been shown to be more desirable than lower but more frequent dosages because of their higher total body water and larger volume of distribution of the drug. The use of a single daily dose of 6.6 mg/kg BW of gentomycin may be advantageous since lower through concentrations should reduce the risk of toxicity [91]. However, there are no studies comparing the efficacy and toxicity of this regimen compared with the more traditional dosage regimen of 2.2 mg/kg BW, QID. Preliminary studies have demonstrated that single day dosing leads to higher urinary concentrations of GGT (Livesey, personal communication).

One of the earliest signs of aminoglycoside nephrotoxicity is the appearance of tubular cell casts in the urine [87]. This is followed by loss of concentrating ability and increasing serum concentration of creatinine. Toxicity should be suspected in horses receiving aminoglycosides that develop depression and anorexia. Aminoglycoside toxicity can be reversible, provided that is recognized early, the drug is withdrawn and appropriate fluid therapy is provided [88, 90, 92]. Peritoneal dialysis may help to remove aminoglycosides and nitrogenous waste products [92].

Heavy metal, plant and environmental nephrotoxins

Many substances have been implicated in outbreaks and individual cases of equine nephrotoxicosis. There are various reports of oxalate toxicosis [93, 94]. However, oxalate crystals can accumulate in the kidneys secondary to renal disease [5, 18]. Nephrotoxic heavy metals include zinc, cadmium [95] and mercury, which has been used both in an experimental model [63] and caused acute renal failure when used both with and without the solvent dimethyl sulfoxide in leg paints [96, 97]. The administration of synthetic vitamin K [98, 99] and vitamin D [67] and plants containing tannins [100], and tremetol [101], and those contaminated with aflatoxins [102] and cantharidin [103] can induce acute renal failure. In many of these examples, the renal disease is accompanied by other clinical signs, particularly gastrointestinal lesions. Cantharidin (blister beetle) toxicosis produces dramatic lesions on many epithelial surfaces, including skin sloughing, oral mucosal ulcers, gastrointestinal lesions and cystitis (Figure 4). The disease is characterized by a marked hypocalcaemia and hypomagnesaemia [103]. Vitamin D toxicosis and cadmium and zinc toxicity lead to nephrocalcinosis [67, 95]. Most of the other nephrotoxins listed above produce clinical and laboratory findings that are consistent with acute tubular necrosis [8]. The tubular basement membrane often remains intact, therefore the diseases can be reversible and the aims of therapy are to induce diuresis and provide supportive care [8].

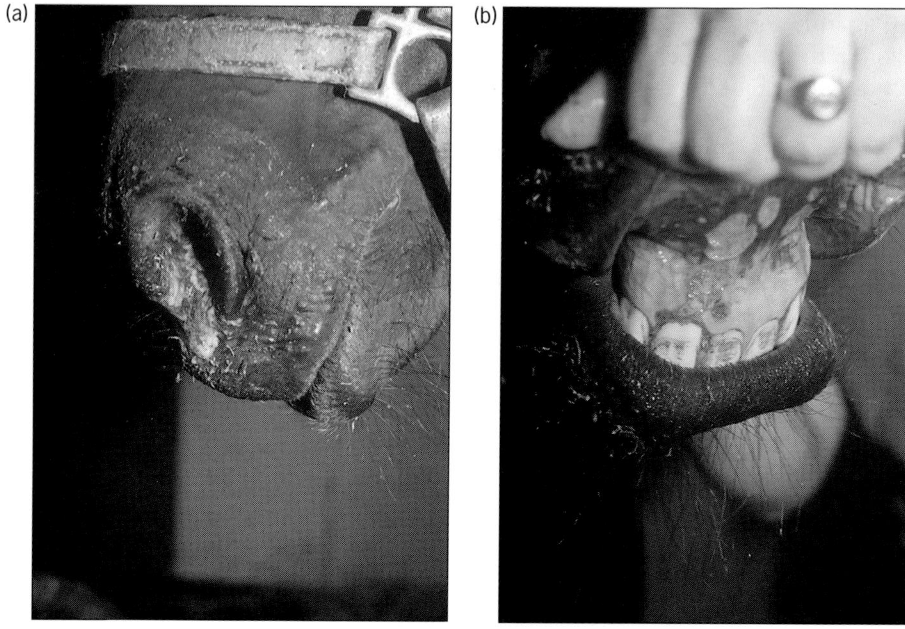

Figure 4. Severe skin crusting (a) and oral mucosal ulcers (b) from an 8-year-old mare with cantharidin toxicosis.

Pigment induced nephropathy

Haemoglobin and myoglobin can cause renal tubular necrosis in horses that are dehydrated or have poor renal perfusion. Myoglobin probably exerts its effect by producing vasoconstriction [8]. Haemoglobin itself is not toxic and the nephropathy associated with haemolysis is the result of erythrocyte stromal elements. Large amounts of myoglobin are released in response to exertional and post-anaesthetic myopathy. In order to prevent nephropathy, large volumes of intravenous fluids should be administered to obtain diuresis in horses with myopathies. In most cases, if addressed early, the renal dysfunction appears to be reversible. Haemoglobin nephropathy results from extensive intravascular haemolysis for example with babesiosis, neonatal isoerythrolysis, liver failure, *Clostridium novei* infection and haemolytic toxins such as phenothiazine, wild onion, and red maple leaf [8]. Haemolytic-uraemic syndrome is a common cause of renal disease of unknown aetiology in children and a similar syndrome has been described in horses [46, 104]. It is characterized by intravascular haemolysis, arteriolar microangiopathy and oliguric renal failure; it carries a poor prognosis [46, 104].

Non-steroidal anti-inflammatory drugs

In acute non-steroidal anti-inflammatory drugs (NSAIDs) toxicity, clinical signs relating to protein-losing enteropathy usually predominate [105, 106]. However,

NSAIDs have been implicated in renal papillary necrosis [5, 107]. Dehydration appears to be a predisposing factor [5]. Renal papillary necrosis is often subclinical but occasionally causes azotaemia and haematuria [107]. A relationship between renal papillary necrosis and the development of nephroliths has been proposed to explain the apparent increasing frequency of occurrence of nephrolithiasis coincident with the introduction of widespread use of NSAIDs [30].

Haemodynamic Nephropathies

Neonatal asphyxia

In asphyxiated foals, renal lesions can be produced by a hypoxic–ischaemic mechanism. Fluid retention is the result of oliguria and the excessive release of antidiuretic hormone. Oedema is exacerbated by increased capillary permeability [53]. This often follows dystocia, prematurity, dysmaturity, Caesarean section, or hypothermia, and the foals present with cardiovascular failure, hypoxia, metabolic acidosis, oliguria, azotaemia and oedema. Oliguria can be dificult to appreciate, but generalized oedema (Figure 5) typically appears at 24–72 hours of age and may be accompanied by signs of neurological dysfunction associated with cerebral oedema, such as depression, aimless wandering, seizures and abnormal posturing. The main alternative differential diagnoses for acute renal failure in

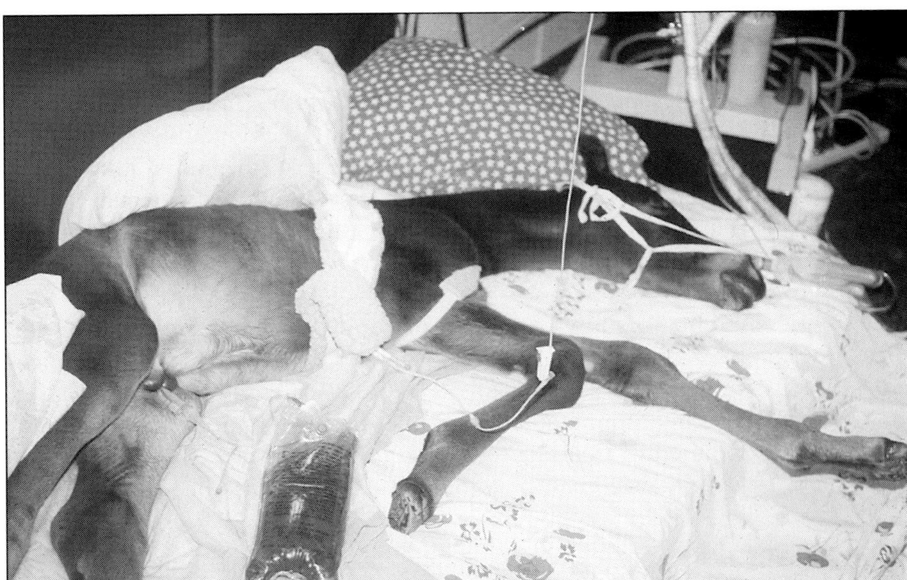

Figure 5. In this 2-day-old foal born by Caesarian section, there is generalized oedema that is most obvious around the prepuce and ventral abdomen. The urine is being collected in a closed system, via a Foley catheter, to monitor urinary output.

foals are pyelonephritis and congenital renal dysplasia [37, 38, 52, 53]. Foals can be treated successfully by fluid therapy, which must be monitored carefully to avoid over hydration in an oliguric, oedematous animal. Frusemide and dopamine can used for diuresis; dobutamine may improve cardiovascular function and intensive supportive care is mandatory. The prognosis is poor without intensive care [53]. A complete recovery can be achieved in some cases. Occasionally, foals will recover from the acute episode but may be left with marginal renal function, poor growth rates and signs of ill-thrift.

Vasomotor renal failure

Blood loss, severe dehydration, and septic or endotoxic shock can lead to acute tubular necrosis. The haemodynamic changes induce renal ischaemia and patchy renal tubular necrosis [7]. In horses, possible predisposing conditions are metritis, enterocolitis, peritonitis, and myositis but in some cases the concurrent disorder is not particularly severe [7]. Bilateral renal cortical necrosis or infarction of the majority of the renal cortex, the generalized Shwartzmann reaction, can be induced experimentally by administration of endotoxin and staphylococcal toxin [108]. In horses, it has occurred in association with enterocolitis [108] and with streptococcal cellulitis (Figure 2). The clinical signs and laboratory abnormalities are not specific and are similar to the other forms of acute renal failure. Marked renal enlargement and perirenal oedema are poor prognostic indicators [7] that can be demonstrated ultrasonographically [82].

Bacterial Infections and Leptospirosis

In foals with neonatal septicaemia, renal involvement is common. *Escherichia coli*, *Klebsiella*, and *Actinobacillus* are the organisms most frequently implicated. Frequently, this is part of generalized infection. Early diagnosis, intravenous antibiotics and intensive supportive care are essential [53]. In adult horses, pyelonephritis is less common and usually more chronic. Gram-negative organisms, *Streptococcus* spp., *Staphlococcus* spp. and *Corynebacterium* spp. are potential causative organisms [19, 109].

Leptospirosis in horses causes a number of conditions including abortion, still births, pyrexia and uveitis [47]. Renal leptospirosis has occurred in a neonatal foal [47], a weanling [11] and a stallion [10]. All cases presented with fever, leukocytosis, azotaemia, and isothenuria. The foal also had gross haematuria. These cases responded to treatment with penicillin with trimethoprim sulfa or amikacin or ticarcillin/clavulonic acid followed by streptomycin.

Hyperlipaemia

Hyperlipaemia is a disturbance of lipid metabolism characterized by excessive mobilization of fatty acids and subsequent fatty infiltration of body tissues. Clinical signs are non-specific and can be attributed to liver and kidney failure.

Eleven of 14 cases in a recent survey had azotaemia, although this was mild in seven of the ponies [12].

Treatment of Acute Renal Failure

The main goal of treatment of acute renal failure is to establish effective diuresis while preventing fluid overload, particularly if the horse is oliguric. Arterial blood pressure and central venous pressure should be used as a guide to fluid therapy and it can be very helpful to measure urinary output. It is most practical to measure arterial blood pressure from the coccygeal artery using an indirect manometer. Central venous pressure is obtained using a catheter, which is long enough to reach the cranial vena cava, placed in the jugular vein [110]. A water manometer consisting of a fluid-filled length of tubing is used to measure the pressure. Ideally, central venous pressure should not rise above 10 cm H_2O to avoid over hydration. One of the first clinical signs that fluid administration is excessive is that the conjunctiva become oedematous [109]. Jugular distension and increased pulses also indicate volume overload. Acid–base and electrolyte disorders should be corrected and monitored frequently. Peritoneal dialysis has been used successfully in aminoglycoside nephrotoxicosis [92].

In oliguric horses, dopamine and furosemide can help to improve urinary output. At low doses (2–5 μg/kg BW.min) dopamine acts directly on the renal vascular bed leading to vasodilation and improved renal blood flow and urinary output. The infusion rate of dopamine must be carefully controlled and arterial blood pressure should be monitored during administration because at higher doses, dopamine can cause deleterious vasoconstriction [109, 110]. Furosemide (1 mg/kg BW q2h) can be used alone but it is frequently more effective when used in conjunction with dopamine infusions. In non-oliguric horses, sodium chloride (0.9%) or balanced polyionic solutions are administered at 40–80 mL/kg BW.day until the serum creatinine concentration improves, and continued at a lower rate until the serum creatinine concentration is normal [110]. Hypertonic saline solutions should be avoided in horses with renal dysfunction.

Causes of Chronic Renal Failure

Glomerulonephritis

Chronic glomerulonephritis can occur in horses as young as 3 years of age but appears to be more common in older animals [15, 111]. Glomerular disease is immunologically mediated with antigen–antibody complexes either being deposited in a subendothelial location, or forming *in situ*. This activates complement, causing platelet aggregation and sequestration of neutrophils leading to cellular injury. An association with Group-C steptococcal antigen has been documented [16]. Glomerulonephritis can be found incidentally at post-mortem examination [6], or cause signs of nephrotic syndrome [15, 16] or chronic failure (polydipsia, polyuria and azotaemia) [13, 18].

Interstitial Nephritis

The majority of the types of acute renal failure described above can progress to chronic interstitial nephritis and fibrosis [109]. The critical factor in determining whether renal failure is reversible or not appears to be the status of the basement membrane [8]. A history of a previous episode of acute renal failure is not always recognized and interstitial nephritis often presents with an insidious onset [112]. Frequently, by presentation, markedly fibrosed end-stage kidneys have developed and the prognosis is poor. Renal biopsy can help the clinical to determine the prognosis in individual cases.

Nephrolithiasis

Urinary calculi usually represent mineralization of an organic nidus, that can be necrotic or inflammatory debris. Calcium carbonate is the major component of equine urinary calculi [113]. Renal papillary necrosis may be a predisposing factor. The apparent increasing incidence of nephroliths may be related to the increasing use of NSAIDs and consequent increase in frequency of renal papillary necrosis [30]. Nephrolithiasis has been reported in horses both with [29–31] and without concurrent interstitial fibrosis. Concurrent pyelonephritis occurs less commonly [30]. It has been speculated that the renal parenchymal disease is the consequence of obstruction by the nephrolith [114]. However, it may be the cause and frequently, bilateral renal interstitial fibrosis is found in horses with unilateral calculi. On the other hand, it is possible that previous obstruction has been relieved prior to examination [30]. Unilateral nephrectomy has been successful in a colt with unilateral nephrolithiasis, normal serum chemistry and normal ultrasonographic findings in the contralateral kidney [48]. However, bilateral nephrolithiasis and the possibility of concurrent interstitial nephritis in the contralateral kidney should be investigated before surgery, to ensure a favourable prognosis.

Renal Neoplasia

Adenocarcinoma is the most frequently diagnosed primary renal tumour [20, 21, 24]. The tumour is usually unilateral and may metastasize widely, with the lung, liver, and regional lymph nodes being common sites for metastases [24]. Carcinoma and adenoma of the renal pelvis [22, 23] have been reported in one case each. Rarely, the kidney can be involved in generalized or multicentric lymphosarcoma [82, 115, 116]. The clinical signs relating to renal neoplasia are non-specific but may include haematuria, polydipsia and polyuria.

Renal Tubular Acidosis

Renal tubular acidosis develops when there are abnormalities of tubular function that lead to loss of bicarbonate and its replacement by chloride. It is characterized by severe hyperchloraemic acidosis with normal serum creatinine concentration. The dysfunction can occur when distal renal tubule is unable to excrete hydrogen ions against a pH gradient (Type 1), when there is a reduction in reabsorption of bicarbonate ions in the proximal renal tubule (Type 2), a combination of these (Type 3), or when the secretion of hydrogen and potassium ions in the distal renal tubule decreases (Type 4) [117]. Types 1 and 2 have been reported in horses [117–119]. The clinical signs are of non-specific depression, weakness and mild abdominal pain [118]. Type 1 is diagnosed if, in response to acid loading by the administration of ammonium chloride, the pH of the urine does not fall [117], while Type 2 is diagnosed if, in response to bicarbonate administration, the urinary pH increases in the presence of systemic acidosis [119]. In humans, renal tubular acidosis can be a genetic disorder as well as arising secondary to systemic disease [120]. The pathogenesis in horses is unknown. Two horses with Type 1 renal tubular acidosis responded to treatment with bicarbonate and ultimately the condition resolved spontaneously [118]. Bicarbonate therapy will not be helpful in Type 2 renal tubular acidosis [119].

References

1. Koterba AM & Coffman JR. Acute and chronic renal disease in the horse. *Comp Cont Educ Pract Vet.* 1981; **3**, S461–S469.
2. MacDougall DF & Ricketts SW. Progress in equine nephrology. *Equine Vet J.* 1987; **19**, 172–173.
3. Pringle J. Pathophysiology and diagnosis of Urinary Disease. In: Kobluk CN, Ames TR & Goer RJ (eds). *The Horse Disease and Clinical Management.* Philadephia: WB Saunders 1995; 575–582.
4. Cotran RS, Kumar V & Robbins SL. The Kidney. In: *Robbins Pathologic Basis of Disease,* 5th edn. Philadephia: WB Saunders 1994; 927–990.
5. Gunson DE. Renal papillary necrosis in horses. *JAVMA.* 1983; **182**, 263–266.
6. Banks KL & Henson JB. Immunologically-mediated glomerulonephritis of horses. II. Glomerular basement membrane antibody and other mechanisms in spontaneous disease. *Lab. Invest.* 1992; **26**, 708–715.
7. Divers TJ, Whitlock RH, Byars TD *et al.* Acute renal failure in six horses resulting from haemodynamic causes. *Equine Vet J.* 1987; **19**, 178–184.
8. Schmitz DG. Toxic nephropathy in horses. *Comp Cont Educ Pract Vet.* **10**, 104–111.
9. Brobst DF, Grant BD, Halberd BJ *et al.* Blood biochemical changes in horses with prerenal and renal disease. *J. Equine Med Surg.* 1977; **1**, 171–177.
10. Divers TJ, Byars TD & Shin SJ. Renal dysfunction associated with infection of *Leptospira interrogans* in a horse. *JAVMA.* 1992; **201**, 1391–1392.
11. Hogan PM, Bernard WV, Kazakevicius PA & Fitzgerald MR. Acute renal disease due to *Leptospira interrogans* in a weanling. *Equine Vet J.* 1996; **28**, 331–333.

12. Watson TDG, Murphy D & Love S. Equine hyperlipaemia in the United Kingdom, clinical features and blood biochemistry of 18 cases. *Vet Rec.* 1992; **131**, 48–51.
13. Brobst DF, Lee HA & Spencer GR. Hypercalcemia and hypophosphatemia in a mare with renal insufficiency. *JAVMA.* 1978; **173**, 1370–1372.
14. Pringle J & Ortenburger A. Diseases of the kidneys and ureters. In: Kobluk CN, Ames TR & Goer RJ (eds). *The Horse. Disease and Clinical Management.* Philadelphia: WB Saunders 1995; 583–596.
15. Sabnis SG, Gunson DE & Antonovych TT. Some unusual features of mesangioproliferative glomerulonephritis in horses. *Vet Pathol.* 1984; **21**, 574–581.
16. Divers TJ, Timoney JF, Lewis RM & Smith CA. Equine glomerulonephritis and renal failure associated with complexes of Group-C streptococcal antigen and IgG antibody. *Vet Immunol Immunopathol.* 1992; **32**, 93–102.
17. Alders RG & Hutchins DR. Chronic nephritis in a horse. *Aust Vet J.* 1987; **64**, 151–154.
18. Roberts MC & Seiler RJ. Renal failure in a horse with chronic glomerulonephritis and renal oxalosis. *J Equine Med Surg.* 1979; **3**, 278–283.
19. Carrick JB & Pollitt CC. Chronic pyelonephritis in a brood mare. *Aust Vet J.* 1987; **64**, 252–254.
20. Brown PJ & Holt PE. Primary renal cell carcinoma in four horses. *Equine Vet J.* 1985; **17**, 473–477.
21. Owen Rh ap Rh, Haywood S & Kelly, DF. Clinical course of renal adenocarcinoma associated with hypercupraemia in a horse. *Vet Rec.* 1986; **119**, 291–294.
22. Penninck DG, Eisenber HM, Teuscher EE & Virins A. Equine renal ultrasonography, normal and abnormal. *Vet Radiol.* 1986; **27**, 81–84.
23. Servantie J, Magnol JP, Regnier A *et al.* Carcinoma of the renal pelvis with bony metaplasia in a horse. *Equine Vet J.* 1986; **18**, 236–238.
24. West HJ, Kelly DF & Ritchie HE. Renal carcinomatosis in a horse. *Equine Vet J.* 1987; **196**, 548–551.
25. Marr CM, Love S & Pirie, HM. Clinical, ultrasonographic and pathological findings in a horse with splenic lymphosarcoma and pseudohyperparathyroidism. *Equine Vet. J.* 1989; **21**, 222–226.
26. Mair TS, Yeo SP & Lucke VM. Hypercalcaemia and soft tissue mineralisation associated with lymphosarcoma in two horses. *Vet Rec.* 1990; **126**, 99–101.
27. Divers TJ. Chronic renal failure in horses. *Comp Cont Educ Pract Vet.* 1983; **6**, S310–S317.
28. Macharg MA, Foerner JJ, Phillips TN & Barclay WP. Two methods for the treatment of ureterolithiasis in a mare. *Vet Surg.* 1984; **13**, 95–98.
29. Hope WD, Wilson WD, Hager JH *et al.* Chronic renal failure associated with bilateral nephroliths and ureteroliths in a two-year-old Thoroughbred colt. *Equine Vet J.* 1989; **21**, 228–231.
30. Ehnen SJ, Divers TJ, Gillette D & Reef VB. Obstructive nephrolithiasis and urterolithiasis associated with chronic renal failure in horses, eight cases (1981–1987). *JAVMA.* 1990; **197**, 249–253.
31. Hillyer MH, Mair TS & Lucke VM. Bilateral renal calculi in an adult horse. *Equine Vet J.* **2**, 1990; 117–120.
32. Laverty S, Pascoe JR, Ling GV *et al.* Urolithiasis in 68 horses. *Vet Surg.* 1992; **21**, 56–62.
33. Johnson BD, Klingborg DJ, Heitman JM *et al.* A horse with one kidney, partially obstructed ureter and contralateral urogenital anomalies. *JAVMA.* 1976; **169**, 210–218.
34. Andrews FM, Rosol TJ, Kohn CW *et al.* Bilateral renal hypoplasia in four young horses. *JAVMA.* 1986; **189**, 209–212.
35. Anderson WI, Picut CA, King JM & Pergrizet JA. Renal dysplasia in a Standardbred colt. *Vet Pathol.* 1988; **25**, 179–180.
36. Brown CM, Parks AH, Mullaney TP *et al.* Bilateral renal dysplasia and hypoplasia in a foal with an imperforate anus. *Vet Rec.* 1988; **122**, 91–92.
37. Jones SL, Langer DL, Sterner-Kock A *et al.* Renal dysplasia and benign ureteropelvic polyps associated with hydronephrosis in a foal *JAVMA.* 1994; **204**, 1230–1234.

38. Zicker SC, Marty GD, Carlson GP *et al.* Bilateral renal dysplasia with nephron hypoplasia in a foal. *JAVMA.* 1990; **196**, 2001–2004.
39. Scott PC & Vasey J. Progressive polycystic renal disease in an aged horse. *Aust Vet J.* 1986; **63**, 92–93.
40. Bertone JJ, Traub-Dargatz JL, Fettmen MJ *et al.* Moniotoring the progression of renal failure in a horse with polycystic kidney disease: use of the reciprocal of serum creatinine concentration and sodium sulfanilate clearance half-time. *JAVMA.* 1987; **191**, 565–568.
41. Ramsay G, Rothwell TLW, Gibson KT *et al.* Polycystic kidneys in an adult horse. *Equine Vet J.* 1987; **19**, 243–244.
42. Houlton JEF, Wright IM, Matic S & Herrtage ME. Urinary incontinence in a Shire foal due to ureteral ectopia. *Equine Vet J.* 1987; **19**, 244–247.
43. Rantanen NW. Diseases of the kidneys. *Vet Clin N Am [Equine Pract.]* 1986, **2**, 89–103.
44. Harris P. Collection of urine. *Equine Vet J.* 1988; **20**, 86–88.
45. Behm RJ & Berg IE. Hematuria caused by renal medullary crest mecrosis in a horse. *Comp Cont Educ Pract Vet.* 1987; **9**, 698–703.
46. Morris CF, Robertson JF, Mann PS *et al.* Hemolytic uremic-like syndrome in two horses. *JAVMA.* 1987; **191**, 1453–1454.
47. Bernard WV, Williams D, Tuttle PA & Pierce S. Hematuria and leptospiruria in a foal. *JAVMA.* 1993; **203**, 276–278.
48. Juzwiak JS, Bain FT, Slone DE *et al.* Unilateral nephrectomy for treatment of chronic hematuria due to nephrolithiasis in a colt. *Can Vet J.* 1988; **29**, 931–933.
49. Schott HC, Hodgson DR & Bayly WM. Ureteral catheterization in the horse. *Equine Vet Educ.* 1990; **2**, 140–143.
50. Kohn CW & Strasser SL. 24 hour renal clearance and excretion of endogenous substances in the mare. *Am J Vet Res.* 1986; **47**, 1332–1337.
51. Kohn CW & Chew DJ. Laboratory diagnosis and characterization of renal disease in horses. *Vet Clin N Am [Equine Pract.]* 1987; **3**, 585–615.
52. Brewer BD. Renal conditions of the newborn and older foal. *Equine Vet Educ.* 1990; **2**, 127–129.
53. Brewer BD. Renal Disease. In: Koterba AM, Drummond WH & Kosch PC (eds) *Equine Clinical Neonatology.* Philadelphia: Lea and Febiger 1990; 447–458.
54. Finco PR & Groves C. Mechanism of renal excretion of creatine by the pony. *Am J Vet Res.* 1985; **46**, 1625–1628.
55. Koterba AM, Adams R, McClure J & Cudd T. Renal and urinary tract function and dysfunction in the neonatal foal. *Proc Am Ass Equine Pract.* 1985; **31**, 659–671.
56. Thurmon JC, Steffey EP, Zinkl JG *et al.* Xylazine causes transient dose-related hyperglycaemia and increased urine volumes in mares. *Am J Vet Res* 1984; **45**, 224–227.
57. Trim, CM, Hanson, RR. Effects of xylazine on renal function and plasma glucose in ponies. *Vet Rec. 1986;* **118**, 65–67.
58. Carlson GP, Rumbaugh GE & Harrold D. Physiologic alteration in the horse produced by food and water deprivation during periods of high environmental temperatures. *Am J Vet Res.* 1979; **40**, 982–985.
59. Rambaugh GE, Carlson GP & Harrold D. Urinary production in the healthy horse and in horses deprived of feed and water. *Am J Vet Res.* 1982; **43**, 753–758.
60. Edwards DJ, Brownlow MA & Hutchins DR. Indices of renal function, values in eight normal foals from birth to 56 days. *Aust Vet J.* 1990; **67**, 251–254.
61. Adams R, McClure JJ, Gossett KA, Evaluation of a technique for measurement of gamma glutamyl transpeptidase in equine urine. *Am J Vet Res.* 1985; **46**, 147–150.
62. Brobst DF, Carroll RJ & Bayly WM. Urinary enzyme concentrations in healthy horses. *Cornell Vet.* 1986; **76**, 299–305.
63. Bayly WM, Brobst DF, Elfers RS & Reed SM. Serum and urinary biochemistry and enzyme changes in ponies with acute renal failure. *Cornell Vet.* 1986; **76**, 306–316.
64. Richardson DW & Kohn CW. Uroperitoneum in the foal. *JAVMA.* 1983; **182**, 267–271.

65. Tennanet B, Bettleheim P & Kaneko JJ. Paradoxic hypercalcaemia and hypophosphataemia associated with chronic renal failure in horses. *JAVMA.* 1982; **180**, 630–633.
66. Elfers RS, Bayly WM, Brobst DF *et al.* Alterations in calcium, phosphorus and C-terminal parathyroid hormone levels in equine acute renal disease. *Cornell Vet.* 1986; **76**, 317–329.
67. Harrington DD & Page EH. Acute vitamin D_3 toxicosis in horses, case reports and experimental studies of the comparative toxicity of vitamins D_2 and D_3. *JAVMA.* 1983; **182**, 1358–1369.
68. Grossman BS, Brobst DF, Kramer JW *et al.* Urinary indices for differentiation of prerenal azotemia and renal azotemia in horses. *JAVMA.* 1982; **180**, 284–288.
69. Morris DD, Divers TJ & Whitlock RH. Renal clearance and fractional excretion of electrolytes over a 24-hour period. *Am J Vet Res.* 1984; **45**, 2431–2435.
70. Traver DS, Salem C, Coffman JR *et al.* Renal metabolism of endogenous substances in the horse, volumetric clearance ration methods. *J Equine Med Surg.* 1977; **1**, 378–382.
71. Clark LL, Argenzio RA & Roberts MC. Effect of meal feeding on plasma volume and urinary electrolyte clearance in ponies. *Am J Vet Res.* 1990; **51**, 571–576.
72. Kinslow P, Harris P, Gray J & Allen WR. Influence of the oestrus cycle on electrolyte excretion in the mare. *Equine Vet J.* 1995; **18**, 388–391.
73. King C. Practical use of urinary fractional excretion. *J Equine Vet Sci.* 1994; **14**, 464–468.
74. Brewer BD, Clement SF, Lotz WS & Gronwall R. Single injection inulin/PAH method for the determination of renal clearances in adult horses and ponies *J. Vet Pharmacol Therap.* 1988; **11**, 409–412.
75. Brewer BD, Clement SF, Lotz WS & Gronwall R. A comparison of inulin: para-aminohippuric acid and endogenous creatine clearance as measures of renal function in neonatal foals. *J Vet Int Med.* 1990; **4**, 301–305.
76. Knudson E. Renal clearance studies on the horse 1. Inulin: endogenous creatine and urea. *Acta Vet Scand.* 1959; **1**, 52–66.
77. Brobst DF, Bramwell K & Kramer JW. Sodium sulfanilate clearance as a method of determining renal function in the horse. *J Equine Med Surg.* 1978; **2**, 500–502.
78. Taylor FGR, Hillyer MH & Lowrey PA. The assessment of glomerular filtration rate in ponies and horses by sodium sulphanilate clearance. *Equine Vet Educ.* 1990; **2**, 137–139.
79. Walsh DM & Royal HD. Evaluation of a single injection of 99mTc-labelled diethylenetriaminepentacetic acid for measuring glomerular filtration rate in horses. *Am J Vet Res.* 1992; **53**, 776–780.
80. Hoffman KL, Wood AKW & McCarthy PH. Sonographic–anatomic correlation and imaging protocol for the kidneys of horses. *Am J Vet Res.* 1995; **56**, 1403–1411.
81. Rantanen NW. Renal ultrasound in the horse. *Equine Vet Educ.* 1990; **2**, 135–136.
82. Marr CM. Equine abdominal ultrasonography. In: Goddard PJ (ed.) *Veterinary Ultrasonography.* Wallingford: CAB International 1995; 185–206.
83. Bayly WM, Liggitt HD, Brobst DF *et al.* A reproducible means of studying acute renal failure in the horse. *Cornell Vet.* 1986; **76**, 287–298.
84. Divers TJ & Yeager AE. The value of ultrasonographic examination in the diagnosis and management of renal disease in horses. *Equine Vet Educ.* 1995; **7**, 334–341.
85. Kiper ML, Traub-Dargatz JL & Wrigley RH. Renal ultrasonography in horses. *Comp Cont Educ Pract. Vet.* 1990; **12**, 993–998.
86. Barratt-Boyes SM, Spensely MS, Nyland TG & Olander HJ. Ultrasound localisation and guidance for renal biopsy in the horse. *Vet Radiol.* 1991; **32**, 121–126.
87. Edwards DJ, Love DN, Raus J & Baggott JD. The nephrotoxic potential of neomycin in the horse. *Equine Vet J.* 1989; **21**, 206–210.
88. Riviere JE, Traver DS & Coppoc GL. Gentamycin toxic nephropathy in horses with disseminated bacterial infection. *JAVMA.* 1982; **180**, 648–651.
89. Sojka JE & Brown SA. Pharmacokinetic adjustment of gentamycin dosing in horses with sepsis. *JAVMA.* 1986; **189**, 784–789.
90. Sweeney RW, Divers TJ & Rossier Y. Disposition of gentamycin administered intravenously to horses with sepsis. *JAVMA.* 1992; **200**, 503–506.

91. Nordstrom L, Ringberg H, Cronberg S *et al.* (1990) Does administration of an aminoglycoside in a single daily dose affect its efficiacy and toxicity? *J Antimicrobial Chemotherapy*. 1990; **25**, 159–173.
92. Sweeney RW, Macdonald M, Hall *et al.* Kinetics of gentamycin elimination in two horses with acute renal failure. *Equine Vet J.* 1988; **20**, 182–184.
93. Andrews EJ. Oxalate nephropathy in a horse. *JAVMA*. 1971; **159**, 49–51.
94. Webb RF & Knight PR. Oxalate nephropathy in a horse. *Aust Vet J.* 1977; **53**, 554–555.
95. Gunson DE, Kowalczvk DF, Shoop CR & Ramberg CF. Environmental zinc and cadmium pollution associated with generalized osteochondrosis, osteoporosis and nephrocalcinosis in horses. *JAVMA*. 1982; **180**, 295–299.
96. Markel MD, Dyer RM & Hattel AL. Acute renal failure associated with application of a mercuric blister in a horse. JAVMA. 1984; 185, 92–94.
97. Schuh JCL, Ross C & Meschter C. Concurrent mercuric blister and dimethyl sulphoxide (DMSO) application as a cause of mercury toxicity in two horses. *Equine Vet J.* **20**, 68–71.
98. Rebhun WC, Tennant BC, Dill SG & King JM. Vitamin K_3-induced renal toxicosis in the horse. *JAVMA*. 1984; **184**, 1237–1239.
99. Maxie G, van Dreumel T & McMaster D. Methadione (vitamin K_3) toxicity in six horses. *Can Vet J.* 1992; **22**, 756–757.
100. Anderson GA, Mount ME, Virins AA & Ziemer EL. Fatal acorn poisoning in a horse, pathologic findings and diagnostic considerations. *JAVMA*. 1983; **182**, 1105–1110.
101. Olsen CT, Keller WC, Gerken DF & Reed SM. Suspected tremetol poisoning in horses. *JAVMA*. 1984; **185**, 1001–1003.
102. Angsubhakorn S, Poomvises P, Romruen K & Newberne PM. Aflatoxicosis in horses. *JAVMA*. 1981; **178**, 274–278.
103. Schmitz DG. Canthardin toxicosis in horses. *J Vet Int Med.* 1992; **3**, 208–215.
104. MacLachlan NJ & Divers TJ. Hemolytic anemia and fibrinoid change of renal vessels in a horse. *JAVMA*. 1982; **181**, 716–717.
105. Snow DH, Bogan JA, Douglas TA & Thompson H. Phenylbutazone toxicity in ponies. *Vet Rec.* 1979; **105**, 26–30.
106. Snow DH, Douglas TA, Thompson H *et al.* Phenylbutazone toxicosis in equidae, a biochemical and pathophysiologic study. *Am J Vet Res.* 1981; **42**, 1754–1759.
107. Read WK. Renal medullary crest necrosis associated with phenylbutazone therapy in horses. *Vet Pathol.* 1983; **20**, 662–669.
108. Nordstoga K. Spontaneous bilateral renal cortical necrosis in animals. *Path Vet.* 1967; **4**, 233–244.
109. Divers TJ. Chronic renal failure. In: Smith BP (ed.) *Large Animal Internal Medicine*, 2nd edn. St. Louis: Mosby 1996; 958–962.
110. Vaala WE, Johnson JK Marr CM & Orsini JA. Intensive care. In: Higgins AJ & Wright IM (eds) *The Equine Manual.* London: WB Saunders 1995; 725–796.
111. McCausland IP & Milestone BA. Diffuse mesangioproliferative glomerulonephritis in a horse. *NZ Vet J.* 1976; 24, 239–241.
112. Buntain B & Greig WA. Chronic nephritis in a pony. *Vet Rec.* 1979; **104**, 307–309.
113. Mair TS. Crystalline composition of equine urinary calculi. *Res Vet Sci.* 1986; **40**, 288–291.
114. Divers TJ. Nephrolithasis and ureterolithiasis in horses and their association with renal disease and failure. *Equine Vet J.* 1989; **21**, 161–162.
115. Van den Hoven R & Franken P. Clinical aspects of lymphosarcoma in the horse: a clinical report of 16 cases. *Equine Vet J.* 1983; **15**, 49–53.
116. Mair TS & Hillyer MH. Clinical features of lymphosarcoma in the horse, 77 cases. *Equine Vet Educ.* 1991; **4**, 108–113.
117. Ziemer EL, Parker HR, Carlson GP & Smith BP. Clinical features and treatment of renal tubular acidosis in two horse. *JAVMA*. 1987; **190,** 294–296.
118. Ziemer EL, Parker HR Carlson GP *et al.* Renal tubular acidosis in two horses, diagnostic studies. *JAVMA*. 1987; **190**, 289–293.

119. Trotter GW, Miller D, Parks A & Arden W. Type II renal tubular acidosis in an mare. *JAVMA*. 1986; **188**, 1050–1051.
120. Coe FL & Kathpalia S. Hereditary tubular disorders. In: Wilson JD, Braunwald E, Isselbacher KJ, Petersdorf RG, Martin JB, Fauci AS & Root RK (eds). *Harrison's Principles of Internal Medicine*, 12 edn. New York: McGraw-Hill, Inc. 1991; 1196–1202.

10

Endotoxaemia

James N Moore and Michelle H Barton

Key Points

- Endotoxin is the toxic lipolysaccharide component of the outer cell envelope of enteric Gram-negative bacteria.
- Circulating levels of endotoxin are normally kept low by an effective mucosal barrier and elimination by fixed macrophage and circulating antibodies.
- Endotoxaemia is a consequence of certain diseases of the gastrointestinal tract, Gram-negative bacterial infections, and septicaemia of neonates.
- Clinical manifestations include abdominal pain, reduced gastrointestinal sounds, alterations in circulatory status, tachycardia and tachpnoea, dehydration, and increased mortality.
- The deleterious effects of endotoxin are effected by pro-inflammatory mediators, principally eicosanoids, platelet activating factor, tumour necrosis factor, interleukins and tissue factor.
- Targets for therapy include the prevention of transmural movement of endotoxin, neutralization of endotoxin before it interacts with inflammatory cells, prevention of endotoxin-induced cellular activation, and prevention of the synthesis, release and action of inflammatory mediators.
- Recognition of patients with, or at risk of, endotoxaemia is essential for effective therapy and reduction of mortality.

Introduction

Over the past two decades, there have been numerous studies dealing with various aspects of endotoxaemia in horses. The basis for the initial studies was the fact that the effects of endotoxin in laboratory animal species were very similar to clinical findings noted in horses with naturally occurring diseases characterized by acute abdominal pain (colic). The subsequent studies have included evaluation of the effects of administration of widely divergent amounts of endotoxin in horses and ponies, determination of plasma concentrations of endotoxin in horses clinical diseases characterized by clinical evidence of endotoxaemia, investigation of specific interactions between endotoxin and equine cells *in vitro*, and assessment of the efficacy of individual treatment regimens.

As a result of these studies, endotoxaemia now is firmly associated with diseases involving the gastrointestinal system, Gram-negative bacterial infections, and septicaemia in equine neonates. Endotoxaemia has also been implicated in the pathogenesis of laminitis, although this has been questioned by the results of clinical and experimental studies (see Chapter 1). The aim of this chapter is to review the basic nature of endotoxin, discuss methods used to detect endotoxin in circulation, and highlight the most clinically relevant information from existing studies of endotoxaemia in horses.

Endotoxin: Structure, Source and the Intestinal Mucosal Barrier

Endotoxin is the toxic lipopolysaccharide component of the outer cell envelope of enteric Gram-negative bacteria. Endotoxin is comprised of three parts: a variable outer polysaccharide component, termed the 'O-antigenic' region, a unique core region consisting primarily of monosaccharides, and a fatty acid-rich portion known as 'lipid A'. Strains of Gram-negative bacteria containing all three portions of endotoxin are termed smooth strains. In contrast, strains lacking the O-antigenic portion are termed rough. Based on numerous studies using purified portions of endotoxin from these strains of bacteria, most of the toxic properties of endotoxin have been linked to the lipid A moiety [1–3].

The horse's intestinal tract normally harbours extremely large numbers of Gram-negative bacteria. Because endotoxins are released from the cell membrane when these bacteria die or multiply rapidly, the intestinal lumen normally contains a large amount of endotoxin. These endotoxins are restricted to the intestinal lumen by an extremely complex and efficient mucosal barrier (Table 1) [2]. This barrier is composed of the mucosal epithelial cells and their tight junctions, enzymes and antibodies secreted by these cells and the adjacent resident bacteria. Endotoxins that manage to traverse this barrier are either bound to high density lipoproteins in plasma, neutralized by circulating antibodies or cleared from the circulation by fixed marcophages in the liver.

Table 1. **Mucosal barrier to endotoxin in health and disease**

Components of mucosal barrier function
• epithelial cells and tight junction
• secreted enzymes and antibodies
• adjacent resident bacteria
Factors that reduce barrier function
• intestinal inflammation
• restriction of intestinal blood flow
• overwhelming Gram-negative infection

***Table 2.* Conditions associated with clinical signs of endotoxaemia**

- Intestinal strangulation and obstruction
- Carbohydrate overload
- Colitis
- Proximal enteritis
- Septicemia in neonates

The situation changes markedly if the intestinal wall is inflamed or blood flow to the bowel is restricted. The results of several morphological studies have documented sloughing of the mucosal epithelial cells after relatively short periods of intestinal ischaemia. Under such circumstances, the efficiency of the mucosal barrier is greatly reduced and the amount of endotoxin entering the portal circulation exceeds the liver's ability to remove it. Endotoxin also moves across the damaged intestinal wall and into the peritoneal cavity, from which it enters the systemic circulation via the peritoneal lymphatics. Clinical conditions commonly associated with clinical signs of endotoxaemia in horses are listed in Table 2 [3–6].

Detection of Endotoxin in Plasma

Nearly 40 years ago, it was discovered that minute quantities of endotoxin resulted in death of the horseshoe crab, *Limulus polyphemus*, by widespread thrombosis [7]. Subsequent studies revealed that this was due to profound stimulation of coagulation enzymes located in the crab's multi-functional circulating amoebocytes. These findings led to the development of a highly sensitive assay for the detection of endotoxin in fluids, namely the *Limulus* amoebocyte lysate assay [8]. Initially, the end-point of this assay was the formulation of a gel, and the detection limit for endotoxin was approximately 100 pg/ml. The results of early studies indicated that plasma contains certain substances that interfere with the detection of endotoxin. Consequently, methods were developed to reduce the concentration and effect of these substances. This was achieved primarily by diluting the plasma sample with endotoxin-free water and heating [9]. Subsequently, the effects of endotoxin on the coagulation enzymes of the horseshoe crab were linked to a substrate containing a chromophore, allowing the development of a chromogenic assay for detection of endotoxin. Finally, techniques have improved that allow the production of syringes and collection tubes containing heparin that are endotoxin-free. These latter improvements have increased the reliability and importance of data regarding the detection of endotoxin in blood from patients suspected of having diseases associated with endotoxaemia.

There have been several clinical studies performed in horses in which the *Limulus* amoebocyte lysate assay was used to determine the prevalence of endotoxaemia. Although differences in sample handling techniques and the detection limits of the assay make it difficult to compare plasma concentrations of endotoxin among the studies, the overall results suggest that 35–45% of horses presented to veterinary schools with gastrointestinal disease are endotoxaemic [4, 5, 10–12].

Clinical Effects of Endotoxaemia

Endotoxaemia may increase the likelihood that a horse with gastrointestinal disease will be acutely painful, as often occurs when horses have intestinal strangulation obstructions or acute colitis. Alternatively, endotoxaemia may cause the horse to exhibit clinical signs indicative of mild or moderate abdominal pain (i.e., pawing, looking at the flank region, stretching out, lying down) or appear depressed. Presumably, these effects are due to the synthesis and release of proinflammatory substances that reduce the threshold for painful stimuli and alter intestinal blood flow [6]. Some of the more common findings on physical examination of endotoxaemic horses include hyperaemic mucous membranes, alterations in capillary refill time, decreased gastrointestinal sounds, increased heart and respiratory rates, and evidence of dehydration (Table 3). If the horse has ischaemic intestine, the onset of circulatory shock may be rapid and the ischaemic intestine must be removed surgically as rapidly as possible. Because the adverse effects of endotoxaemia are not restricted to the ischaemic portion of intestine, the mucosal barrier function of the 'normal' intestine may be impaired. Thus, horses with ischaemic intestine may exhibit clinical signs of endotoxaemia for several days after the ischaemic intestine has been removed. Similarly, transmural movement of endotoxin across the inflamed intestinal wall may persist for several days in horses with enteritis or colitis.

Table 3. **Clinical effects of endotoxin**

- Depression
- Mild–moderate abdominal pain
- Decreased gastrointestinal sounds
- Dehydration
- Hyperaemic mucus membranes
- Altered capillary refill time
- Increased heart and respiratory rates

Interaction of Endotoxin with Plasma Proteins and Inflammatory Cells

Once endotoxin enters the circulation, it may interact with plasma components, circulating blood cells or be removed by tissue-fixed macrophages in the liver, spleen and pulmonary vasculature. There is a considerable amount of information indicating that the hydrophobic nature of endotoxin causes it to enter the blood stream in aggregates. These aggregates then disperse, allowing endotoxin to interact with high density lipoproteins and a unique plasma protein named lipopolysaccharide binding protein [13, 14]. The binding of endotoxin with high density lipoproteins prolongs the half-life of endotoxin in circulation, but reduces its ability to interact with pro-inflammatory cells [15].

In contrast, binding of endotoxin with lipopolysaccharide binding protein markedly enhances its ability to interact with the cells. Lipopolysaccharide binding protein is a small, 60-kDa glycoprotein synthesized by the liver [13]. This protein normally exists in trace amounts in plasma ($<0.5\ \mu g/mL$), but its concentration may increase by 100-fold in response to stimuli that initiate the acute phase response. Lipopolysaccharide binding protein interacts strongly with the lipid A portion of endotoxin, an effect that is heat sensitive. Thus, serum samples heated to 56°C lose more than 70% of their ability to bind endotoxin, suggesting that lipopolysaccharide binding protein may account for some of the inhibitory properties of undiluted plasma in the *Limulus* amoebocyte lysate assay.

Lipopolysaccharide binding protein binds with endotoxin from a wide variety of Gram-negative bacteria. In plasma the association between lipopolysaccharide binding protein and endotoxin is transient, with some of the endotoxin being transferred to lipoproteins or mononuclear phagocytes. The protein has a unique and clinically important effect of substantially increasing the sensitivity of mononuclear phagocytes to endotoxin. The combination of endotoxin with lipopolysaccharide binding protein markedly increases the sensitivity of these cells to endotoxin when compared with the effect of incubation of the cells with endotoxin in serum-free media.

In the past decade a substantial body of evidence has indicated that most of the early deleterious effects of endotoxaemia are mediated by inflammatory mediators synthesized and released by mononuclear phagocytes (monocytes and macrophages) [6]. Thus, it is vitally important to recognize that, in addition to binding to endotoxin, lipopolysaccharide binding protein also binds avidly to a cell surface antigen on mononuclear phagocytes termed CD14 [14]. In doing so, lipopolysaccharide binding protein markedly accelerates the rate of binding of endotoxin to these cells and promotes cellular activation. This interaction between endotoxin, lipopolysaccharide binding protein and CD14 increases the sensitivity of these cells to endotoxin, and results in the synthesis of pro-inflammatory mediators. This latter effect of endotoxin can be inhibited by pre-incubation of the cells with monoclonal antibodies directed against CD14 or by enzymatically removing CD14 from the surface of the cells [13]. These results suggest a central and important role of CD14 in the cellular response to endotoxin. Furthermore, there is evidence that endotoxin and lipopolysaccharide binding protein may interact with a soluble form of CD14 that has been released from the surface of mononuclear phagocytes. Through these interactions, the endotoxin-soluble CD14 complex may interact with cells lacking CD14 and otherwise unable to respond to endotoxin. The importance of soluble CD14 during endotoxaemia remains to be elucidated [16].

Proinflammatory Mediators during Endotoxaemia

Based largely on the results of studies with monocytes and macrophages from a variety of species, including the horse, it has been shown that binding of endotoxin to CD14 via lipopolysaccharide binding protein mobilizes intracellular messengers. These messengers in turn interact with the nucleus to induce genes encoding pro-inflammatory substances. Although there is a considerable amount of debate about which cellular signalling systems are involved, there is agreement for the time being that many of the deleterious effects of endotoxin are mediated by cytokines and proinflammatory substances synthesized and released by the mononuclear phagocytes. These cells generate many of the inflammatory mediators that have been detected in the circulation of horses administered endotoxin under experimental conditions and in horses with naturally occurring gastrointestinal disease [6, 17–19]. The most widely studied of these mediators include the eicosanoids (arachidonic acid metabolites), platelet activating factor, tumour necrosis factor, the interleukins, and tissue factor.

Eicosanoids

Arachidonic acid is a 20-carbon fatty acid in cell membrane phospholipids. Arachidonic acid is released by the enzyme phospholipase A2 and then metabolized by cyclooxygenase or lipoxygenase. Based largely on the availability of sensitive radioimmunoassays which detect the metabolites of the cyclooxygenase-derived products and the stability of these metabolites in plasma, more information is available about cyclooxygenase-derived metabolites of arachidonic acid in horses than lipoxygenase-derived metabolites. The most widely studied cyclooxygenase-derived metabolites include thromboxane A2, prostaglandin I2, prostaglandin E2, and prostaglandin F2α.

The cyclooxygenase-derived metabolites of arachidonic acid are best known for their vasoactive properties. Thromboxane A2 and prostaglandin F2α cause vasoconstriction by decreasing cAMP concentrations in vascular smooth muscle cells, whereas prostaglandins I2 and E2 cause vasodilation by increasing cAMP. Many of the early haemodynamic effects of endotoxaemia are mediated by these cyclooxygenase-derived metabolites of arachidonic acid [3]. Specifically, the dyspnoea, hypoxaemia, and pulmonary hypertension that occur within minutes of endotoxin administration in horses are closely correlated with substantial increases in plasma concentrations of the stable metabolite of thromboxane A2. These findings corroborate the vasoconstrictive and bronchoconstrictive effects of thromboxane A2 reported in other species. Plasma concentrations of the stable metabolite of prostaglandin I2 subsequently increase, reaching peak values approximately 90 minutes after administration of endotoxin [3, 6]. Plasma concentrations of this eicosanoid are associated with discoloration of the horse's mucous membranes, prolongation of the capillary refill time and the onset of hypotension.

In contrast to the wealth of knowledge concerning the cyclooxygenase-derived metabolites of arachidonic acid, considerably less is known about the lipoxygenase-derived metabolites in endotoxaemic horses. Some of these metabolites, most notably leukotriene B4, are potent chemoattractant agents and cause vasoconstrition. The complex metabolic pathways involved in metabolism of arachidonic acid by lipoxygenase enzymes, the extremely short plasma half-lives of the products and difficulties with assays for their detection have thwarted efforts to study the role of lipoxygenase-derived products in horses [6].

Platelet Activating Factor, Tumour Necrosis Factor, and Tissue Factor

A similar situation exists regarding the involvement of platelet activating factor in equine endotoxaemia. This lipid-derived mediator of inflammation was originally named because of its effect as a stimulator of platelet aggregation. Platelet activating factor is synthesized and released by a variety of cells in response to various stimuli, including endotoxin and tumour necrosis factor. In addition to its effects on platelets, platelet activating factor increases vascular permeability, and causes bronchoconstriction, hypotension, neutropaenia and haemoconcentration. The precise role of platelet activating factor in endotoxaemia remains undetermined, as pretreatment of horses with a potent platelet activating factor receptor antagonist delayed, but did not prevent, many of the deleterious effects of endotoxin [20].

Tumour necrosis factor is a 17 kDa polypeptide cytokine that is synthesized by mononuclear phagocytes exposed to endotoxin and other proinflammatory stimuli [21, 22]. Synthesis of tumour necrosis factor is increased after the endotoxin–lipopolysaccharide binding protein complex binds to CD14 on the cell surface. Serum concentrations of this cytokine increase shortly thereafter *in vivo* and administration of recombinant tumour necrosis factor intiates a cascade of responses indistinguishable from those caused by endotoxin [23, 24]. These responses include hypotension, haemoconcentration, metabolic acidosis, and disseminated intravascular coagulation. The central role of tumour necrosis factor in the pathogenesis of endotoxaemia is substantiated by the fact that exposure to tumour necrosis factor stimulates the synthesis of other inflammatory mediators (including the interleukins, eicosanoids, and tissue factor), the acute phase response and fever [23, 24]. Administration of anti-tumour necrosis factor antibodies also significantly increases the survival rate of animals subjected to either endotoxic or septic shock, thereby exemplifying the pivotal role this cytokine plays in these complex syndromes.

Tissue factor ('procoagulant activity' or thromboplastin) is a glycoprotein synthesized by monocytes, macrophages and to a lesser degree by endothelial cells in response to endotoxin. Greater than 85% of the tissue factor synthesized by these cells remains on their surface and thus comes in contact with coagulation factor VII in plasma. As a result of this interaction, the extrinsic arm of the coagulation cascade is stimulated and recalcification time of whole blood is shortened. Consequently, this test is used as an indirect measure of tissue factor activity or the cells can be lysed and cellular lysates used directly to test their ability to shorten the recalcification time of pooled plasma. Using both of these assays, tissue factor activity has been shown to increase significantly in horses administered endotoxin and in horses with naturally occurring gastrointestinal disease [5, 25]. Furthermore, in the clinical study the magnitude of the increase in tissue factor activity correlated inversely with the animal's prognosis for survival.

Methods of Treatment

Endotoxaemia often provides the equine practioner with a difficult therapeutic challenge, due primarily to the horse's very rapid response to endotoxin and the effects of such a diverse array of mediators. Information gleaned from studies about the development of endotoxaemia, interactions between endotoxin and the host's inflammatory cells, and the synthesis and release of the various mediators suggests that there are four primary therapeutic targets: (1) prevention of the transmural movement of endotoxin; (2) neutralization of endotoxin before it interacts with CD14 on the inflammatory cells; (3) prevention of endotoxin-induced cellular activation; and (4) prevention of the synthesis, release or action of the inflammatory mediators (Table 4).

Prevention of Transmural Movement of Endotoxin

The first goal for treating endotoxaemia in horses is to decrease the translocation of endotoxin into the circulation by identifying the underlying disease process. Although it may not be possible to prevent the occurence of endotoxaemia in horses with intestinal ischaemia or inflammatory intestinal diseases, all efforts should be expended to identify the underlying condition and initiate appropriate therapy as soon as possible. For horses with intestinal ischaemia, this means making the decision for surgery early and removing the affected intestine.

***Table 4.* Primary therapeutic targets for horses with, or at risk from, endotoxaemia**

- Prevention of the transmural movement of endotoxin
- Neutralization of endotoxin before it interacts with inflammatory cells
- Prevention of endotoxin-induced cellular activation
- Prevention of the synthesis, release or action of inflammatory mediators
- Maintenance of circulatory function, prevention of metabolic acidosis and electrolyte abnormalities

Neutralization of endotoxin

The veterinarian must decide rapidly if attempts will be made to neutralize endotoxin before it activates the horse's inflammatory cells. This can be accomplished with antibodies directed against either the core region of endotoxin, lipid A, or the O-antigenic chains [26–34]. Appropriately administered antibodies may enhance opsonization of intact bacteria, removal of endotoxin from the blood, and interfere with the interaction of endotoxin with the inflammatory cells [32, 33]. Because the core and lipid A regions are well conserved among Gram-negative bacteria, antibodies against these regions are usually utilized in clinical situations.

Commercially available antiendotoxin antibodies are harvested from horses vaccinated against the exposed core regions of rough strains of J5 *Escherichia coli* or a Re *Salmonella* mutant. These antibodies have been used in several clinical and experimental trials, often with conflicting results. In some studies, treatment of horses with plasma or serum containing antiendotoxin antibodies resulted in reduced mortality and fewer days of hospitalization, when compared with horses that did not receive antibodies or received plasma from non-vaccinated horses [27–29]. In contrast, the effects of antiendotoxin antibodies in other studies have been equivocal [26, 30, 31, 33]. There are several potential reasons for these discrepancies, not the least of which is the timing of treatment. Because the interaction between endotoxin and the horse's inflammatory cells occurs rapidly, the antibodies may have been administered too late in some of the studies. It is also feasible that the anti-core antibodies are unable to penetrate the O-antigenic chains of intact smooth endotoxin to neutralize the core region [33]. Finally, the failure of the antiendotoxin antibodies to produce beneficial effects in clinical situations may reflect the inability of the host's compromised inflammatory systems to opsonize or phagocytose bacteria [32]. From our perspective, the concerns about this form of treatment can be addressed only by additional controlled clinical trials in which antiendotoxin antibodies or nonspecific immunoglobulins are administered to horses very early in the course of the disease.

An alternative immunological approach to endotoxaemia is through active immunization of horses with vaccines against the core region of mutant Gram-negative bacteria. This approach has been tried and has provided some, but not complete, protection against subsequent challenge with endotoxin [29]. These vaccines are now commercially available, however, questions remain concerning the degree of protection afforded against naturally occurring diseases associated with endotoxaemia and the duration of the antibody response.

Rather than use antibodies directed against endotoxin, other investigators have used drugs that avidly bind endotoxin and thus prevent it from interacting with the inflammatory cells. One of these drugs is polymixin B, an antibiotic that forms an extremely stable complex with lipid A. The clinical usefulness of this approach is limited, however, by polymixin B's inherent toxicity. Although pretreatment of horses with polymixin B (2.5 mg/kg BW) did not alter the development of shock, acidosis, and lameness in a carbohydrate overload model of acute laminitis [35], the results have been more promising in a less severe model of endotoxaemia in foals. In that study, pretreatment with polymixin B (6000 u/kg BW) ameliorated clinical signs, prevented leucopaenia, and resulted in significantly lower serum concentrations of tumour necrosis factor and interleukin-6-activity, when compared with values for foals not receiving polymixin B and foals receiving J5 hyperimmune serum (1.5 mL/kg BW [36]. Additional studies are underway with less toxic pharmaceuticals [37].

Prevention of Endotoxin-induced Cellular Activation

The third therapeutic target is to prevent or interfere with cellular activation by endotoxin. This form of therapy has tremendous potential for producing beneficial effects in the clinical arena. Not only would it potentially protect animals that are developing endotoxaemia, it could inhibit the synthesis and release of inflammatory mediators by cells that have interacted with endotoxin. This method of treatment for endotoxaemia remains a goal of researchers in this area, as the precise mechanisms by which endotoxin activates the inflammatory cells have not been identified.

Prevention of Synthesis, Release or Action of Inflammatory Mediators

Once the horse's inflammatory cells have interacted with endotoxin and become activated, the therapeutic aim must be to prevent or reduce the synthesis, release or effect of the inflammatory mediators (Table 5). Numerous studies have been performed to evaluate various types of treatments for endotoxaemia in horses. These include administration of non-steroidal anti-inflammatory drugs, corticosteroids, monoclonal antibodies directed against cytokines, platelet activating factor receptor antagonists, methylxanthine derivatives, and omega-3 polyunsaturated fatty acids [38–48].

Non-steroidal anti-inflammatory drugs have been used in the treatment of endotoxaemia in horses for more than 15 years. The results of several experimental studies and clinical experience indicate that the most efficacious of these

***Table 5.* Potential strategies for preventing the synthesis, release or activation of inflammatory mediators**

- Non-steroidal anti-inflammatory agents, e.g. flunixin meglumine, ketoprofen
- Monoclonal antibodies to equine tumour necrosis factor
- Platelet activating factor receptor antagonists
- Methylxanthine derivatives, e.g. pentoxifylline
- Omega-3 polyunsaturated fatty acids, e.g. linseed oil, marine fish oil

drugs in this regard is flunixin meglumine. When compared with phenylbutazone, dipyrone, or ibuprofen, flunixin meglumine (1.1 mg/kg BW) was most effective at preventing endotoxin-induced synthesis of prostaglandins and thromboxane and the clinical signs of endotoxaemia [48]. Furthermore, administration of flunixin meglumine (0.25 mg/kg BW) more effectively prevented synthesis of prostaglandins and thromboxane than phenylbutazone (2 mg/kg BW) [48]. Purported advantages associated with the lower dose of flunixin meglumine include reduced risk of toxic side effects associated with non-steroidal anti-inflammatory drugs (gastrointestinal ulceration and renal papillary necrosis) and effective inhibition of prostaglandin and thromboxane synthesis without completely masking clinical signs of endotoxaemia. Consequently, many veterinary clinicians prefer to administer flunixin meglumine at 0.25 mg/kg BW, IV, q8h to endotoxaemic horses.

One of the potential adverse effects of cyclooxygenase inhibition is the redirection of arachidonic acid metabolism to the lipoxygenase pathway, with the subsequent synthesis of the pro-inflammatory leukotrienes. In the past few years, a purported inhibitor of both cyclooxygenase and lipoxygenase, ketoprofen, has become available for use in horses. In an experimental study of endotoxaemia in horses ketoprofen (0.5 mg/kg BW) and flunixin meglumine (0.25 mg/kg BW) were equally effective in preventing the measured responses to endotoxin [41]. We are not aware of any studies defining the effect of ketoprofen on leukotriene synthesis in horses or the effects of cyclooxygenase inhibition on leukotriene synthesis in horses.

Rather than prevent the synthesis of a particular mediator, it is also possible to prevent the mediator from interacting with its own receptor on target cells. This approach has been utilized recently with monoclonal antibodies directed against tumour necrosis factor and with specific receptor antagonist for platelet activating factor. Miniature ponies were pretreated with monoclonal antibodies against equine tumour necrosis factor (2 mg/kg BW) and then challenged with endotoxin. Pretreatment with the antibodies reduced the severity of the clinical signs of endotoxaemia, reduced endotoxin-induced systhesis of tumour necrosis factor, interleukin-6 and thromboxane B2, and prevented the development of leucopaenia and lactic acidosis [39]. Based on the fact that peak serum concentrations of tumour necrosis factor occur approximately 90 minutes after administration of endotoxin, this method of therapy may have limited clinical use in horses.

In the second set of studies, platelet activating factor receptor antagonists were evaluated during endotoxaemia. In these studies these receptor antagonists reduced endotoxin-induced ileus, fever, leucopaenia, tachycardia, and lactic acidaemia [20, 42]. In an experimental study, a platelet activating factor antagonist reduced the degree of leucopaenia and thrombocytopaenia associated with colonic ischaemia-reperfusion, but had no effects on the effects on the cardiovascular system and actually exacerbated the development of metabolic acidosis [40]. These drugs are not available for clinical use.

Despite the documented complexity of endotoxaemia, most studies performed to date to evaluate the efficacy of treatment modalities have been directed towards a single type of mediator. Consequently, it is not surprising that many of the treatments have failed to some degree or another. Because many of the pathophysiological effects of endotoxin are ultimately associated with alterations in intracellular messengers, it seems logical that therapy directed towards these messengers might affect more than one type of mediator. Pentoxifylline is a methylxanthine derivative used in humans as a rheological agent for the treatment of intermittent claudication. Pentoxifylline's mechanism of action has been associated with inhibition of phosphodiesterase and subsequent increased intracellular concentrations of cAMP. Presumably through its effects on cAMP concentrations, pentoxifylline inhibits endotoxin-induced cytokine, thromboxane, and thromboplastin production [47]. Studies are now underway to evaluate pentoxifylline in experimentally induced endotoxaemia in horses.

A novel approach to modulate the host's response to endotoxin has been by altering the fatty acid composition of the host's inflammatory cell membranes, thereby reducing the synthesis of the mediators of endotoxaemia. This has been achieved by increasing the proportion of omega-3 fatty acids, such as eicosapentaenoic acid and its parent molecule alpha-linolenic acid, in the animal's diet [44–46]. Eicosapentaenoic acid then becomes incorporated into cell membrane phospholipids, replacing arachidonic acid to some extent. Such alterations in the fatty acid composition of the cell membrane modify certain cellular functions, including phagocytosis, receptor binding, and the actions of membrane bound enzymes. Additionally, when the omega-3 fatty acids are metabolized by cyclooxygenase and lipoxygenase, the end-products have markedly different effects from the metabolities of arachidonic acid. Specifically, rather than cause vascoconstriction and platelet aggregation like thromboxane A2, the cyclooxygenase-derived metabolite of eicosapentaenoic acid, thromboxane A3, produces vasodilation and inhibits platelet aggregation. Similarly, the lipoxygenase derived metabolites of the omega-3 fatty acids induce less pronounced proinflammatory responses than the leukotrienes derived from arachidonic acid.

To evaluate the potential positive effects of omega-3 fatty acids in horses, a ration enriched with 8% linseed oil, as a source of alpha-linolenic acid, was fed to horses. Monocytes were then isolated from these horses and incubated with endotoxin. Ingestion of the omega-3 fatty acid enriched diet reduced endotoxin-induced synthesis of thromboxane B2 and expression of tissue factor by 71% and 51%, respectively, when compared with values for monocytes from horses fed a control ration [44]. Furthermore, peritoneal macrophages obtained from the horses consuming the omega-3 fatty acid enriched ration produced significantly less tumour necrosis factor activity upon exposure to endotoxin than did macrophages from control horses [46]. Although the results of these *in vitro* studies were very encouraging, clinical signs of endotoxaemia for horses fed the omega-3 fatty acid enriched ration were not different from those exhibited by horses fed the control ration [45].

A cornerstone in the treatment of endotoxaemic horses is the administration of isotonic polyionic fluids, with special attention being paid to addressing metabolic acidosis and any electrolyte abnormalities. In certain situations, small volumes (4 mL/kg BW) of hypertonic (7%) saline solution may be used to rapidly increase the circulating volume and improve tissue perfusion [49]. This form of treatment must be used with caution in horses with electrolyte abnormalities and total body fluid deficitis must be replaced with isotonic fluids. Tissue perfusion can also be improved with vasoactive compounds. The results of studies performed in anaesthetized horses suggest that administration of dopamine at a dose rate of 2.5 μg/kg BW.min will increase cardiac output and blood pressure during endotoxaemia [50].

References

1. Moore JN, Garner HE & Shapland JE. Equine endotoxemia: an insight into cause and treatment. *J Am Vet Med Assoc.* 1981; **179**, 573–576.
2. Moore JN. Endotoxemia: Definition, characterization, and host defences. *Compend Cont Educ.* 1981; **3**, 355–359.
3. Moore JN & Morris DD. Endotoxemia and sepsis in horses, Experimental and clinical correlates. *J Am Vet Med Assoc.* 1992; **200**, 1903–1914.
4. King J & Gerring E. Detection of endotoxin in cases of equine colic. *Vet Rec.* 1988; **123**, 269–271.
5. Henry M & Moore J. Endotoxin-induced procoagulant activity in equine peripheral blood monocytes. *Circ Shock.* 1988; **26**, 297–309.
6. Morris DD. Endotoxemia in horses. A review of cellular and humoral mediators involved in its pathogenesis. *J Vet Intern Med.* 1991; **5**, 167–181.
7. Bang FB. A bacterial disease of *Limulus polyphemus. Bull Johns Hopkins Hosp.* 1958; **98**, 325–351.
8. Levin J & Bang FB. A description of cellular coagulation in *Limulus. Bull Johns Hopkins Hosp.* 1964; **115**, 337–345.
9. Sturk A, Joop K, Cate JW & Thomas LL. Optimization of a chromogenic assay for endotoxin in blood. In, Cate JAW, Buller HR, Sturk A & Levin J (eds). *Bacterial Endotoxins. Structure, Biomedical Significance and Detection with the Limulus Amoebocyte Lysate Test.* New York: Alan R. Liss 1985; 117–136.
10. Meyers KM, Reed SM & Keck M. Circulating endotoxin-like substance(s) and altered hemostasis in horses with gastrointestinal disorders. *Am J Vet Res.* 1982; **43**, 2233–2235.
11. Fessler JF & Bottoms GD. Plasma endotoxin concentrations in experimental and clinical equine subjects. Equine subjects. *Equine Vet J.* 1989; **S7**, 24–28.
12. Steverink PJ, Salden JH, Sturk A *et al.* Laboratory and clinical evaluation of a chromogenic endotoxin assay for horses with acute intestinal disorders. *Vet Quart.* 1994; **16**; **S2**, 117–121.
13. Tobias PS & Ulevitch RJ. Lipopolysaccharide binding protein and CD14 in LPS dependent macrophage activation. *Immunobiol.* 1993; **187**, 227–232.
14. Ulevitch RJ, Mathison JC, Schumann RR & Tobias PS. A new model of macrophage stimulation by bacterial lipopolysaccharide. *J Trauma.* 1990; **30**, 189–192.
15. Ulevitch RJ, Johnston A & Weinstein DB. New function for high density lipoproteins. *J Clin Invest.* **67**, 1981; 827–837.

16. Wurfel M, Hailman E & Wright S. Soluble CD14 acts as a shuttle in the neutralization of lipopolysaccharide by LPS binding protein and reconstituted high density lipoprotein. *J Exp Med.* 1995; **181**, 1743–1754.
17. MacKay RJ, King RR, Dankert JR *et al.* Cytotoxic tumor necrosis factor activity produced by equine alveolar macrophages, preliminary characterization. *Vet Immunol Immunopath.* 1991; **29**, 15–30.
18. MacKay RJ & Lester GD. Induction of the acute phase cytokine, hepatocyte-stimulating factor/interleukin 6, in the circulation of horses treated with endotoxin. *Am J Vet Res.* 1992; **53**, 1285–1289.
19. Morris D, Moore J & Fischer J. Endotoxin-induced production of tumour necrosis factor activity by equine peritoneal macrophages. *Circ Shock.* 1990; **30**, 229–236.
20. Carrick JB, Morris DD & Moore JN. Administration of a receptor antagonist for platelet activating factor during equine endotoxemia. *Equine Vet J.* 1993; **25**, 152–157.
21. Beutler B & Cerami A. Cachectin: More than just a tumor necrosis factor. *New Eng J Med.* 1987; **316**, 379–385.
22. Michie HR, Manogue KR, Spriggs DR *et al.* Detection of circulating tumor necrosis factor after endotoxin administration. *N Eng J Med.* 1988; **318**, 1481–1486.
23. Tracey KJ, Beutler B, Lowry SF *et al.* Shock and tissue injury induced by recombinant human cachectin. *Science*, 1986; **234**, 470–474.
24. Turner CR, Esser KM, Wheeldon EB *et al.* Cardiovascular and pulmonary effects of human recombinant tumor necrosis factor in the conscious rat. *Circ Shcok.* 1989; **28**, 369–384.
25. Henry MM & Moore JN. Clinical relevance of monocyte procoagulant activity in horses with colic. *J Am Vet Med Assoc.* 1991; **198**, 843–848.
26. Divers T. The use of hyperimmune plasma against endotoxin in horses with colic. *Proceedings, New Perspectives on Equine Colic.* 1994.
27. Spier SJ, Lavoie JP, Cullor JS *et al.* Protection against clinical endotoxemia in horses by using plasma containing antibody to an Rc mutant of *E. coli* (J5). *Circ Shock.* 1989; **28**, 235–248.
28. Garner HE, Sprouse RF & Lager K. Cross protection of ponies from sublethal *Escherichia coli* endotoxemia by *Salmonella typhimurium* antiserum. *Equine Pract.* 1988; **10**, 10–17.
29. Sprouse RF, Garner HE & Lager K. Protection of ponies from heterologous and homologous endotoxin challenges via *Salmonella typhimurium* bacterin-toxoid. *Equine Pract.* 1989; **11**, 34–40.
30. Morris DD, Whitlock RH & Corbeil LB. Endotoxemia in horses, Protection provided by antiserum to core lipopolysaccharide. *Am J Vet Res.* 1986; **47**, 544–550.
31. Morris DD & Whitlock RH. Therapy of suspected septicemia in neonatal foals using plasma containing antibodies to core lipopolysaccharide. *J Vet Intern Med.* 1987; **1**, 175–182.
32. Tyler J, Cullor JS, Spier SJ *et al.* Immunity targeting common core antigens of Gram-negative bacteria. *J Vet Intern Med.* 1990; **4**, 17–25.
33. Morris DD. Antiendotoxin serum: Therapeutic rationale and clinical perspectives. *Comp Cont Ed Pract Vet.* 1989; **11**, 1096–1099.
34. Bonen Clark GD, MacKay RJ & Ward RE. Elicitation of anti-lipid A antibody response in horses inoculated with A4, a murine monoclonal anti-idiotypic antibody. *Proceedings, Fifth Equine Colic Research Symposium.* 1994; 15.
35. Raisbeck MF, Garner HE, Osweiler GD *et al.* Effects of polymixin B in selected features of equine carbohydrate overload. *Vet Hum Tox.* 1989; **31**, 422–426.
36. Durando MM & MacKay RJ. Evaluation of two potential treatments of equine endotoxemia. *Proceedings, 10th Annual ACVIM Forum.* 1992; 816.
37. Coyne CP, Fenwick BW & Cox J. Nonimmunologic neutralization of lipopolysaccharide from gram-negative bacteria. *Proceedings, 9th Annual ACVIM Forum, New Orleans, LA.* 1991; 876.
38. Semrad SD, Hardee GE, Hardee MM *et al.* Low-dose flunixin meglumine, Effects on eicosanoid production and clinical signs induced by experimental endotoxemia in horses. *Equine Vet J* 1987; **19**, 201–206.
39. Cargile J & MacKay R. Monoclonal antibodies to isolated serum equine tumor necrosis factor. *J Vet Intern Med.* 1993; **7**, 142.

40. Wilson DV, Stick JA & Eberhart SW. The use of a specific platelet activating factor antagonist in equine large colon torsion. *Proceedings, Fourth Equine Colic Research Symposium.* 1991; p. 34.
41. Merrit AM, MacKay RJ, Burrow JR *et al.* Anti-endotoxin effect of ketoprofen in horses. *Proceedings, Fourth Equine Colic Research Symposium.* 1991; 56.
42. King JN & Gerring EL. Antagonism of endotoxin induced disruption of equine gastro-intestinal motility with platelet activating factor antagonism. *J Vet Pharmacol Ther.* 1990; **13**, 333–339.
43. Lochner F, Sangiah S, Burrows G *et al.* Effects of allopurinal in experimental endotoxin shock in horses. *Res Vet Sci.* 1989; **47**, 178–184.
44. Henry MM, Moore JN, Feldman EB *et al.* The effect of dietary alpha linolenic acid on equine monocyte procoagulant activity and eicosanoid synthesis. *Circ Shock.* 1990; **32**, 173–188.
45. Henry MM, Moore JN & Fischer JK. Influence of an omega-3 fatty acid-enriched ration on *in vivo* response of horses to endotoxin. *Am J Vet Res.* 1991; **52**, 523–527.
46. Morris DD, Henry MM, Moore JN *et al.* Dietary alpha linolenic acid reduced endotoxin induced production of tumor necrosis factor activity by equine peritoneal macrophages. *Am J Vet Res.* 1991; **52**, 528–532.
47. Barton MH & Moore JN. Pentoxifylline inhibits mediators synthesis in an equine *in vitro* whole blood model of endotoxemia. *Circ Shock.* 1994; **44**, 216–220.
48. Semrad S. Update on endotoxemia. *Proceedings, 5th Annual ACVIM Forum.* 1987; 785–788.
49. Bertone J, Gossett KA, Shoemaker KE *et al.* Effect of hypertonic saline solution on response to sublethal *Escherichia coli* endotoxemia in horses. *Am J Vet Res.* 1990; **51**, 999–1007.
50. Trim CM, Moore JN, Hardee MM *et al.* Effects of infusion of dopamine on the cardiovascular effects of *Escherichia coli* endotoxin in anesthetized horses. *Res Vet Sci.* 1991; **50**, 54–63.

11

Fluid and Electrolyte Abnormalities: The Role of Exercise and Oral Fluids

Leopoldo A Sosa León and Reuben J Rose

Key Points

- A major threat to horses undertaking prolonged exercise, especially when performed under hot and humid environmental conditions, is dehydration and its potential adverse effects such as hyperthermia.
- The proper administration of oral fluid and electrolytes during exercise can help to avoid or minimize the deleterious effects of dehydration.
- The aim of fluid and electrolyte administration is to promote the maintenance of an adequate hydration status of the exercising horse so that it can perform at its best while also minimizing potential health risks such as heat stroke.
- The provision of fluid and electrolytes during exercise should be based on the fluid and electrolyte deficits that result from a given time of exercise.
- In general, the use of isotonic fluid containing Na, K and Cl is preferred as it is absorbed quickly without causing major plasma fluid and electrolyte alterations.
- Fluid can be administered at different stages of exercise; before, during or after the ride or a combination of these, taking into account the distance and environmental conditions during the ride.

Introduction

Many years of clinical experience and research have demonstrated that in biological systems, fluid and electrolyte balance are essential for all the basic events that sustain life. However, either as a consequence of pathological processes such as diarrhoea or as a physiological response to requirements for thermoregulation, such as may occur during prolonged exercise, horses often lose large amounts of fluid and electrolytes that require close clinical attention if health is to be maintained.

Equine clinicians have been well aware of the need for fluid and electrolyte treatment related to problems such as diarrhoea and severe colic, as the massive quantities of fluid required intravenously are a therapeutic challenge. More recently, there has been an increasing awareness of the potential problems for horse performance resulting from disturbances to fluid and electrolyte balance in the apparently 'normal' horse. This particularly applies to those horses involved in athletic endeavours such as racing, endurance riding and eventing. The importance of fluid and electrolyte disorders is acknowledged by many equine clinicians and riders, who give routine 'saline drenches' as part of their management of athletic horses. Unfortunately, the assistance given to the horses is mostly empirical as very little research has been done to evaluate the response to such treatment, which is seldom based on the reported fluid and electrolyte alterations associated with exercise and training.

This article will concentrate on disturbances to fluid and electrolyte balance that can arise from exercise, the management of these and the role of oral fluid and electrolyte administration. Our aims are to present fluid and electrolyte abnormalities caused by exercise as central to the problem of homeostasis, thermoregulation, exercise performance and health of the equine athlete. Also, we have tried to provide the necessary information for a rational approach to treatment. The acute major fluid and electrolyte disturbances, such as acute severe diarrhoea or duodenitis-proximal jejunitis, that compromise the circulatory status of the horse will not be considered as these are well covered in a number of other publications [1–4].

Anatomy of Body Fluid and Electrolytes – Rest

To understand the abnormalities that may be imposed by an external stimulus such as exercise, it is important to discern body fluid composition and distribution, as well as the mechanisms that govern the dynamics of solutes and water transport at rest. For ease of understanding, the traditional approach to fluid and electrolyte distribution has been based on different compartments [5, 6]. This compartmental concept was developed in the 1930s [6] and prevails as a useful model for analysis of fluid and electrolyte alterations. Although this model was initially developed for humans, it is known that the same principles that govern the compartmental distribution and dynamics of fluid and electrolytes in this species also hold true to many others and certainly to the horse.

The Fluids

Generally, two major body fluid compartments are recognized: the intracellular fluid (ICF) and the extracellular fluid (ECF). This distribution has arbitrarily been established as water shifts freely in and out of the cells [7]. Each fluid compartment, however, presents some anatomical boundaries and, more importantly, characteristic electrolyte patterns [5–8] that makes it useful to identify them separately.

The ICF is inside the cells and in contact with the ECF through the pores of the cell membrane. The ECF, on the other hand, is further subdivided into plasma volume (PV) and interstitial lymph fluid volume. The PV is contained in the cardiovascular space and is in close relationship and in equilibrium with the interstitial fluid at the capillary level [6, 9]. Other extracellular fluid (ECF) compartments have also been identified and grouped separately. They are: dense connective tissue, cartilage and bone water, and transcellular fluid. The last, according to Edelman and Liebman [5] describes a number of extracellular fluid collections that are not simply transudates and have the common property of being formed by the transport activity of cells. In the horse, the gastrointestinal fluid is the largest of the transcellular fluids and may be an important reservoir when fluid deficits occur [1]. However, the role of fluid absorption from the gastrointestinal tract during exercise has not been established and may not be available owing to diversion of blood flow from the gastrointestinal tract during exercise [10]. It may be that movement of fluid from the gastrointestinal tract to the effective circulating blood volume does occur during periods of rest in competitive situations such as endurance riding.

The relationship between the ECF and transcellular fluid of the gastrointestinal tract has been recognized by clinicians in the treatment of large intestinal impactions. Large volume intravenous fluid therapy results in softening of the impacted mass because of fluid movement into the gastrointestinal tract. The rest of the transcellular fluid (fluid contained in glands and some organs), athough in smaller quantities, can also support contractions of PV that occur in situations such as shock and dehydration caused by prolonged exercise [8].

Quantification of Body Fluid Compartments

The total body water (TBW) in the horse is about 60% of the bodyweight [11] from which two-thirds is in the ICF and one-third is distributed to the ECF. The total of ECF expressed as percentage of body weight is 4–6, 8–10, and 6–10% for plasma, interstitial lymph, and transcellular fluid, respectively [1, 7]. Table 1 shows an approximated quantification of the compartmental body fluid distribution in a 500 kg horse.

In humans, there is a difference in the percentage of TBW between sexes. The variation is primarily the consequence of differences in the total body fat content between the two sexes, since adipose tissue, which is normally accumulated in higher quantities in women, contains little water [5]. In the horse, no significant differences of TBW between sexes have been reported. Age, however, does affect the TBW. The TBW relative to body weight in foals is greater than adults [12], primarily as a consequence of a higher ECF volume [13]. However, by 6 months of age, foals reach a body fluid status similar to adults [13].

***Table 1.* Fluid distribution and electrolyte composition of the major fluid compartments**

		Extracellular Fluid			
Item	*Intracellular Fluid*	*Plasma*	*Interstitial Fluid*	*Connective Tissue*	*Transcellular Fluid*
Water (L)†	200	17	44	17	22
Electrolyte (mEq/L)‡					
Cations					
Na^+	12.0	142	145.1		
K^+	140.0	4.3	4.4		
Ca^{2+} (ionized)	4.0	2.5	2.4		
Mg^{2+} (ionized)	34.0	1.1	1.1		
Total	190	149.9	153		
Anions					
Cl^-	4	104	117.4		
HCO_3^-	12	24	27.1		
$HPO^{2-}{}_4$, $H_2PO_4^-$	40	2	2.3		
Proteins	50	14	0		
Other	84*	5.9	6.2		
Total	190	149.9	153		

† Adapted from Rose RJ [7].
‡ Adapted from Rose BD [9].
* This largely represents organic phosphates such as ATP.

The Electrolytes

The electrolyte composition in the ECF and ICF vary considerably (Table 1). However, there is equilibrium, as the total of organic and inorganic solutes inside and outside the cells is equal – a function of the law of equal charges [9]. There are a number of other particles in both fluid compartments that, although in small quantity, exert important metabolical and physiological effects, such as proteins [9]. Some others, such as the minor electrolytes, do not exert important responses to fluid movement as their negligible quantities have no significant osmotic effect.

The ECF Electrolytes

The sodium ion is the single most important osmotically active solute of the extracellular fluid [14] and represents the main determinant of this volume [7]. The total exchangeable sodium is found mostly in the ECF, with a larger proportion in the interstitial lymph fluid (41%) than plasma (16%) [5]. This is an important consideration because, in most instances, deficiencies in Na ions are borne largely by this compartment and there is a complex relationship between plasma sodium values and ECF sodium balance [15].

Plasma Cl and HCO_3 constitute the major anions of the ECF, with plasma proteins, which are essentially intravascular, also constituting an important fraction of the total extracellular anions. The total exchangeable body chloride is almost exclusively extracellular and moves passively in and out of the cells by exchange with HCO_3 ions.

There are important differences between the electrolyte concentrations of plasma and interstitial fluids, with plasma Na concentration being higher and the concentrations of Cl and proteins lower, when compared with interstitial fluid [9]. These important differences are largely attributed to the effects of the Gibbs–Donnan equilibrium that helps in maintaining an even distribution of fluid between compartments [9]. The transcellular fluid electrolytes of the gastrointestinal tract are also readily exchangeable with other ions of the ECF [16, 17].

The ICF Electrolytes

The potassium ion is the counterpart of the sodium ion, representing the osmotic skeleton of the intracellular fluid [7]. The total exchangeable body potassium is about 95%, of which about 99% is intracellular and mainly intramuscular [5]. The rest is found in the ECF (less than 2%), mainly in the plasma and interstitial lymph fluid, and it is therefore impossible to assess the total body potassium balance by measurements of plasma potassium [5, 7]. The potassium plus magnesium ions represent the major cations, while organic phosphates and proteins are the major anions.

Fluid and Electrolyte Balance

The body fluids and electrolytes are so intrinsically interwined that they should not be observed as separate substances. Fluids and electrolytes must be in equilibrium for the physiological and biochemical events that maintain life [18]. This equilibrium involves: (1) an external balance which is maintained by intake and output, and (2) an internal balance which comprides both balance between the major fluid compartments as well as balance at a cellular level.

External Balance

External electrolyte balance is intimately related to water balance [19] and its constancy is based upon the equilibrium between intake and output [1, 19]. Body water is obtained from oral fluid ingestion and the water content of food, and metabolic water, while losses occur through the expired air, sweat, faeces and urine [1, 20]. The ingestion of water is affected by environmental factors such as temperature, humidity and type of food [21–23]. Likewise, the excretion of water by expiration, sweating and faeces is not under tight physiological control

Table 2. **Daily water intake and output in horses comparing two studies carried out at different ambient temperatures**

Study	*Ambient Temperature (°C)*	*Water Intake (ml/kg BW)*	*Output (ml/kg BW)*			
			Urine	*Faeces*	*Insensible Losses*	*Total*
Tasker [22]	4.4–21	56.5	12	34	10.5	56.5
Groenendyk *et al.* [23]	16–25	64	23.2	16.9	23.4	63.5

and its magnitude is determined by environmental factors such as temperature and humidity [20]. Only renal losses can be regulated precisely, helping to maintain the volume and composition of the body fluids, despite wide variation in the daily intake of water and solutes [20].

Unfortunately, there are very few data on external balance of fluids and electrolytes in the horse. The results of two studies on the external balance of fluid and electrolytes are shown in Table 2. Tasker [22] reported the results of a study carried out in four horses over a period of 7 days. Horses were fed with a daily ration of alfalfa–timothy hay and water was provided *ad libitum*. Urine and faeces were collected and samples taken every 24 hours for fluid and electrolyte determinations. More recently, a similar study investigated the external balance of fluids and electrolytes in five horses over a period of 14 days [23]. Horses were fed with chaffed lucerne and watered twice daily. Urine and faecal samples were collected every 24 hours for fluid and electrolyte measurements. Although the data are limited and there are some methodological differences between the two studies, some general conclusions can be drawn:

- There is a tight physiological control between input and output.
- Water intake is greatly affected by ambient temperature. In the study by Groenedyk *et al.* [23], a direct relationship was found between water intake and evaporative loss (insensible losses), the latter being smallest when ambient temperature was lowest.

Dietary composition and particularly the electrolyte content of ingested food and water are important in determining water intake and output. Cymbaluk [21] reported that the type of food affects the route through which fluids are excreted. Most of the differences between the studies of Tasker [22] and Groenendyk *et al.* [23] could be attributed to the total electrolyte intake, mainly sodium, which was greater in the latter study (Table 2).

The most striking aspect of most horse diets is the large amount of potassium that is ingested and excreted each day. This contrasts with sodium, which is usually in much smaller amounts and is more tightly regulated (Table 3). Regulation of urinary potassium losses is not as precise as those of sodium, with the possibility of substantial potassium losses continuing in the event of anorexia [24–26].

Table 3. **Electrolyte input and output (mmol) with different diets**

	Electrolyte Input			*Electrolyte Output*						
				Urine			*Faeces*			
Source	*Na*	*K*	*Cl*	*Na*	*K*	*Cl*	*Na*	*K*	*Cl*	*Ref. No.*
Hay	329	3930	–	7	2196	nm	101	985	mm	[22]
Lucerne chaff	986	3320	3008	527	2661	2347	253	504	174	[23]
Cubes + hay	nm	nm	nm	180	2220	1750	nm	nm	nm	[55]
None	–	–	–	818	1393	971	nm	nm	nm	[25]
None	–	–	–	72	534	nm	35	106	nm	[26]

nm = not measured

Internal Balance

Water and electrolytes are in continuous movement and this movement is regulated, in principle, by the movement of electrolytes [27]. Interaction between water and electrolytes allows a continuous exchange of water and solutes across fluid compartments. Solute movement occurs by active and passive mechanisms. The former requires metabolic energy while the latter does not and its movement across membranes follows down concentration or electrical gradients. In contrast, all water movement is passive and follows down osmotic gradients.

The passive movement of water is determined by two forces: hydrostatic and osmotic pressures. The former takes place exclusively in the vascular space and is maintained by the heart pump. At a capillary level, it forces plasma out of the vascular space into the interstitial space.

Cellular Balance

At a cellular level, the Na^+-K^+ATPase pump and the diffusion of fluid across the cellular membranes are the main mechanisms of intracellular fluid balance [28]. Alterations of the activity of the ionic pump or changes in the osmotic gradient in the interstitial fluid will alter this balance [29]. Cellular mechanisms are important but difficult to study in the whole animal.

Overview

There are two major compartments in which water and electrolytes interact to maintain a steady state system. The movement of water between these two compartments is accomplished by the active and passive transport of ions which produce an osmotic gradient causing a net movement of water. Also, changes in the amount of organic metabolites in the cells produce fluid shifts by means of passive osmotic transfer.

The rapid and free movement of water across cell membranes occurs to establish equality of osmotic concentrations of intra- and extracellular fluid. The relative intra- and extracellular fluid volume depend on the quantities of ions contained within these compartments. Sodium is the main cation of the ECF while Cl and HCO_3 constitute the major anions. In the ICF, K is the major cation and organic PO_4 and proteins are the major anions. The primary difficulty in assessment of fluid and electrolyte balance is accurately determining changes in the composition of the ICF. We can readily assume ECF changes from determination of plasma composition but there is no simple technique for measuring alterations in the ICF compartment.

Fluids and Electrolytes – Exercise

Exercise brings about important changes in the body fluid and electrolyte balance. When exercising at high intensities, such as racing, rapid but transient fluid and electrolyte shifts occur, without substantial losses. In contrast, prolonged exercise at low intensities, such as endurance riding, might result in major fluid and electrolyte losses. In either case, and to varying degrees, fluid shifts occur enabling an appropriate blood flow distribution to working muscle while increments in cutaneous blood flow occur to promote dissipation of metabolic heat. In the face of these changes, maintenance of an adequate circulating blood volume is essential if equilibrium between these dynamic responses is to be maintained during exercise. When exercise results in losses of large amounts of fluid and electrolytes, this dynamic equilibrium is most likely to be compromised. Thus, the intensity and duration of exercise will determine magnitude of response.

Because prolonged exercise, especially in the heat, often results in various degrees of dehydration, thermoregulatory stability can be compromised in proportion of the degree of dehydration. In addition to fluid losses, dehydration also results in large electrolyte losses since sweating, being the main mechanism for heat dissipation, contains substantial quantities of electrolytes, particularly sodium, potassium and chloride [30, 31].

Fluid Shifts

The redistribution of body fluid (fluid shifts) during exercise is basically the same at low and high intensities but more marked in the latter. At the start of exercise, there is a rapid movement of fluid and electrolytes from the vascular to the interstitial space as a result of changes in hydrostatic and oncotic pressure gradients across the capillary membranes. This response is characterized by increases in haematocrit (PCV), total plasma protein concentration (TP), decreases in PV and increases in arterial and capillary pressures. The increases in PCV are mainly the result of the addition of red cells into the circulation caused by the splenic contraction that occurs during exercise. Plasma proteins, however, are mainly limited to the vascular space as their large size is an impediment to crossing the capillary wall, reflecting a net fluid movement out of the vascular space that results in reduction of PV. The result of this escape of fluid into the interstitium is a better fluid perfusion to working muscles and to the skin, which promotes heat dissipation.

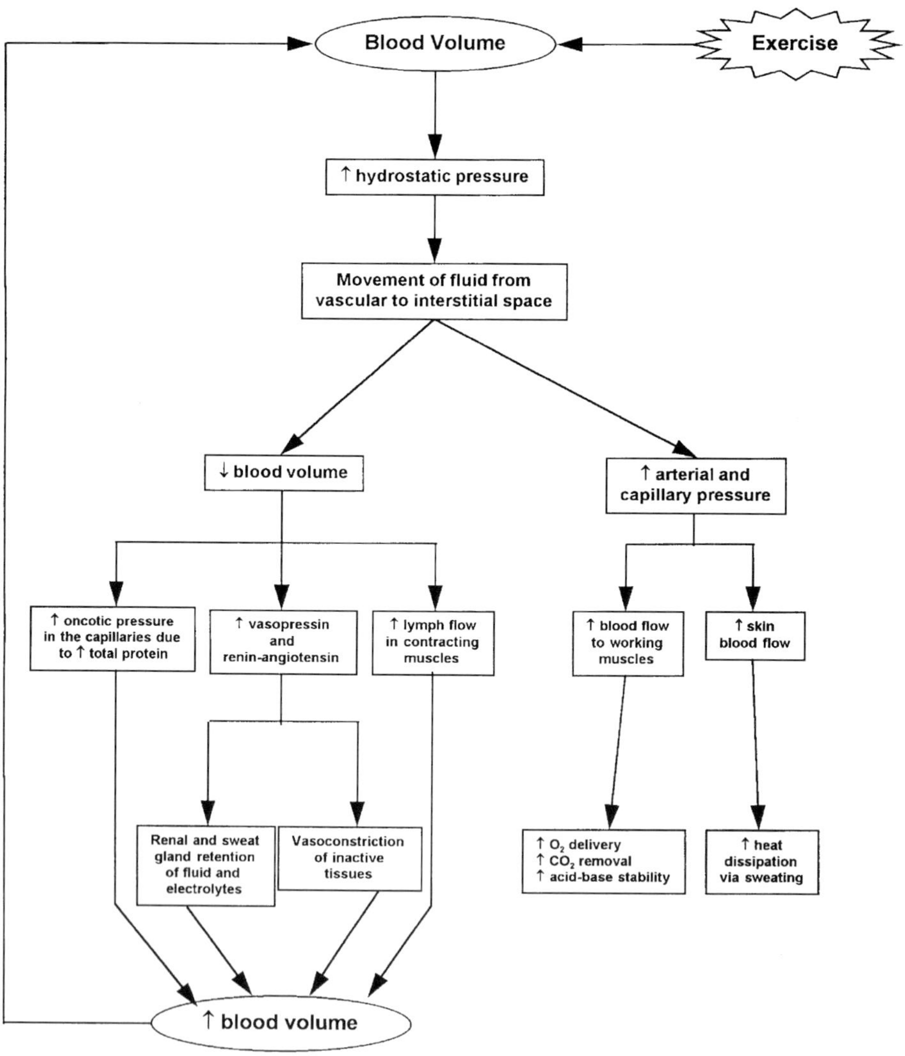

Figure 1. Counterbalance mechanisms during exercise to maintain adequate circulating fluid in the vascular space. Adpated from Convertino [27].

As PV decreases, so does the effective circulating volume which is essential for an adequate tissue perfusion. However, early in exercise, a counterbalancing response to the fluid shifts out of the vascular space takes place so an effective circulating volume can be established. This protective mechanism involves Starling forces characterized by increases in plasma oncotic pressure at capillary levels as a result of increments in TP. Also, exercise induced increases in plasma vasopressin and renin–angiotensin cause vasconstriction in inactive tissues, resulting in net fluid movement from inactive interstitial spaces into the general circulation. In addition, increases in lymph flow in contracting muscles can contribute to the maintenance of PV during long-term exercise. Some of these interacting-processes are shown in Figure 1.

Therefore, fluid shifts out of the vascular space and the protective counterbalancing mechanisms that bring back fluid into the circulation maintain an orderly dynamic distribution of fluid that benefits muscle metabolism and thermoregulation during exercise. Finally, these dynamic responses are facilitated by the cardiovascular system with the heart propelling blood, which in turn is distributed by the blood vessels.

The most important clinical point is that, with acute, short-term exercise, the fluid shifts are transient and no substantial deficits occur. Most of the changes that occur return to normal within 60 minutes after completion of exercise. However, with more prolonged exercise, in addition to the fluid shifts which are less extreme than with high intensity exercise, substantial fluid losses from sweat can occur.

Electrolyte Shifts

Major electrolyte shifts occur during exercise and these shifts differ in various parts of the circulation. Carlson [32] noted that when arterial and mixed venous blood were compared, intense exercise resulted in a profound decrease

Table 4. **Plasma fluid and electrolyte changes after high and low intensity exercise**

Item	*Racing*	*3-Day Event*	*Endurance*
PCV	↑↑↑	↑↑	↑
TP	↑↑↑	↑↑	↑↑
PV	↓↓↓	↓↓	↓↓
Na	↑	N	↓
K	↑	↓	↓
Cl	↑	↓	↓↓
HCO_3	↓↓↓	↓↓	N

↑ or ↓ minor change
↑↑ or ↓↓ moderate change
↑↑↑ or ↓↓↓ severe change
N – no change

in bicarbonate concentration in arterial blood, whereas bicarbonate concentration increased slightly in mixed venous blood. This is because more than 70% of the CO_2 produced during high intensity exercise is transported as bicarbonate in the venous circulation. Chloride values in mixed venous blood during maximal exercise are substantially lower than those in arterial blood. In contrast, there are few differences in sodium and potassium values between mixed venous and arterial blood. During maximal exercise, there is a modest increase in plasma sodium and substantial increase in plasma potassium, with values as high as 10 mmol/L [33]. Similar, but less dramatic changes occur with the major electrolytes during low intensity exercise. These changes are summarized in Table 4.

Thermoregulation – Effects on Fluid and Electrolytes

Exercise results in increments in metabolic heat production that are proportional to the intensity of exercise. If health is to be maintained, there must be a balance between production, gain and loss of heat. There are four main mechanisms by which heat losses are accomplished: (1) conduction, (2) convection, (3) radiation and (4) evaporation [10]. Evaporative cooling, especially under hot environmental conditions, is the most efficient and important means for heat dissipation during exercise in the horse. The cardiovascular system carries the heat load in the blood from the production sites, mainly muscles, to the skin and respiratory tract from where heat is liberated [34, 35].

When exercising for prolonged periods, such as with endurance rides, there is a continuous necessity to dissipate heat. As a result of evaporative cooling, large amounts of fluid are lost in sweat, estimated to be up to 15 L/h [31, 36]. If these losses are not replaced, dehydration and in extreme cases, shock, will ensue with a reduction in effective circulating volume. This results in a compromise between central and peripheral blood flow distribution [27, 37, 38]. At a central level, blood supply is required to maintain stroke volume and blood flow to working muscles. At a peripheral level, there is a reduction in skin blood flow to help maintain central blood volume despite the necessity for heat dissipation.

In humans, the thermoregulatory responses to exercise are known to be affected by the state of training. The threshold for the onset of sweating appears to be higher when the individuals are better trained. Also, the rate of sweat production as well as the electrolyte composition in sweat seem to be affected by the state of training [39]. In contrast, limited studies performed in the horse indicate that there are few changes in the production or composition of sweat caused by training [35].

Exercise, Dehydration and Rehydration

Prolonged exercise, especially in the heat, inevitably leads to dehydration as large amounts of sweat are required for heat dissipation. In addition to fluid losses, large electrolyte losses also occur because equine sweat is hypertonic. This reduces the TBW and decreases the effective circulating volume, which in turn leads to compromised cardiovascular and thermoregulatory function. Therefore, fluid supplementation is essential to maintain circulatory stability and effective thermoregulation.

The wealth of information related to exercise-induced dehydration in humans has allowed for the development of strategies to combat problems of dehydration occurring under different levels of physical activity [40]. In contrast, the current recommendations to replenish fluid and electrolyte alterations associated with exercise in the horse are largely empirical. Nevertheless, the need to assist the hydration status of the exercising horse is well recognized by trainers and riders who often use 'saline drenches' in an attempt to limit the level of dehydration during exercise. While a huge variety of oral fluid and electrolyte mixtures are available commercially, there is little research in the horse that allows a rational approach to fluid and electrolyte replacement during exercise.

With the available information, we will discuss some of the key factors that can affect fluid absorption in the horse. In particular, we will address considerations relating to the use of oral fluids prior to, during or after exercise.

Gastric Emptying of Oral Rehydration Solutions

In humans, gastric emptying is delayed by exercise. Thus, in exercising humans, gastric emptying determines the rate at which fluids can be available to the absorption sites in the intestine and into circulation [41, 42]. In theory, the sooner the fluid is emptied from the stomach, the more rapidly it will be available for absorption. However, studies in humans have shown that the characteristics of the fluid affects the rate of gastric emptying both at rest and during exercise. Fluid tonicity, glucose concentration, fluid temperature and exercise, affect the rate of gastric emptying [41, 43, 44]. We have studied these issues in horses deprived of food overnight. All horses received 8 L of fluid via nasogastric tube and gastric fluid samples were collected every 15 minutes for a period of 1 hour. We found that about 80–90% of the stomach fluid content was emptied 15 minutes after its administration regardless of its composition and temperature [45]. Only when tonicity was highly hypertonic ($\approx$1500 mOsm/kg) did we observe reductions in the gastric emptying rate, up to 50% over 1 hour. When fluid was administered after a bout of exercise at moderate intensity, gastric emptying was even greater [45]. So, the few available data suggest that the gastric emptying rate in the horse is not a critical obstacle to fluid and electrolyte supplementation, provided that the fluid is not highly hypertonic.

Oral Fluid Administration

A range of questions will be addressed, relating to oral fluid administration and its use in the horse following exercise.

What is the optimum oral rehydration solution (ORS)?

The optimum ORS, when given, should replenish all the water and substrates that are lost. Provision of all substrates is not possible as adequate availability of an energy source is not possible in an ORS for horses. Water and electrolyte losses are mainly from sweating, so knowing the sweating rate and composition is helpful in matching the relative fluid demands. Owing to technical difficulties in the collection of horse sweat, sweating rate and composition have not properly been established. However, changes in body weight after exercise give a good indication of fluid losses and in relation to electrolytes, most studies agree that horse sweat is hypertonic in relation to plasma and the major electrolytes are Na, K and Cl [30, 35, 36]. While sweat Na and Cl concentrations are between 10 and 50% higher than those in plasma, the sweat K concentration is around 10-fold greater than the value in plasma [30, 35, 36]. Thus, ORS in the horse should approximate the concentrations of electrolytes lost in sweat. This can be achieved by the use of 1 tablespoon (about 20 g) of Lite salt and 1 tablespoon of table salt in 4 L of water [46].

What is the optimum fluid tonicity?

Fluid tonicity appears not to affect absorption rate in the horse. However, administration or water of hypertonic fluids (twice the normal tomicity) at a volume equivalent to 4% body weight does cause major plasma electrolyte disturbances and therefore renal fluid and electrolyte elimination [47]. Isotonic fluid does not alter plasma osmolality and therefore would appear to be the most suitable option to ensure maximum fluid and electrolyte absorption.

How much fluid can be given?

The maximum amount of fluid that a horse (450–500 kg) can tolerate well is about 8–10 L in a single dose. After about 30 minutes, another dose can be given and most horses will tolerate the same amount without showing signs of abdominal pain. We have administered 25–30 L over a period of 1 hour given in 8–10 L doses, 20 minutes apart. This fluid was well tolerated and there were no major signs of abdominal discomfort.

Does fluid have to be given via a drench?

It is clearly the best option that horses rehydrate themselves by drinking a solution containing electrolytes. However, many horses will not voluntarily drink all that has been lost. Thus, in most horses, fluid administration by nasogastric intubation provides the best results. It is important to ensure that there is normal gastrointestinal function as many exhausted horses will have ileus following exercise.

Is fluid temperature important?

The belief exists among horse trainers that cold fluid will cause colic. Our observations indicate that this must be rare and we have not observed signs of abdominal discomfort in horses administered large volumes of fluid (up to 30 L), given at a temperature of 4°C. We have also shown that fluid temperature does not have major effects on fluid absorption [47].

Can fluid uptake be enhanced by inclusion of glucose in the ORS?

The inclusion of glucose in ORS has been shown to increase fluid uptake in humans [42]. It appears that glucose may have minimal effects on fluid and electrolyte absorption in the horse [47]. Additionally, when glucose is included in a solution, the total electrolyte concentration is reduced if the solution is to be isotonic and so administration of such solutions will be less ideal in replacing electrolyte deficits.

Fluid Administration Prior to Exercise

The administration of fluid in advance of exercise (hyperhydration) has been shown to be beneficial in humans exercising for prolonged periods [48]. Increases in plasma volume, lower heart rate, and lower core temperature, together with increases in sweat rate, are some of the responses observed in hyperhydrated athletes [48]. These features are desirable for horses involved in endurance events. The data available to address this issue in the horse are limited, with the exception of some experiments conducted under controlled conditions of treadmill exercise. Recently, we found that horses treated orally with hypotonic fluid equivalent to 4% body weight 90 minutes prior to exercise, maintained higher plasma volume throughout exercise than their counterparts exercising without fluid [49]. In another study, we observed similar responses when isotonic fluid equivalent to 6% body weight was given prior to 2 hours of low and moderate intensity exercise alternatively [50]. Signs of gastrointestinal disturbance immediately before and during exercise, such as mild diarrhoea, were also observed when fluid was given at a volume equivalent to 6% body weight. In these two studies, heat dissipation was not improved with fluid prior to exercise. While this is difficult to achieve under laboratory conditions, in the field evaporative cooling is more easily accomplished. Thus, hyperhydration prior to exercise may have benefits under field conditions that are not evident in the laboratory as a routine procedure. Nonetheless, hyperhydration, while offering some benefits, is not a practice that is easy to justify in the horse.

Perhaps, among the range of the equine athletic endeavours, the second day of a 3-day event could be the type of exercise where horses may receive the most benefit from hyperhydration prior to exercise. This is because this part of the event requires continuous exercise for about 2 hours with only 10 minutes rest. However, administering fluids at the 10 minute rest stage could be detrimental for the horse because of the extra weight carried. Additionally, fluid administered by nasogastric tube will not be absorbed until horses complete the next 30 minutes of the competition. Thus, the only opportunity to assist the hydration status of a horse competing in this event is before exercise. In other words, the approach to treatment is prophylactic and the aim is to offset most, if not all, of the fluid and electrolyte losses that occur throughout the event. Body weight losses up to 20 kg or more, mainly as sweat, are normally found [51], accompanied by cation losses (Na^+, K^+) of up to 3000 mmol. While it is difficult to administer this amount of fluid before exercise, volumes of 10–15 L can be given safely. The total amount of fluid can be split into two or three doses, 20 minutes apart, and given approximately 2 hours before exercise, which is the best time for maximum fluid absorption to occur. The fluid has to be administered by nasogastric tube as a normally hydrated horse will not drink a fluid solution that contains electrolytes. The solution used can be commercial or home made as long as it is isotonic and contains sodium, chloride and potassium. The formula of Carlson [46] is the most simple mixture available.

Fluid Replacement during Exercise

The replacement of fluid and electrolytes during high intensity exercise clearly is not as important as with longer duration exercise. The fluid and electrolyte losses that occur during the warm up period and exercise appear not to affect either the health of the horse or its performance. The practice of 'assisting' the fluid and electrolyte status of the horse before competition by means of 'jugs' or 'saline drenches' is unlikely to be of benefit. The administration of 1 or 2 L of an electrolyte solution with or without vitamins would appear to be of little help for a horse that has a total body water of 300 L. The practice of administering pre-race electrolytes, while a good source of income for equine practitioners, does not fulfil its purposes and should therefore probably be discontinued.

The other source of fluid and electrolyte losses in racehorses is the use of frusemide to treat horses with exercise-induced pulmonary haemorrhage. Horses may excrete a fluid volume up to an equivalent of 4% of body weight [52]. These fluid and electrolyte losses induced by frusemide could compromise performance. From a physiological standpoint, the higher the contraction of plasma volume, the greater the compromise of cardiovascular and thermoregulatory function [27]. Nevertheless, these is some evidence that frusemide enhances performance [53], although the issue remains controversial.

When horses exercise for long distances such as endurance rides and 3-day events, three key elements should be provided: (1) water, (2) electrolytes and (3) energy. It is impossible to provide energy in a readily available form without gastrointestinal disturbances and laminitis. However, water and electrolytes can be administered, particularly during check points of endurance rides. For each hour of exercise, up to 10–15 L of water can be lost accompanied by electrolyte losses (mmol) of Na (1000–1500), K (400–600) and Cl (1300–2000). These extensive losses do not continue and in most circumstances total fluid deficits after an 80 km ride are about 20–25 L. During endurance rides, most riders normally allow horses to drink as often as they can. Generally, this is beneficial as offsetting fluid deficits is fundamental to the maintenance of fluid balance. However, the electrolyte deficits may be overlooked and, therefore, the addition of water could worsen the abnormal plasma electrolyte concentrations. Some endurance riders administer electrolytes in the form of a paste concentrate. We have studied the effects of administering concentrated electrolytes via paste in a group of frusemide-dehydrated horses. On one occasion, 88 g (about 4 tablespoons) of each Lite salt and table salt mixed with custard was given and water was supplied *ad libitum*. On another occasion, only water was given *ad libitum*. The group given the paste had a higher water consumption than when paste was not administered and restored body weight at the end of 6 hours. The fluid, electrolyte and acid–base alterations caused by frusemide administration (1 mg IM) were reversed 2–3 hours after the administration of the paste. In contrast little change was observed when water only was given (Sosa Leon *et al.* unpublished). The study showed that electrolyte administration in the form of paste can have beneficial effects. However, care is needed because if the concentration of the paste is too high, it can result in further fluid movement out of the circulating fluid volume, into the gastrointestinal tract. Conversely, if the concentration is too low, it may fail to replenish adequately fluid and electrolyte losses.

Fluid Administration Post-Exercise

Fluid administration post-exercise sometimes is overlooked, as it might be thought that the endeavour has finished and the horse is about to rest. In fact, fluid administration post-exercise may be as critical as during exercise.

Fluid replacement without electrolytes results in hyponatraemia which can be maintained for several hours if electrolytes, particularly sodium, are not replaced [47]. Hyponatraemia decreases the stimulus for thirst, thus delaying the rehydration process. This syndrome has been recognized in humans and it is characterized by the lack of weight gain several hours post-exercise, even with water intake [54]. Whether this happens in the horse is not known but horses do fail to replenish fluid losses up to 24 hours post exercise [51] which may imply that involuntary dehydration also happens in horses.

Some horses will not drink, despite dehydration, unless they have food first. In this case, the addition of salts in the meal could help to replenish electrolyte losses while also increasing the thirst.

Conclusions

The body fluid and electrolyte balance is vital to maintain the normal function of the different body systems. Strenuous exercise, particularly in the heat, can seriously affect this equilibrium, as large amounts of fluid and electrolyte often are lost. As a result, health and performance can be compromised owing to reductions in cardiovascular and thermoregulatory function. Thus, assisting the hydration status of the equine athlete is essential, particularly for the more prolonged events.

Because of the wide range of physical activities that horses undertake, the approach to treatment of fluid and electrolyte losses is best based on the approximation of the total sweat losses that occur during exercise. The use of oral fluid to replenish these losses is safe, effective, easy to administer and relatively cheap, especially if home made. Fluid composition appears not to affect the rate of absorption. However, isotonic fluid should be given as it does not alter plasma osmolality and has less dramatic effects on fluid and electrolyte excretion. Fluid temperature appears not to affect fluid absorption and we have found no adverse effects, such as colic, when administering cold fluid.

The use of fluid in advance of exercise could be advantageous in maintaining higher plasma volume in horses during the second day of the 3-day event or before and at the mid points of endurance rides. During exercise, care should be taken in matching the fluid and electrolyte losses in sweat. Similarly, after exercise, fluid and electrolytes should be replaced as some horses may experience some degree of involuntary dehydration. Whenever possible, horses should be encouraged to voluntarily replenish fluid and electrolyte losses. However, some horses will not drink and administration by nasogastric tube is advisable. Otherwise, concentrated electrolytes in the form of a paste are easy to administer and can be very effective in restoring fluid and electrolyte losses. Post exercise, electrolytes can also be supplied in the meal. However, overall, we need to remember the old saying 'you can lead a horse to the water but you can't make it drink'.

References

1. Carlson GP. Fluid therapy in horses with acute diarrhea. *Vet Clin N Am: Large Anim Pract.* 1979; **1**, 313–329.
2. Michell AR, Bywater RJ, Clarke KW *et al. Veterinary Fluid Therapy*. Oxford: Blackwell Scientific Publications 1989; 263.
3. Murray MJ. Alimentary tract disease. In: Robinson NE (ed). *Current Therapy in Equine Medicine.* Philadelphia: WB Saunders 1992; 167–263.
4. Rose RJ & Hodgson DR. Alimentary system. In: Rose RJ & Hodgson DR (eds). *Manual of Equine Practice.* Mexico: WB Saunders 1993; 192–249.

5. Edelman IS & Leibman MD. Anatomy of body water and electrolytes. *Am J Med.* 1959; **27**, 256–277.
6. O'Connor WJ. Normal sodium balance in dogs and man. *Cardiovasc Res.* 1977; **11**, 375–408.
7. Rose RJ. A physiological approach to fluid and electrolyte therapy in the horse. *Equine Vet J.* 1981; **13**, 7–14.
8. Carlson GP. Hematology and body fluids in the equine athlete, a review. In: Gillepsie JR & Robinson NE (eds). *Equine Exercise Physiology* 2. Davis: ICEEP Publications, 1987; 393–425.
9. Rose BD. *Clinical Physiology of Acid-base and Electrolyte Disorders.* 3rd ed. New York: McGraw-Hill 1989; 853.
10. McConaghy FF. Aspects of thermoregulation in the exercising horse. PhD thesis, University of Sydney, 1995.
11. Robb J, Harper RB, Hintz HF *et al.* Chemical compositon and energy value of the body, fatty acid composition of adipose tissue, and liver and kidney size in the horse. *Anim Prod.* 1972; **14**, 25–34.
12. Kami G, Merritt AM & Duelly P. Preliminary studies of plasma and extracellular fluid volume in neonatal ponies. *Equine Vet J.* 1984; **16**, 356–358.
13. Spensley MS, Carlson GP & Harrold D. Plasma, red blood cell, total blood, and extracellular fluid volumes in healthy horse foals during growth. *Am J Vet Res.* 1987; **48**, 1703–1707.
14. Leaf A. The clinical and physiological significance of serum sodium concentration. *N Engl J Med.* 1962; **267**, 24–30, 77–83.
15. Edelman IS, Leibman J, O'Meara MP *et al.* Interrelations between serum sodium concentration, serum osmolarity and total exchangeable sodium, total exchangeable potassium and total body water. *J Clin Invest.* 1958; **37**, 1236–1256.
16. Edelman IS & Sweet NJ. Gastrointestinal water and electrolytes. I. The equilibration of radiosodium in gastrointestinal contents and in the proportion of exchangeable (Nae) in the gastrointestinal tract. *J Clin Invest.* 1956; **35**, 502–511.
17. Nadell J, Sweet NJ & Edelman IS. Gastrointestinal water and electrolytes. II. The equilibration of radio potassium in gastrointestinal contects and the proportion of exchangeable potassium (Ke) in the gastrointestinal tract. *J Clin Invest.* 1956; **35**, 512–521.
18. Carlson GP. Fluid, electrolyte, and acid-base balance. In: Kaneko JJ. (ed). *Clinical Biochemistry of Domestic Animals.* 4th ed. San Diego: Academic Press Inc. 1989; 543–575.
19. Rose RJ. Electrolytes, clinical applications. *Vet Clin N Am, Equine Pract.* 1990; **6**, 281–293.
20. Kinsey EM & Smith MD. *Fluids and Electrolytes, a Conceptual Approach.* 2nd edn. New York: Churchill Livingstone Inc. 1991; 166.
21. Cymbaluk NF. Water balance of horses fed various diets. *Equine Prac.* 1989; **11**, 19–24.
22. Tasker JB. Fluid and electrolyte studies in the horse. III. Intake and output of water, sodium and potassium. *Cornell Vet.* 1967; **57**, 649–657.
23. Groenendyk S, English PB & Abetz I. External balance of water and electrolytes in the horse. *Equine Vet J.* 1988; **20**, 189–193.
24. Carlson GP, Rumbaugh GE & Harrold D. Physiological alterations in the horse produced by food and water deprivation during periods of high environmental temperatures. *Am J Vet Res.* 1979; **40**, 982–985.
25. Rumbaugh GE, Carlson GP & Harrold D. Urinary production in the healthy horse and in horses deprived to feed and water. *Am J Vet Res.* 1982; **43**, 735–737.
26. Tasker JB. Fluid and electrolyte studies in the horse. IV. The effects of fasting and thirsting. *Cornell Vet.* 1967; **57**, 658–667.
27. Convertino VA. Fluid shifts and hydration state: Effects of long term exercise. *Can J Sport Sci.* 1987; **12**, 136S–139S.
28. Sweadner KJ & Goldin SM. Active transport of sodium and potassium ions, mechanism, function, and regulation. *N Engl J Med.* 1980; **302**, 777–783.
29. Senay LC Jr & Pivarnik JM. Fluid shifts during exercise. *Exerc Sports Sci Rev.* 1985; **13**, 335–387.

30. Carlson GP & Ocen PO. Composition of equine sweat following exercise in high environmental temperatures and in response to epinephrine administration. *J Equine Med Surg.* 1979; **3**, 27–32.
31. Carlson GP. Physiological responses to endurance exercise. *Proc Annu Conv Am Assoc Equine Pract Conf.* 1979; 459–468.
32. Carlson GP. Interrelationships between fluid, electrolyte and acid-base balance during maximal exercise. *Equine Vet J.* 1995; **Suppl. 18**, 261–265.
33. Harris PA & Snow DH. The effects of high intensity exercise on plasma concentration of lactate, potassium and other electrolytes. *Equine Vet J.* 1988; **20**, 109–113.
34. Hodgson DR, Davis RE & McConaghy FF. Thermoregulation in the horse in response to exercise. *Br Vet J.* 1994; **150**, 219–235.
35. McConaghy FF, Hodgson DR, Evans DL & Rose RJ. Equine sweat composition: effects of adrenaline infusion, exercise and training. *Equine Vet J.* 1995; **Suppl. 20**, 158–164.
36. Kerr MG & Snow DH. Composition of sweat of the horse during prolonged epinephrine (adrenaline) infusion, heat exposure, and exercise. *Am J Vet Res.* 1983; **44**, 1571–1577.
37. Naylor JRJ, Bayly WM, Gollnick PD *et al.* Effects of dehydration on thermoregulatory responses of horses during low-intensity exercise. *J Appl Physiol.* 1993; **75**, 994–1001.
38. Hodgson DR, McCutcheon LJ, Byrd SK *et al.* Dissipation of metabolic heat in the horse during exercise. *J Appl Physiol.* 1993; **74**, 1161–1170.
39. Daly C & Dill DB. Salt economy in humid heat. *Am J Physiol.* 1937; **118**, 285–289.
40. Gisolfi CV & Duchman SM. Guidelines for optimal replacement beverages for different athletic events. *Med Sci Sports Exerc.* 1992; **24**, 679–687.
41. Costill DL & Saltin B. Factors limiting gastric emptying during rest and exercise. *J Appl Physiol.* 1974; **37**, 679–683.
42. Ramsbottom N & Hunt JN. Effect of exercise on gastric emptying and gastric secretion. *Digestion.* 1974; **10**, 1–8.
43. Coyle EF, Costill DL, Fink WJ & Hoopes DG. Gastric emptying rates for selected athletic drinks. *Res Quart.* 1978; **49**, 119–124.
44. Fordtran JS & Saltin B. Gastric emptying and intestinal absorption during prolonged severe exercise. *J Appl Physiol.* 1967; **23**, 331–335.
45. Sosa León LA, Hodgson DR & Rose RJ. Gastric emptying of oral rehydration solutions (ORS) at rest and after exercise in the horse. *Res Vet Sci.* 1997 (in press).
46. Carlson GP. Response to oral or intravenous fluid. *Proc 5th Annu Sci Meet Assoc Equine Sports Med.* 1985; 82–90.
47. Sosa León LA, Davie AJ, Hodgson DR & Rose RJ. The effects of tonicity, glucose concentration and temperature of an oral rehydration solution on its absorption and elimination. *Equine Vet J.* 1995; **Suppl. 20**, 140–146.
48. Greenleaf JE & Castle BL. Exercise temperature regulation in man during hypohydration and hyperhydration. *J Appl Physiol.* 1971; **30**, 847–853.
49. Sosa León LA, Davie AJ, Hodgson DR *et al.* Effects of oral fluid on cardiorespiratory and metabolic responses to prolonged exercise. *Equine Vet J.* 1995; **Suppl. 18**, 274–278.
50. Sosa León LA, Hodgson DR, Evans DL *et al.* Effects of hyperhydration on cardiorespiratory and metabolic responses to exercise during a simulated 2nd day of the 3-day-event. *Pferdeheilkunde.* 1996; **12**, 459–462.
51. Andrews FM, Ralston SL, Williamson LH *et al.* Weight loss, water loss and cation balance during the endurance test of a 3-day event. *Equine Vet J.* 1995; **Suppl. 18**, 294–297.
52. Freestone JF, Carlson GP, Harrold DR & Church G. Influence of furosemide treatment on fluid and electrolyte balance in horses. *Am J Vet Res.* 1988; **49**, 1899–1902.
53. Sweeney CR, Soma LR, Maxson AD *et al.* Effects of furosemide on the racing times of Thoroughbreds. *Am J Vet Res.* 1990; **51**, 772–778.
54. Greenleaf JE. Problem: thirst, drinking behaviour, and involuntary dehydration. *Med Sci Sports Exerc.* 1992; **24**, 645–656.

12

Clinical Assessment of Nutritional Status of the Horse

David Kronfeld

Key Points

- Clinical assessment of nutritional status addresses those procedures that a clinician may be reasonably expected to perform in a practice, on a farm, or in a hospital.
- Clinical assessment of nutritional status is needed for four main purposes:
  - Enhance performance of healthy horses,
  - Guide nutritional support of sick horses,
  - Identify nutritional component of certain important diseases,
  - Document humane and legal actions.
- A common cause of emaciation is the reliance of inexperienced horse owners on products advertized to improve digestion and metabolism. This often leads to underfeeding of hay during the winter.
- The first decision to be made in the nutritional support of a sick horse is whether it is hypo- or hyper-metabolic.
- Stall confinement, stationary feeding, and two starchy meals a day are alien to the horses's nutritional heritage.
- The customary approaches to nutritional assessment are dietary, morphometric, biochemical, physiological, behavioral and clinical. For equine practice, additional emphasis is placed on adding body weight, body condition score, dietary history and ration evaluation to the clinical or physical examination of the animal.
- The body condition score is crucial and should be standardized.
- Muscle wasting and loss of strength are signs of protein depletion. Loss of muscle (wasting) is even more serious clinically than loss of fat (condition).
- The mathematical drudgery of ration evaluation has been eliminated by the availability of numerous inexpensive, user-friendly computer software.
- A set of equine *recommended dietary allowances* would be about 1.4 times the mean minimum nutrient requirements specified by the National Research Council (NRC) [1]. Equine 'RDAs' are more likely than the NRC requirements to reach the lower regions of optimal ranges for nutrients and hence to be useful goals for practical nutrition.

Introduction

Clinical assessment of nutritional status addresses those procedures that a clinician may be reasonably expected to perform in a practice, on a farm or in a hospital. In every case, the clinician will prioritize these procedures, deciding on those to be done and, just as deliberately, the others to be left undone. In every case, the short list should include the type of animal, its intended use and level of performance, its body weight and body condition score. Any longer list is discretionary, but none of the optional methods of assessment (See Methods of Assessment) should be overlooked for legal as well as veterinary purposes. The day when a veterinarian can say in court that the patient's body weight was unknown (or guessed) has passed with the advent of inexpensive, convenient electronic scales.

Purposes

Clinical assessment of nutritional status is needed to achieve a desired level of performance in healthy horses, to provide nutritional support to sick horses, to identify and evaluate the nutritional component of several important diseases, and to document humane and legal actions. An appreciation of the purposes in hand may influence the selection of methods to be applied in a particular case, dealing with an individual or a group.

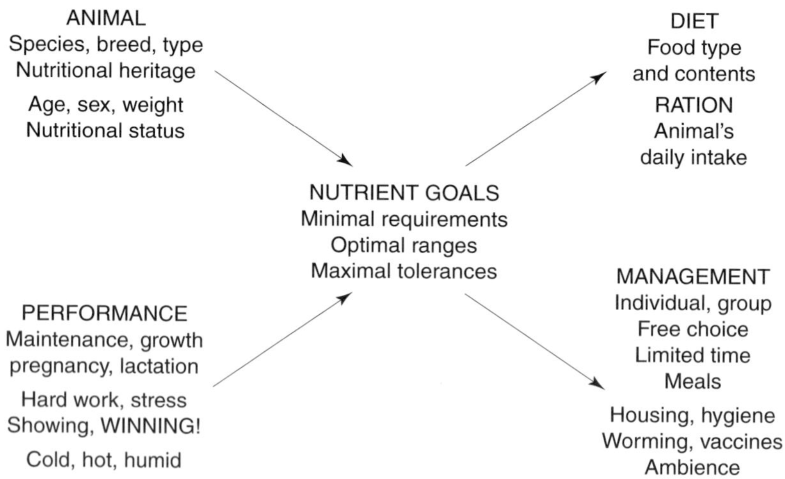

Figure 1. An orientation of nutritional practice focuses initially on setting nutritional goals for energy and nutrients in keeping with an animal's nature, state of health, and desired level of performance. The second step is to design a diet and feeding management program likely to achieve these goals. Suitable goals are optimal ranges or target zones (Figure 2).

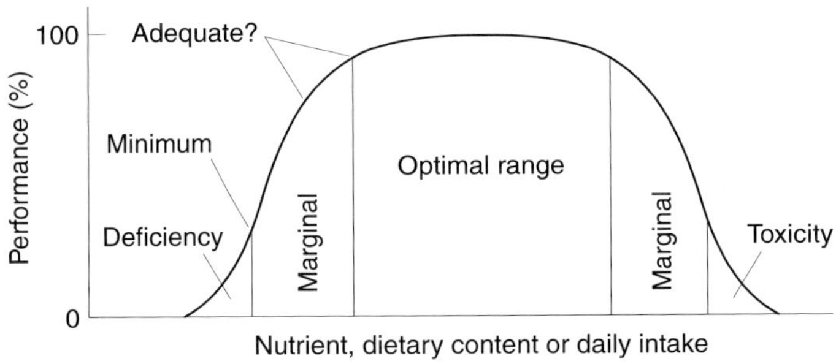

Figure 2. The influence of dietary content or nutrient intake on a specified measure of performance rises to a plateau, the optimal range, then declines [46]. Traditionally, performance is measured as energetic efficiency in production animals, but other measures of reproductive efficiency (e.g. conception rate, live foaling rate, foal weight), growth (e.g. weight, size, bone mineral content) and athletic fitness (e.g. speed, times, lactate threshold, maximal oxygen capacity) may be used for the horse. Minimum requirements (e.g. National Research Council [1]) are usually set to avoid an adverse effect, and optimal function may be reduced before such an adverse effect becomes evident. For practical purposes, nutritional goals (allowances or target zones) should be in optimal ranges rather be restricted to the minimum requirement.

An orientation of nutritional practice (Figure 1) has been successfully used by the author and associates for many species, including the horse. The focus is the setting of goals for intakes of energy and nutrients. These goals are not specified as single numbers or requirements, but rather as optimal ranges, with upper and lower limits as well as a median value (Figure 2).

Clients tend to ask questions about the diet or ingredients in the diet, but the practitioner should not be distracted from evaluating the whole system. This paper focuses on nutritional status, which is placed in the top left corner of Figure 1, but the whole picture must be kept in mind.

Nutritional Condition of Healthy Horses

Optimal body condition

In healthy horses, the need for nutritional assessment increases with the level of desired performance. Just as important as body weight is the degree of fatness [1], the fat:lean ratio or *body condition score* (Table 1). On a scale from 1 (emaciated) to 9 (obese), most horses should score 4–6.

Usual goals for body condition scores are about 4 for sport, 5 for growth and 6 for reproduction. In each case, the goal should be adjusted according to the individual's performance, and this capability may be a good index of a trainer's competence. Deviations from an optimal body weight and condition are more tolerable in a horse at maintenance than in a horse for reproduction, growth or hard work.

Table 1. Body condition scores of horses

1. *Extreme emaciation.* No fatty tissue. Protruding bones. Wasted muscles especially noticeable over bones: flat shelf over transverse processes.
2. *Emaciation.* Slight fat cover. Prominent bones. Wasted muscles.
3. *Thin.* Fat covers transverse processes and half-way up spinous processes; tailhead prominent but individual vertebrae not seen: ribs seen sharply.
4. *Moderately thin.* Slight back ridge; ribs barely discernible.
5. *Moderate.* Back is flat (no crease or ridge), ribs easily felt but not seen.
6. *Moderately fleshy.* Fat feels spongy over ribs and around tailhead; back crease slight or absent.
7. *Fleshy.* Back crease definite. Ribs covered but individual ribs can be palpated. Fat is palpable in neck, rump.
8. *Fat.* Back creased, neck thick, fat along withers, behind shoulders, and inside thighs.
9. *Too fat.* Back crease is deep: fat bulging on neck, along withers, behind shoulders, around tailhead, inside thighs.

Modified from Kronfeld (1993) [2]

Underweight and emaciation

Underweight and emaciation have many causes in addition to underfeeding or malnutrition (Table 2), so require a careful differential diagnosis [2]. In my experience, the most common cause of emaciation has been the trust that neophytes place in alleged digestive and nutritional aids. Reliance on such aids often leads to the underfeeding of hay during the winter when pastures have declined. Such aids may improve the efficiency of utilization of roughages, but they do not replace the staple sources of energy. Moreover, improving efficiency may not be the goal, because inefficient utilization of roughages generates heat, which is not wasted in winter.

In contrast, excessively hot and humid conditions may reduce appetite. In this case, digestive aids and nutrient supplements may benefit the horse. In my experience, judicious supplementation with corn oil, gradually introduced, is helpful. Studies in beef cattle have suggested that probiotics may improve heat tolerance.

Table 2. Causes of emaciation in horses

Deprivation of food, total or partial – bad teeth, bad feet, bad feed, bad people.
Deprivation of energy or protein or both – abuse of supplement, abuse of wobbler candidate.
Seasonal declines of energy and nutrients in pasture.
Malnutrition – protein deficiency, fluorosis.
Malabsorption, chronic diarrhea.
Intestinal parasites, also severe lice or ticks.
Cancer – melanoma, adenoma, lymphoma, etc.
Diabetes mellitus.
Chronic disease of liver, pancreas, kidney, heart.
Chronic infectious disease – pneumonia, abscesses, equine infectious anaemia.
Lactation, pregnancy.
Old age, senescence and senility.

Modified from Kronfeld [2]

Overweight and obesity

Overweight and obesity also have many causes, although overconsumption is by far the most likely. Fatness impairs athletic and reproductive performance. It also predisposes to hyperlipaemia, especially in ponies. Heaviness in a horse or pony is often stated to be associated with laminitis; it may exacerbate distal dislocation of the distal phalanx. The main danger of obesity in humans, mature-onset diabetes mellitus, is uncommon in the horse.

Attribution of overweight, a thick neck and sluggishness to hypothyroidism needs confirmation with an appropriate test (see Chapter 5). Cushinoid horses also need to be differentiated, by appropriate tests (see Chapter 3).

Grazing versus meals

The horse evolved as an herbivorous, hind-gut fermenter – browsing and grazing. It has a more or less continuous intake of fibrous plant materials, consisting mainly of carbohydrates (Figure 3). Most of the nutrients resist hydrolytic digestion in the small intestine and are fermented in the large bowel

NON-STRUCTURAL CARBOHYDRATES	• *HYDROLYZABLE* ✓ Monosaccharides ✓ Disaccharides ✓ Some starches • *FERMENTED* ✓ Oligosaccharides ✓ Resistant starches ✓ Gums, mucilages, pectins
NEUTRAL DETERGENT FIBRES	✓ Hemicellulose
ACID DETERGENT FIBRES	✓ Cellulose ✓ Lignin

• *HYDROLYZABLE* → glucose
✓ Sugars and some starches

• *FERMENTED RAPIDLY* → lactic acid – / → acetic
✓ Resistant starches, oligosaccharides
✓ Gums, mucilages, pectins
✓ Hemicellulose

• *FERMENTED SLOWLY* → acetic acid, etc
✓ Cellulose
✓ Ligno-cellulose

Figure 3. Current proximate analysis usually measures acid detergent fiber (lignin and cellulose) and neutral detergent fiber (lignin, cellulose and hemicellulose), then calculates nonstructural carbohydrate by difference. The latter includes hydrolyzable carbohydrates (monosaccharides, disaccharides and some starches) and nonhydrolyzable or fermented carbohydrates (oligosaccharides, resistant starches, gums, mucilages and pectins). The common assumption in livestock nutrition – that all nonstructural carbohydrate is hydrolyzable – is acceptable for ruminants, in which hydrolyzable counts as rapidly fermented, but misleading for hind-gut fermenters, such as the horse.

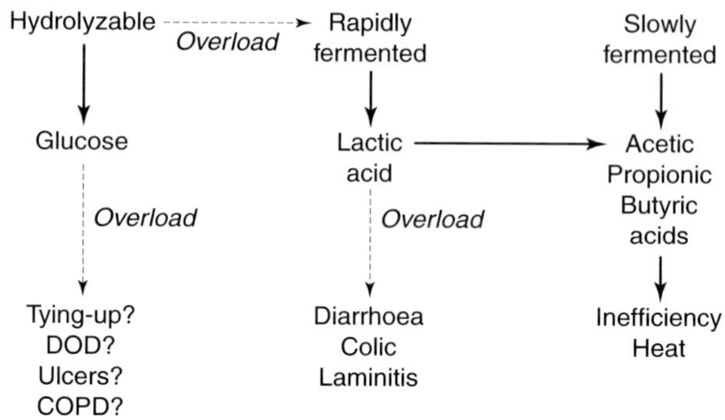

Figure 4. Carbohydrates may be hydrolyzed in the small intestine or fermented, rapidly or slowly, in the large intestine. Hydrolysis of sugars and non-resistant starches yields hexoses, mainly glucose. Rapid fermentation of hydrolyzable overload plus resistant starches, oligosaccharides, soluble fibers and some hemi-celluloses often allows lactic acid to accumulate. Slow fermentation of some hemicelluloses, cellulose and ligno-cellulose yields acetic, propionic and butyric acids. An overabundance of glucose following a starch meal may lead to certain disorders, although the pathogenic links are not well determined at present. More secure is the impact of lactic acid on osmotic diarrhea and laminitis. Both excess gas and excess lactic acid, which attracts water into the lumen, could contribute to some types of colic. The mixture of short-chain fatty acids is utilized inefficiently, the heat being useful in cold climates but not under hot and humid conditions.

(Figure 4). The products of fermentative digestion, mainly acetic, propionic and butyric acids, are metabolized relatively inefficiently. This inefficient digestive–metabolic strategy limits the working capacity and athletic performance of the horse.

To provide more food energy in a form that is digested and metabolized more efficiently, grain concentrates are supplied as two meals a day to horses kept in stalls. These meals establish the feeding–fasting cycle (Figure 5), which is alien to the horse's nutritional heritage. The substitution of starch for fibre is confounded by meal-feeding, confinement in a stall and not being able to take a step while eating.

Nutritional Support of the Sick Horse

The first decision to be made in the nutritional support of a sick animal is whether it is hypo- or hyper-metabolic [3]. If it is eu-metabolic, the horse is probably not a candidate for nutritional support. If a mistake is made in determination of hypo- versus hyper-metabolism, the patient is likely to receive far too much or far too little nutritional support. In human hospitals, the energy expenditure of a patient is readily determined by respirometry at bedside, with the instruments set on a metabolic cart. Until such a service is available in equine hospitals, the attending veterinarian must reach a global decision based on a physical examination and history, weighing both against metabolic–hormonal

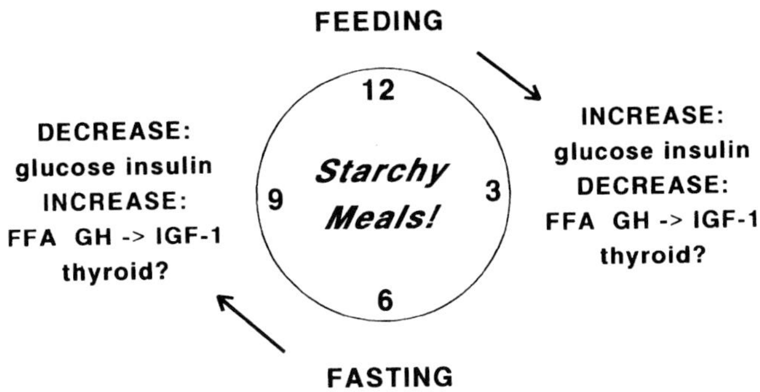

Figure 5. The feeding–fasting cycle of metabolic and hormonal changes, which is evident in plasma concentrations of metabolites and hormones, as it would occur in animals consuming two starchy meals. It would not be expected in horses grazing more or less continuously on roughages or fed meals consisting mainly of fibre and fat. It may be involved in several ways in the aetio-pathogenesis of certain diseases, as discussed in the text. Prolongation of the fasting stage leads to hypometabolism. FFA = free fatty acids, GH = growth hormone, IGF-1 = insulin-like growth factor 1.

descriptions such as the following, which are based mainly on metabolic studies in other species and clinical observations on the horse.

Hypometabolism

The daily feeding–fasting, glucose–fatty acid, or insulin–growth hormone cycle of meal-fed humans and animals presumably occurs in horses fed two meals of starch-rich concentrate a day (Figure 5). This cycle is the usual starting point for consideration of metabolism in the sick animal, with extension of the fasting phase becoming hypometabolism. The fire of life burns low and may approach basal or minimal metabolism, often about 50–70% of maintenance. (*Maintenance* is the daily energy intake needed to maintain a healthy adult at a constant body weight in a comfortable environment; it is usually about 1.5 times the basal or fasting metabolic rate.)

Glucose utilization falls to the same or a larger extent than energy metabolism, and the blood glucose concentration may be low or in the normal range. Certain tissues remain obligatory glucose users, notably brain, renal medulla and blood cells – also repairing tissues and certain cancers. The body mobilizes fatty acids for oxidation. It also mobilizes tissue protein to sustain gluconeogenesis, but this is kept to a minimum – in general protein is conserved. Plasma insulin falls, and the counter-regulatory hormones, especially growth hormone, rise and retard glucose utilization.

A hypometabolic horse eats and drinks little if at all. It is relatively inactive. The horse's ears may feel cold. Rectal temperature may be low or in the normal range. Immune competence subsides [4].

In this down-regulated, hypometabolic state, nutrition support should be introduced gradually and at a low level, perhaps 25–50% of maintenance per day, divided into several small meals. Excessive alimentation may lead to hyperglycemia and, perhaps, the *re-feeding syndrome* [5]. Although this hypophosphataemic, hypokalaemic syndrome has not been described in the horses, the common observation of death supervening after 3 days of re-feeding a starved horse suggests that careful monitoring of blood glucose, phosphorus and potassium should be used to guide the rate of re-alimentation.

Hypermetabolism

Hypermetabolism is likely to develop in horses suffering from trauma, sepsis and stress [3]. The metabolic rate may reach three times maintenance, supported by mobilization of nutrients, mainly fatty acids, from tissues. Intake is unable to match energy expenditure, so loss of weight and condition is usually much faster than in the hypometabolic animal. The release of cortisol tends to maintain blood glucose through promoting gluconeogenesis from amino acids; it also diminishes immune competence. The protein-sparing mechanisms of hypometabolism are missing, and muscle wastage may be evident within 2–3 days of the onset of hypermetabolism.

The hypermetabolic animal usually has an elevated temperature and a warm or hot skin. It exhibits physical and behavioral signs of stress. Its level of activity depends on the degrees of systemic involvement and sepsis. On the other hand, hypermetabolism may attend a severe local injury, such as a long bone fracture or head injury.

In contrast to hypometabolism, the introduction of nutrition support needs to be vigorous for hypermetabolic patients. Administration remains frequent and amounts start small but soon build, often to twice maintenance on the second or third day. Slurries have been developed for oral administration [6]. Inclusion of corn oil and dehydrated cottage cheese helps to achieve the desired high levels of energy density and protein quality.

Convalescence

Convalescence requires the repletion of tissue protein losses that have impaired functions of vital organs. Muscle wasting is evident as weakness, but losses of enzymes from the brain, liver and kidneys are equally serious although less readily evident. Restoration of immune competence is crucially important. Cumulative protein losses are likely to be greater following hypermetabolism than hypometabolism.

As a general guide, nutritional support for convalescence should last for about 2 weeks for uncomplicated surgeries, 2–4 weeks uncomplicated trauma, and up to 12 weeks for complicated trauma and sepsis. Rehabilitation from neglect and starvation is likely to take about 6 weeks, although compensatory growth following a prolonged period of undernutrition or malnutrition may continue for up to 6 months. (In our studies of vitamin A depletion of the dam and foal until weaning, compensatory growth was incomplete at 14 months.)

During stall rest, horses may lose 0.5–1% of metacarpal bone mineral content per week. Because bone mineral content is related to bone strength, rested horses should be re-introduced gradually to training. Our studies indicate that double the standard recommendation of 0.35% calcium on a dry matter (DM) basis is needed for bone mineral content to increase during training [7].

Nutritional Components of Diseases

Simple nutritional diseases are rare today (Table 3). Instead, nutritional components may be conditional factors in environmental domains of aetiologic complexes, such as host–heredity–pathogen–environment interactions. Such nutritional components may not be the proximate cause or the most important factor, but they should be identified because they are usually amendable to intervention or correction.

The term *production disease* was coined by Jack Payne, the English veterinarian who popularized metabolic profiles. It was applied to man-made diseases of livestock deriving from breeding, feeding and management for high production. The list started with milk fever, hypomagnesaemia and ketosis in dairy cattle and soon extended to bloat, laminitis and mastitis. The animal bred, fed and pushed for high production or performance reveals certain constitutional predispositions that approach a brink as performance increases, then give way and become manifested by lesions – structural or functional – and clinical signs.

The horse is the exempler for a type of production disease or *performance disease* that results from the convergence of multiple aetiologies on a single locus or

Table 3. **Specific signs of malnutrition in horses**

Crooked bones and large joints – calcium deficiency or excess; possibly copper and zinc deficiencies, vitamin D deficiency, vitamin A deficiency or excess, manganese deficiency.
Shifting lameness and softening and enlargement of jaw bones and facial crest – phosphorus excess.
Nervousness, muscle tremors and incoordination – depletion of magnesium and calcium, plus stress (transit).
Discoloured teeth, bone lesions, unthriftness – fluorine excess.
Goitre, enlarged thyroid gland, stillbirths, abnormal oestrus cycles – iodine deficiency or excess in pregnant mare.
Anaemia in foals – iron deficiency.
White muscle disease, possibly tying-up, possible abortion – deficiencies of selenium and vitamin E.
Blind staggers, colic, diarrhoea – acute selenium intoxication.
Loss of hair, mane, tail, cracked coronets – chronic selenium intoxication.
Incoordination, slow heart, missing beats – thiamine deficiency induced by bracken fern or Amprolium (a coccidiostat).
Poor hooves – possibly biotin deficiency.

Modified from Kronfeld [2]

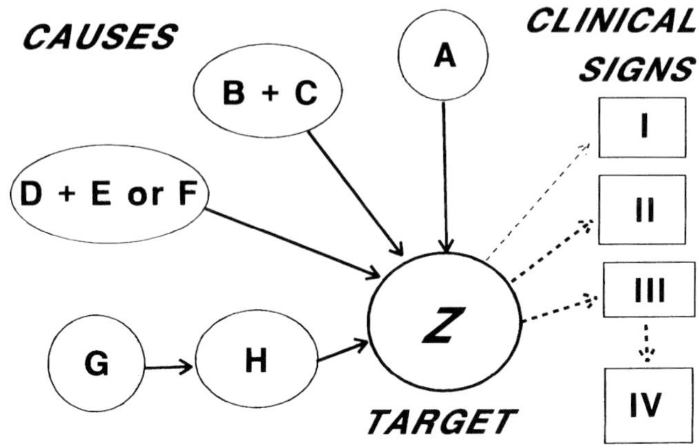

Figure 6. This aetio-pathogenic paradigm of several *performance diseases* proposes a central role for constitutional weaknesses or targets that have been accentuated by breeding, feeding and management for high levels of production and performance. Each target is susceptible to multiple etiologies, simple or multifactorial. In this illustration, cause A is direct, necessary and sufficient. Causes B and C are necessary but neither one is sufficient. Cause D is necessary but not sufficient. Cause G is indirect. Clinical manifestations of a deranged target may be direct (I, II and III) or indirect (IV). This paradigm is applied to production or performances diseases in the text.

target – an inherited or constitutional weakness of the species (Figure 6). Each of these disparate aetiologies may be simple or multifactorial in nature. For a concise exposition on the characterization of causality, see Rothman, 1986 [8].

The several characteristics of casual conditions include consistency. Apparent inconsistency, however, tends to confound studies of a disease – and clinical experiences with a disease – in which multiple aetiologies are possible but not differentiated. For example, if some horses presenting with intermittent equine rhabdomyolysis syndrome (ERS) do not respond to a specified nutritional intervention, that does not mean that all horses with ERS will not respond to this prophylactic measure – not always does not mean never. Different cases may have different aetiologies, so respond to different treatments – to each its own.

Another characteristic of causality is time's arrow. If A is associated with B, and A always preceds B, then A may be the cause of B, but B cannot be the cause of A. This condition is among the strongest characteristics of causality. In the case of some production–performance diseases, however, the existence of a constitutional weakness may precede the ostensible cause, and the target may be willing and ready to expose itself to any of the numerous causes that comes its way. The predisposition for mastitis in the dairy cow is a notable example. The target, a large udder, has hosted about 40 cases per 100 cows per year for the last 50 years, despite successful efforts to eradicate first one organism then another.

A less well documented example in the horse is the failure of widespread, threefold copper supplementation to deter the march of developmental orthopaedic disease (DOD). Horses carrying the predisposition for DOD apparently are ready to settle for any of several causes other than copper deficiency [9].

In this aetiologic paradigm, the horse has a set of target weaknesses, exaggerated by breeding and feeding for high performance, and each target is promiscuously susceptible to a variety of aetiologies or sets of causes. If we control one cause, another is almost sure to happen along. Multiple aetiologies, inadequate differential diagnosis, and inconsistent clinical responses bedevil practice as much as research.

The clinician cannot wait for the biochemist is an aphorism usually attributed to Elliot Joslin, the Boston physician who ameliorated diabetes mellitus by dietetics before the advent of insulin. His example is our guide. The practical nutritional task is not to unravel metabolic mysteries or aetiologic enigmas, but simply to detect the presence of a correctable nutritional component in a case. If this is a necessary causal factor, its correction will alleviate the disease. If it is not necessary, the rule-out will at least enable attention to be focused on other aspects of the disease.

Hyperkalaemic periodic paralysis

Many of the clinical manifestations of this inherited disease are associated with an elevated plasma potassium concentration. The episodes may be reduced in frequency and severity by depletion of body potassium through the gradual introduction of a low potassium diet, grass hay and oats, or a special dietary product (avoid legumes, alfalfa and soybean meal) (see Chapter 7).

Rationally, sodium restriction (simply halve or omit NaCl) should also depelete body potassium, because the kidney will exchange potassium to conserve sodium. My approach would be to test each diet change separately and observe the horse's response.

Fortunately, the performance of the affected type of Quarter Horse (halter class) is to be statuesque rather than athletic. Restriction of dietary sodium and potassium increases the risk of 'tying-up'.

Equine rhabdomyolysis syndrome (ERS)

This degenerative lesion of muscle fibres has multiple causes, including some apparently preventable by nutritional intervention (see Chapter 6). The horse's predisposition or constitutional weakness may lie in the functional integrity of muscle fiber membranes – the sarcolemma and sarcoplasmic reticulum. Both research and prophylaxis have been hampered not only by failure to discriminate between different etiologies but also by polymorphic clinical manifestations, which range from reluctant performances ('subclinical tying-up') to complete immobility.

In many cases, a casual condition may be inferred from the horse's response to intervention. Thus 'tying-up' may be characterized as dantrolene responsive, phenytoin responsive, thyroxine responsive, or nutritionally responsive.

Nutritionally responsive 'tying-up' is illustrated by two cases (my own hunters). A heavy, Warmblood gelding manifested 'tying-up' of varying degrees at every outing. The syndromes ranged from subclinical loss of impetus to hardened muscles and apparent severe pain, with burgundy urine and highly elevated serum creatine phosphokinase activity. These clinical signs were eliminated by an intravenous injection of selenium and vitamin E (Se-E). The treatment became effective unmistakably after a delay of 4 days. Its effectiveness lasted about 4 months and was repeatable.

A Thoroughbred mare suffered intermittently from 'tying-up' that could be prevented in two ways. The first was to withhold her commercial sweet feed the night before and morning of the hunt. This sweet feed was terminated after an experience with racing sled dogs that exhibited subclinical to severe 'tying-up' associated with carbohydrate-loading [10]. This canine 'tying-up' was eliminated by a change to a high fat diet. Accordingly the 'tying-up' mare was fed every day a mixture of small, light but husky (highly fibrous), lightly crimped oats plus corn oil (a coffee can plus half a cup, or 1200 g and 120 g, respectively). She received alfalfa hay in the morning and timothy hay in the evening. Fat adaptation was effective in preventing 'tying-up' and had the added advantage of improving her stamina.

The absence of hyperlacticacidaemia in a few horses exhibiting 'tying-up' has been taken to refute the glycogen-loading theory of this disease. This reasoning assumes the hyperlacticacidaemia is never present because it is not always present. It assumes the consistency of cause–effect relationships, which may be clouded in diseases with multiple etiologies. By now it should be clear that glycogen loading is not the sole, sufficient cause of all cases of 'tying-up'. Similarly, the early trials of Se-E treatment claimed effectiveness is only one-third of cases. Again, this inconsistency probably reflects multiple aetiologies.

The nutritional status of a horse exhibiting 'tying-up' can be evaluated as discussed below (see Chapter 6) in an attempt to identify a component amenable to intervention. Alternatively, the horse may be subjected to a series of nutritional tests, best taken one at a time, such as injection of Se-E (especially in Se deficient regions), withholding sweet feed before an event, replacement of sweet feed with fat-and-fibre (e.g. light oats and corn oil), supplementing with sodium bicarbonate (120 g twice a day stirred into the concentrate), or changing the cation–anion balance on the basis of blood and urine analysis. The specificity of the response may be tested by withdrawing then re-instituting the corrective procedure. A consistent and repeatable clinical response may be assumed to indicate which of the several possible etiologies is at work in this particular case. If a single nutritional intervention appears to be effective in every case of 'tying-up', perhaps the clinician has become 'the plaything of endless illusions'. (Claude Bernard, translated by Green, 1927) [11].

Developmental orthopaedic disease

The DOD complex appears to have multiple etiologies that converge on a single locus – an equine predisposition or constitutional weakness – the conversion of cartilage to bone, which then has several divergent clinical manifestations [9]. Numerous nutritional conditions may contribute to DOD [12, 13], but only experimentally induced copper deficiency or phosphorus excess, have appeared to be sufficient causes of DOD in the horse. An excess of food energy may be a necessary cause of DOD, but it is certainly not a sufficient cause [12].

In the 1970s, an epidemic of stunted, scruffy yearlings was traced to a point source in Colorado, which recommended feeding too little energy in the form of rough hay in order to prevent DOD. This syndrome was difficult to correct, because compensatory growth resulted in abrupt manifestation of flexural deformities (contracted tendons).

After this unkind practice had dwindled for a decade, it was revived in a more sophisticated form [14]. The young horses were selected from families prone to DOD, usually a wobbler syndrome. Cervical canals were examined radiographically for narrowness of malformation. The ration was restricted to 50–65% of the recommendations of the NRC [1], using a computer programme, and the horse was confined to a small, dark stall to discourage exercise. The claimed success rate was 100%, but details are lacking and names of horses and clients have been protected. The ethics of inducing partial starvation to prevent DOD (the end justifying the means) are questionable in regard to abuse of animals, deception of breeders, and safety of riders.

For the objective of preventing DOD, severe dietary restriction is unnecessary. A controlled study in Victoria revealed that restriction of energy intake to 100% of the NRC recommendation was sufficient to suppress the incidence of DOD evident at 128% of the NRC recommended energy intake [15]. The 128% level was described as 'high' [15], but it was the median in a range from 100 to 280% of the recommendation for growth in the USA [12]. There was no clustering of DOD towards the high end of that range, so overfeeding is not a sufficient cause of DOD, although it may be a necessary cause.

This series of experiments also indicated that DOD incidence was increased by high phosphorus but not high calcium, respectively 3.9 and 3.4 times the standards [1], or 2.1% calcium and 1.3% phosphorus on a DM basis [13]. Such high levels of phosphorus have not been seen in my experience (mainly in Pennsylvania, New Jersey, Maryland and Virgina). On the other hand, 2% calcium is not uncommon, because nearly all commercial concentrates in the USA are designed for use with grass hay and in fear of bran disease (nutritional hyperparathyroidism), which is rare today. The combination of 'grass' concentrates with alfalfa hay has been a common dietary association with DOD [12].

Clinical experience in the USA may be reconciled with the Victoria study on 22 weanling foals, in which the incidence of DOD was doubled on the high calcium diet, an increase that was not statistically significant. The doubling would have been significant with nine times the number of horses (giving 198), and I sense that it has been appreciable in the USA, because the number of yearlings at risk has been in the thousands.

Only one nutritional association with DOD has been identified by field surveys – copper deficiency [16, 17]. This finding led to the widespread use of copper in supplements at three times the national standard [1]. Other repeatable associations in my experience in Pennsylvania, Virginia and nearby states have been high grain feeding (70% or more of total food energy), alfalfa hay fed with a concentrate designed for use with grass hay (too much calcium and protein), concentrates with a high zinc to calcium ratio (more than 5:1), and excessive vitamin A supplementation (100 times the minimum requirement).

Starch-rich meals may influence DOD through exaggeration of the feeding–fasting cycle and interactions with hormones, such as thyroxine, insulin and growth hormone [12]. Growth hormone injections into rats makes the physis grow wider, which is the basis of the tibia bioassay. Selection for precocious growth may incidentally select for excessive growth hormone that may increase the risk of DOD, especially in young horses receiving 70% energy in the form of concentrates (abundant in starch), as recommended by the NRC [1]. In this view, the chemical form of food energy – hydrolyzable carbohydrate versus fermented carbohydrate and fat – should be kept in mind when testing any hypothesis concerning energy intake and DOD.

Gastric ulcers

Gastric ulcers have been found in 90% of 2-year-olds after 3 months of training, but none at the start of training [18]. Stall confinement, stationary feeding, and two starchy meals a day are alien to the horse's nutritional heritage. Would these ulcers be prevented by numerous small meals, by replacing starch with fat-and-fibre, and by allowing the horse to move as it eats?

Chronic obstructive pulmonary disease (COPD)

A potentially important component of the pathogenesis of COPD is *apoptosis*: programmed cell death that requires energy (in contrast to degenerative necrosis). Apoptosis is stimulated by insulin-like growth factor-1, which is released by growth hormone. Thus, one might speculate that a feeding–fasting cycle exaggerated by two starchy meals per day could contribute to COPD. Any such contribution would be confounded, of course, by other aspects of stall confinement.

Fermentative disorders: diarrhoea, colic and laminitis

Overload of hydrolyzable carbohydrates (abundant in grain and molasses) or excessive amounts of rapidly fermentable carbohydrates (abundant in beet pulp) may lead to rapid fermentation in which lactic acid accumulates, especially as the fall in pH kills the small bacteria that convert lactate to acetate (Figure 4).

Lactic acid is absorbed poorly, so attracts water into the large bowel, softening the faeces and sometimes resulting in osmotic diarrhoea. Expansion of bowel contents and rapid production of gas may distend the bowel and contribute to colic. Surveys have associated colic with grain feeding [19]. Acidity may break down bacteria, releasing endotoxin and contributing to laminitis and founder [20 and Chapter 10].

Although diarrhoea, colic and laminitis have causes other than rapid fermentation, the nutritional causes may be the most readily amendable to intervention. Replacement of hydrolyzable and rapidly fermentable carbohydrates (Figure 3) with slowly fermented carbohydrates (abundant in mature hay) and fat has been recommended [21, 22]. High fat-concentrate diets, which have been used to provide 75% of digestible energy (DE) in Texas, have been sustained by fibrous Bermuda grass hay. Complete feeds for exercise studies and fat-and-fibre supplements for pasture studies have been based on mature hay or straw, which are abundant in slowly fermented fibres that ensure slow and constant fermentation [22].

The most common view of good quality roughage is exemplified by young timothy hay. Because it contains considerable rapidly fermentable carbohydrates, young timothy hay is best suited for use with little or no supplementation by grain concentrates. It is less able than mature hay, which contains slowly fermentable fibers, to support a high level of supplementation with grain (abundant in hydrolyzable starch) or beet pulp (abundant in rapidly fermentable carbohydrates), which tend to promote rapid fermentation. Thus, what constitutes a good hay depends on its intended use – young hay is best with little or no supplementation, mature hay is more able to support a high level of supplementary concentrates.

Humane and Legal Implications

Veterinarians may be called as expert witnesses in cases concerning horses that may have been neglected or deliberately abused. A horse may have been left without water, feed or shelter for certain periods. The wholesomeness and nutritional value of the feed and water may be in question. The condition of the horse itself may need to be evaluated by physical examination and analysis of blood and urine, or by post mortem. In some jurisdictions, failure of the person responsible for a horse to call for the assistance of a veterinarian in a timely way is grounds for prosecution.

In one illustrative case, an emaciated Thoroughbred mare was found recumbent in a paddock with six other horses in good condition. The horses had free access to a round bale of good hay, and the down horse had been observed eating by farm employees, who had failed to observe its loss of condition. The referring veterinarian used the word starvation, and the attending clinician wrote malnutrition in the medical record. The mare died after 3 days re-feeding and hospital care. The gross post mortem report declared that no potential cause of death was found except emaciation due to starvation.

A veterinary technician called the county animal welfare officer, and the county prosecutor charged the farm manager with starving the horse and with failing to obtain veterinary assistance in a timely way. Three weeks later the somewhat tardy report of histologic examination described numerous emboli and small abscesses in the lungs. At this point the significance of a large abscess beneath the scapula, which had been found in the gross post mortem examination, became more apparent. Also becoming more emphatic was the need for careful identification of the cause(s) of emaciation (Table 2), a point I made to my professional colleagues before speaking on behalf of the farm manager to the county prosecutor.

Methods of Assessment

The customary approaches to nutritional assessment are dietary, anthropometric (zoometric or morphometric), biochemical, physiological, behavioural and clinical [23]. For equine practice, additional emphasis is placed on adding body weight, body condition score, dietary history and ration evaluation to the clinical or physical examination of the animal. The use of laboratory aids is discretionary, because many are currently more useful in research than in practice. Moreover, use of blood and urine data is fraught with difficulties in execution, timeliness and interpretation. Facility with ration evaluation and re-formulation requires extra training and computer skills, Thus a clinician may often choose to rely on a *subjective global assessment* [23, 24]. Human global assessment emphasizes changes in weight, diet, gastro-intestinal functions, muscle strength and metabolic demands (hypo- or hyper-metabolism).

My orientation of nutrition practice first evaluates the animal's nature and the owner's desired performance in order to set nutritional goals that are achieved through diet formulation and feeding management (Figure 1). Veterinarians know in advance much about the horse's nature. It evolved as a gregarious grazer, with its digestive system and metabolism adapted accordingly. We should not overlook the fact that humans customarily house and feed the horse in ways contrary to its nature. We should not assume in advance that we know exactly what the owner wants of the horse, or what the employees are doing with the horse. Precise and accurate information is not always easy to obtain. One usually starts with the client (the owner, trainer or farm manager), then, if allowed, seek confirmation from employees.

Interviewing

In human clinical and epidemiologic nutrition, questionnaires to estimate nutritional status by interviews are detailed and need to be validated [23]. Similar questionnaires have been validated for dogs and cats but not horses. Nevertheless, most large animal veterinarians who practice nutrition use a spreadsheet with boxes for the data needed to fit a computer program for ration evaluation, and this document is used to guide the interview regarding past and current diet(s). This regimentation has the disadvantage that it imposes its own system upon the client, who may have none or a different one.

Another approach is to offer minimal prompts to start the client describing the performance targets, feeding management and dietics. Using this approach, I have all too often found on breeding farms that are a careful feeding program is in place for the young, growing horses, but the brood mares are fed unsystematically and with relatively less care.

Another common experience is that clients and employees will try to please the interviewer by second-guessing the right or assumed to be desired answers. My approach is to interview three persons independently and locate the truth by trigonometry.

Facilities

If possible, I visit the horse's quarters, because facilities and management often contribute to nutritional problems. Usually, if a crucial item is awry, it is not noticed and not mentioned. Only a visit enables its identification.

One must inspect the buildings, yards, pastures and fences. Then examine the feedbins, watering system, and hay storage. In one case, I visited a stud farm that was standing two of the top Thoroughbred sires in the world. Many incumbents had chronic diarrhoea and were too thin for optimal breeding performance. The recitations of the resident veterinarian had revealed nothing remarkable, indeed nothing short of superior management. A visit revealed pigeons galore, with pigeon droppings abundant on the hay and bedding. The owner liked the pigeons and rejected my recommendation to examine the avian droppings for salmonella.

Animal(s)

Physical examination

The field of nutrition abounds with a variety of volunteers, and the unique advantage of a veterinarian lies in the clinical examination of the animal. It should be viewed first from a distance to evaluate demeanor, behaviour and comportment. The type, breed, sex and age should be noted.

The physical examination should be sufficient for the case. If a nutritional component is suspected, examination of the mouth and gastrointestinal system must be thorough. Prehension, mastication and swallowing should be carefully observed. Food falling out of the mouth during chewing may signify sharp edged teeth or central nervous involvement. The case may also require evaluation of the locomotor system. Bad feet or lameness may reduce the feed or water intake of a grazing animal.

Water status. The horse's access to water should be noted and, if possible, the horse should be observed to drink. It may need to be offered water in a bucket on the floor. Underfeeding reduces water intake, following the usual rule of 1 L/Mcal of energy.

Common signs of dehydration are loss of skin turgor, slow capillary refill rate, a thready or weak pulse, and sunken eyes. Pinching a fold or tent of skin over the point of the shoulder provides a test for skin turgor. Repeated tenting on an endurance horse may confound the test. Older horses may have looser skin.

Unfortunately, clinical signs of dehydration are not prominent until perhaps 7 or 8% of body water has been lost, when performance is already impaired. The impact on performance will depend on the distribution of the water depletion; 24 L is an 8% loss from 300 L of total body water, a 20% loss from 120 L of extracellular water, and a 40% loss from 60 L of plasma water.

Crucially important in regard to the horse's voluntary water intake is the osmotic character of the dehydration. Hypertonic sweat may deplete extracellular electrolytes more than water, and the resulting hypo-osmotic extracellular fluid will inhibit thirst and prolong dehydration.

Metabolic rate and energy balance. Especially important in nutritional assessment are rectal temperature, heart rate and respiration rate as indices of metabolic rate. Also relevant to metabolic rate are the horse's level of spontaneous activity and reactions to handling.

Body weight should be determined with an electronic balance. A load cell is near each corner and should be capable of measuring one-third of the horse's weight, because approximately two-thirds rests on the front feet. If tape measurements of girth and length predict a weight more than the scale weight, then the difference may reflect weight lost or body shape. In humans, attention is given to indices calculated from weight and height, for example, Quetelet's *body mass index*, weight (kg)/height $(cm)^2$. Similar indices, such as weight/length $\times$ girth, could be useful in the horse.

The body condition score is crucial and should be standardized (Table 1). Subcutaneous fat is palpated over the ribs, beside the vertebral column over the rump, around the tailhead, and on the neck. Both weight and condition score are signs of energy balance. They should be recorded weekly for a competitive equine athlete, a sick horse, or a valuable horse, and should be used to adjust the ration to achieve the desired weight and condition.

Losses (or gains) in body weight or condition may be obtained in the history. Increased metabolic needs are inferred from fever, sepsis, trauma and burns, as well as growth, lactation or stress (showing, hunting or racing), or exposure to cold and wind. Increased metabolic losses should be noted, such as water and electrolyte depletions in sweat or persistent diarrhoea, or protein losses in blood or exudates from wounds. Oedema is a sign of water retention, sodium overload, or protein loss.

Protein depeletion. Muscle wasting (cachexia, sarcopaenia) and loss of strength are signs of protein depletion. Wasting is most easily seen and palpated in muscles overlying bone, such as the temporal, masseter and gluteals. Loss of muscle (wasting) is far more serious clinically than loss of fat (condition).

Strength is tested most easily by the horse's ability to stand when pushed sideways. The horse's balance may also be disturbed by pulling its tail sideways. Practiced eyes can detect loss of strength at the walk – the feet are dragged or pushed, placement is imprecise. These subtle signs are lost when the horse is roused to a trot, unless the horse is very weak.

Other signs. More specific forms of malnutrition are seen less often in practice. Specific signs are summarized in Table 3.

Imaging

Radiographic estimation of bone mineral density helps to evaluate the skeletal system's response to age, nutrition and training. Metacarpal bone mineral density reaches its maximal value at 6 years of age [25]. It is highly correlated with breaking load, bone strength and elasticity.

In a study of training, bone mineral density increased about 6% after 12 weeks in horses fed twice the NRC recommended level of Ca but not those fed the standard level [7]. Bone mineral density decreased about the same amount with de-training, keeping the horse in a stall. Stall rest for lameness may have a similar effect on bone density and strength, and this should be kept in mind when the horse returns to work.

Metacarpal bone mineral density was estimated with radiographs, aluminium wedges and an imaging program in our studies [7]. Bone mineral loss can be tracked less precisely by a series of radiographs with wedges, but without the expensive imaging equipment. Our attempts to use ultrasonography to estimate bone density were unsuccessful.

Blood and urine data

Betting versus statistics. What are the odds of blood and urine data being useful? These measures are subject to errors arising from sampling, transport, analysis and interpretation [23]. Unless stated otherwise, blood samples are assumed to have been taken from a quiet, resting horse. Excitement and exercise release adrenaline, which may raise the haematocrit and plasma concentrations of glucose, lactate, free fatty acids and triglycerides. Transport may allow potassium and phosphorus to leak from cells and raise serum concentrations. Splitting samples and obtaining analyses from several laboratories is disquieting; 30% differences between duplicates (poor precision) and between laboratories (dubious accuracy) for Cu, Zn and Se are common and usually tolerated, but 5% differences between duplicates and 10% differences between laboratories for plasma glucose or cholesterol usually go unnoticed. Given these variations or errors, a prudent practitioner will use a laboratory that provides its own reference ranges for all measured variables. Some reference ranges should be age-related, for example, for serum Ca, P, Mg and Se.

The most common reference range is a 95% confidence interval, which is determined parametrically as two standard deviations above and below the mean. With reference to this range, the laboratory data are characterized as normal, high or low (Table 4). Assuming a normal distribution, there are 2.5% of values from normal horses at each end that are called high or low, or odds of one in 20 that a normal value will be declared abnormal. If 20 variables are measured, there are 20 chances in 20 that a value for a normal horse will be declared abnormal.

Many blood variables are not distributed normally (a symmetrical bell-shaped

Table 4. **Potential evaluation of the nutritive status of the horse.**

Nutrient	*Analytical base*	*Substance and dimension*	*Under supply*	*Normal range*	*Over supply*
Water	Plasma	Protein; g/dL	> 7.5[1]	6–7	> 30–40
	Blood	Hematocrit; %		35–42	
Protein	Blood	Urea; mmol/L	< 3.4	3.4–5.1	
Calcium	Urine	Ca; mmol/L	< 6.25		
		Ca:Creatinine[2]	< 0.3		
Phosphorus	Plasma	inorg. P; mmol/L			
		at 2 years	< 1.8	1.8–2.56	
		adult	< 0.96	0.96–1.6	> 6[3]
Magnesium	Plasma	Mg; mg/dl	< 1.5	1.5–2.5	> 2.5
Sodium	Urine	Na; mmol/L	< 8.8	35.2–88	> 300
		Na; Creatinine[2]	< 0.2		
Potassium	Plasma	K; mmol/L	< (12)[4]		
	Urine	K; mmol/L	< 26		
		K; Creatinine[2]	< 1.0		
Iron	Blood	Hb; g/dL[5]		11–17	
	Serum	Fe; μmol/L	< 3.58	17.9–26.85	
Copper	Plasma	Cu; μmol/L	< 7.85	10.99–23.55	
	Liver	Cu; μg/g TS	< 10	25–200	
Zinc	Plasma	Zn; μg/dL Foal	< 70		> 800
		Adult	< 60	130	
Iodine	Serum	PBJ; μg/dL		1.5–2.0	
Selenium	Plasma	Se; μg/dL	7	10–14	
Vitamin A	Plasma	Retinol IE/dL	< 60	80–150	> 150
	Liver	Retinol IE/g uS	< 20	150–500	> 2000
Vitamin D	Plasma	Ca; mmol/L[6]			> 3.5
		inorg. P; mmol/L			> 2.24
Vitamin E	Plasma	Tocopherol; mg/dl		0.2–0.7	
Vitamin C	Plasma	Ascorbic acid; mg/dl		0.7–0.9	
Folic acid	Serum	Folate; μg/dL		0.02–0.015	

1 Renal or enteral loss of protein.
2 After physical strain was discounted.
3 Cu less than 1.65 μmol/L.
4 Possibly only temporary.
5 Not specific.
6 Adult, not specific.
Modified from Reference [32], p. 76.

curve). Such variables should have reference ranges determined non-parametrically around a median value. Clinicians may be helped more if all reference ranges, parametric and non-parametric, were expressed in quintiles rather than the current reference ranges.

Over the last two decades, interpretation of laboratory data has emphasized *sensitivity*, the proportion of individuals with malnutrition who have positive tests for malnutrition, and *specificity*, the proportion of individuals without malnutrition who have negative tests [23]. (This specificity should not be confused with analytical specificity, which refers only to measurement of the component of interest.) Both specificity and sensitivity are based on a binary interpretation of a measurement or test, which must be positive or negative (albeit truly or falsely). But a threshold between normal and abnormal, positive or negative, is seldom sharp and often arbitrary. Instead, the zone between health and ill-health is often fuzzy, uncertain or vague, and better interpreted in terms of *fuzzy logic* [26].

Fuzzy logic is a rigorous, quantitative method of analysing imprecise inputs that have uncertain or vague relationships to outcomes [28]. For example, instead of thinking that a plasma creatinine concentration has a cut-off at 159 μmol/L, so that 150 μmol/L is normal but 168 or 274 μmol/L are abnormal, we might better think that the abnormal: normal odds are 80:20 for 150 μmol/L, 85:15 for 168 μmol/L, and 98:2 for 274 μmol/L. Most equine clinicians do not need the statistical sophistication of formal fuzzy logic to evaluate the diagnostic significance of laboratory data – their experience with odds in betting on races is more than good enough.

In short, instead of classifying a laboratory datum as normal or abnormal, an equine clinician should guess at the odds of it being abnormal – with one eye on the horse, of course.

Physiological versus empirical. Blood analysis in the form of a *metabolic profile* has been shown to predict nutritional status – energy, protein, Ca and P – in dairy cows by means of multiple regression equations [27]. The relationships were empirical; for example, serum cholesterol and inorganic P were the two best indices of energy intake, better than the physiologically appealing blood concentrations of glucose, free fatty acids, and β-hydroxybutyrate. Similarly, the Ca intake was predicted better by serum Mg than by serum Ca, which was closely regulated. No similar predictive relationships have been established for horses. The warning is clear, however: homeostatic regulation of blood concentrations of nutrients and metabolites may preclude finding simple relationships to nutrient intakes.

Energy status. A low energy status is characterized by ketosis in most species but not the horse. Instead, an underfed horse usually develops hyperlipidaemia and hyperbilirubinaemia [28, Chapter 2]. If the hyperbilirubinaemia is in excess of the level predicted from the regression on free fatty acids and triglycerides, concurrent liver damage may be inferred. Hyperlipaemia may be grossly evident as an opalescence of the separated serum (see Chapter 2).

Underfeeding also depresses the D-xylose absorption test [29]. It has been shown in horses to diminish immune tests, such as the neutrophil phagocytosis, lymphocyte transformation and delayed skin hypersensitivity tests [4]. Underfeeding leads to loss of tissue proteins, as well as fat, and depression of immune tests are usually used as signs of protein depletion.

Protein status. A low protein status is characterized by low plasma albumin in most species but not the horse. The protein intake is reflected in the serum urea concentration in the short run, and perhaps to a lesser extent by erythropoietic indices in the long run.

In our studies (Thiers and Kronfeld, unpublished data), the blood variable most responsive to a change in dietary protein has been the urea:creatinine ratio, which has responded as quickly as the fractional excretion of urea. Serum urea concentration is a function of protein intake (deamination of amino acids and urea synthesis) and renal clearance. Creatinine is produced by muscle activity, the breakdown of creatine phosphate, which is assumed to be more or less constant, and renal clearance. So, creatinine can be used to devolve the renal clearance component in urea concentration, hence giving clearer reflection of protein intake.

Daily urine creatinine excretion has been used as an index of muscle mass in humans [23]. Similarly, daily routine excretion of 3-methyl-histidine, which is released during degradation of actin and myosin in muscle, has also been used to estimate muscle mass and any predominance of protein degradation over synthesis that may be associated with the protein depletion in humans. Urinary nitrogen excretion, which largely represents urea, increases when protein is catabolized during exercise, stress, infection, sepsis or trauma.

In short, blood and urine analysis and immune tests may provide useful confirmation, but attention to muscle wasting and loss of strength will usually reveal clinically serious protein depletion, especially in a hypermetabolic horse.

Mineral status. A comprehensive series of studies on water and mineral metabolism in the horse has been published in German, with English summaries and extensive tables and figures that are readily understood with little or no knowledge of the language [30]. Serial analyses of blood and urine are embellished by frequent use of renal clearances and creatinine ratios (see below). The effects of feeding and exercise are described. Some of the simpler data are summarized here (Table 4).

Blood or urine concentrations may reflect the status of certain minerals but not others. Yearlings grazing pastures deficient in P, Cu, Zn and Se have had significant depressions of serum concentrations of these elements [31]. In pregnant mares, however, higher serum inorganic P concentrates were found in those consuming pasture only than in those supplemented with a concentrate containing abundant P [32]. These mares also exhibited paradoxical phosphaturia associated with calciuria, so it was concluded that pregnant mares consuming a phosphorus deficient diet would mobilize P and Ca from bone and provide adequate P to the foetus.

Daily urine collections, hence mineral outputs, are desirable to assess mineral status, but usually inconvenient for the horse. A snap-shot picture is provided by the fractional excretion (FE) or creatinine ratio, which compares simultaneous plasma (P) and urine (U) concentrations of metabolite or mineral (M) and creatinine (C):

$$FE = \{[M_U]/[C_U]\}/\{M_P]/[C_P]\} = M_U \times C_P/M_P \times C_U$$

The common practice of presenting only the simplified cross-product formula obscures the physiological intention of the creatinine ratio. (This mathematical obfuscation also prevails in cross-product calculations of the odds ratio in epidemiology and marker digestibilities in nutrition.) Physiologically, the mineral is expressed on a creatinine basis rather than a water basis because water but not creatinine is reabsorbed by the kidney, and because the kidney's retention of the mineral relative to creatinine is taken to reflect the mineral's status.

A high FE is taken to mean that the kidney is eliminating the mineral, so we infer a surfeit in the body. Similarly, a low FE indicates retention, so we infer a deficit. Physiology may play tricks, however: a high FE for potassium, for example, may indicate a potassium surfeit or a sodium deficit, with K being exchanged for Na to increase Na retention. Measures of FE are affected by feeding, excercise, the handling of the horse and the taking of urine samples [30, Chapter 6]. So once again book values are less useful than one's own reference range to detect deviations from normal.

Function tests for trace elements are not used in equine practice at this time but are not difficult and may soon become available. The pattern is to observe a functional response to a physiological dose of the element [23]. Glucose tolerance tests are conducted before and after a dose of chromium. Serum ceruloplasmin activity is assayed before and after a dose of copper. Superoxide dismutase in serum and carbonic anhydrase in erythrocytes are measured before and after a dose of zinc. Glutathione peroxidase is measured before and after a dose of selenium. Transferrin saturation and serum ferritin are measured before and after a dose of iron. Thyroxine and tri-iodthyronine are measured before and after a dose of iodine.

Dehydration. The simplest aid is a microhaematocrit. The packed cell volume (PCV) is read, the tube broken, and the plasma blown on to the lens of a refractometer. The instrument may be calibrated to read total solids or total protein. The instrument measures total solids, and we want to know total protein, which comprises over 95% of total solids. The vascular system contains the serum proteins, so a high total protein concentration is suggestive of haemo-concentration. The PCV is liable to fluctuate with splenic concentrations in the horse, but since this information is immediately available with the horse in full view, the PCV is likely to be interpreted correctly.

Using laboratory data, water volumes and shifts may be inferred from serum albumin, sodium and urea. These substances distribute respectively in plasma water, extracellular water, and total body water. If all are increased to the same relative degree, a corresponding decrease in total body water may be inferred. If an increase is found in plasma albumin but not sodium or urea, the water loss may be confined to the blood. If plasma albumin is increased but sodium is decreased, water may have shifted to the interstitial space. An increase in serum sodium concentration implies that water will be moving from cells to the extracellular compartment, and vice versa. These indications are used cautiously and with full realization that each of these variables is subject to many influences in addition to water volumes and shifts.

Vitamins. Requirements for vitamins A, D and E, thiamin and riboflavin are specified by the NRC [1]. Other vitamins of interest in the horse are biotin and folic acid. The status of these vitamins is seldom if ever assessed in equine practice.

Erythrocyte transketolase and elevated serum pyruvate are indices of thiamin deficiency and may be measured in horses suspected to have been poisoned by antithiamine agents, such as amprolium (a coccidiostat) or caffeic acid (present in bracken fern, horse tail and yellow star thistle). The history, signs, availability of drug or plant, and response to thiamin administration are usually enough to make a secure clinical diagnosis, but laboratory confirmation may be desired for legal purposes [1, 33].

Assessment of the other vitamins named above remains in research rather than the clinic. Tests for vitamin A and vitamin E status are clinically important, however, and relatively simple.

The relative dose response (RDR) test for vitamin A is calculated from serum retinol concentration before and after an oral dose of vitamin A palmitate [34]. Vitamin A depletion is detected better by the RDR test than by serum retinol concentration in adult horses but not neonatal foals. The RDR test has been used to demonstrate depletion of vitamin A during the winter, which could be alleviated by oral administration of vitamin A palmitate but not by a water-dispersible form of β-carotene. Twice the NRC requirement for vitamin A was needed during repletion to match the vitamin A status of horses on green pastures, which provide abundant β-carotene. Vitamin A depletion was associated with a higher pregnancy loss rate, more retained placentas, lower birth weight foals, and more flexural deformities in young foals [35].

Vitamins E status may be inferred from serum α-tocopherol concentration in horses. More precise information on absorption and depletion may be obtained by an oral vitamin E tolerance test (OVETT), which has been applied to the horse [36]. Serum (or heparinized plasma) concentration of α-tocopherol is assayed three times in 24 hours for a baseline, an oral dose of free α-tocopherol is given, and a series of blood samples are taken at 3, 6, 9, 12 and 24 hours for assay. The concentration–time curve is used to calculate several parameters, such as the peak, the time to the peak, and the area subtended by the increments.

An apparently inherited form of equine degenerative myeloencephalopathy has been characterized by low plasma α-tocopherol and favourable clinical responses to vitamin E administration [37]. The OVETT demonstrates that absorption is not affected [36].

Ration Evaluation

The traditional approach is to determine amounts of concentrates and hays consumed, then estimate pasture intake by difference [38–40]. The cumulative errors are potentially huge, especially for horses with access to pasture, but not generally highlighted by nutritionists or, worse, epidemiologists who construct statistical masterpieces on shoddy data. Current uses of computer programs tend to conceal the errors. This is unfortunate because computer programs could be readily designed to cope with variation, to enable sensitivity analysis (assumption of reasonable ranges including all errors), and to provide a realistic picture of the lack of precision in ration evaluation.

Volumes, weights and samples

In practice, one visits the farm or stable and interviews the staff to determine the volumes of hays, concentrates and other supplements that are offered and, if possible, any amounts not consumed. At least two, preferably five, of these volume measures (cans or cups of concentrates, flakes or bales of hay) are weighed. At least two samples of each concentrate and five samples of each hay are taken. Pastures are usually sampled by walking the two diagonals and clipping the grasses and legumes, neglecting the weeds, every 10 paces. Duplicate sub-samples of concentrates, hays and pastures are submitted for proximate and mineral analyses.

Pasture intake by difference

For a horse that has access to pasture, the daily intakes of all hays and concentrates must be determined, so that the pasture intake can be estimated by difference. To estimate this difference, the individual horse is assumed to consume the mean DE intake specified for its weight, age and physiological condition (maintenance, growth, pregnancy, lactation and light, moderate or hard work) by the NRC [1] or some other authority, and the DE provided by the estimated intakes of hay and concentrate is subtracted to leave the DE intake in the form of pasture:

$$\text{DE pasture} = \text{mean total DE intake (assumed)} - \text{DE hay} - \text{DE concentrate}$$

The amount of pasture estimated by difference is often negative for horses that have been observed to graze, which suggests the presence of errors. Some errors may exist in the estimates of DE provided by hays and concentrates. The two greatest errors, however, relate to the mean DE intake. Some mean DE intakes may be too low, for example, for lactation or hard work. More serious is neglect of the variation between animals, that is, the distribution of DE requirements, such as the 90% confidence interval, around the mean. No estimate of the coefficient of variation (CV), is given for the DE requirement by the NRC, but CVs of 14% for maintenance up to 27% for the weanling foal may be calculated from the table of expected daily consumptions of air-dried feed [1]. Thus the 90% confidence intervals for DE intakes are likely to range from 75–125% to 52–148% of the means for adults at maintenance and for the weanling foal, respectively. These upper and lower limits of reasonable ranges should be employed, as well as the mean, in estimating the pasture intake, and these three estimates of pasture intake should be used in ration evaluation.

This error by difference is exacerbated if the horse that is allowed access to pasture also consumes known amounts of hay and concentrate (Figure 7). Let us say that hay and concentrate provide half of the mean daily DE intake, and that this half is well determined. Now all of the variation in daily DE intake is concentrated into the half derived from pasture and the relative errors in estimation by difference are doubled. Would you believe 8% of the mean DE intake for one

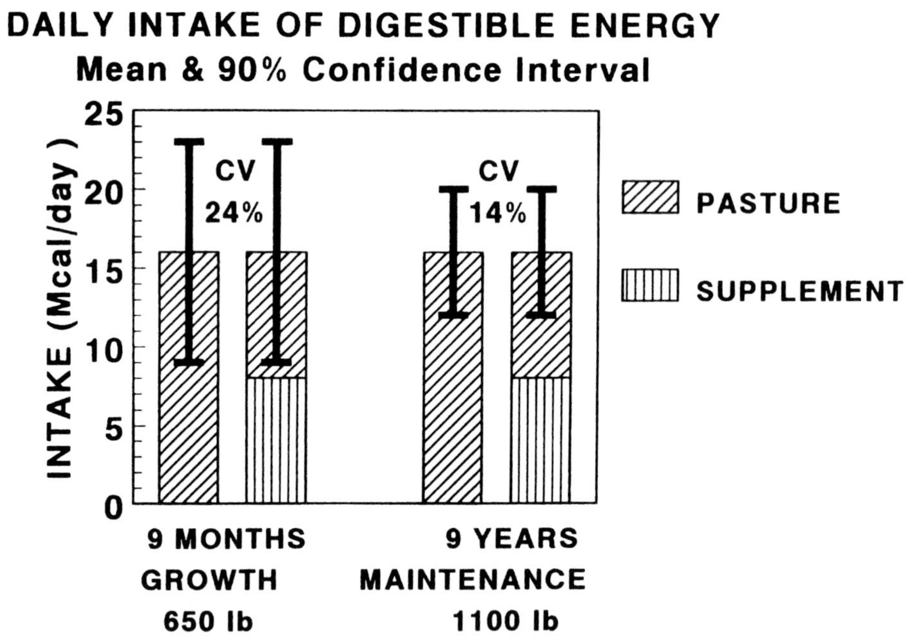

Figure 7. Emphasis in ration evaluation is placed traditionally on the mean intake of digestable energy (DE) (bars), for example, in estimating pasture intake by difference. Virtually overlooked has been the large variation from horse to horse, shown here as the 90% confidence interval (flags on bars). A mean intake of 16.0 Mcal DE/day is shared by an adult at maintainance (right pair of bars) and by the young growing horse (left pair of bars), but the variation is much greater for the latter, which is at risk of DOD and other complaints. If pasture is being estimated, the absolute variation remains the same when a supplement is fed, but the relative variation increases; for example, the percentage variation doubles if the supplement provides half of the daily DE intake (right bars in each pair).

out of 20 weanling foals and 196% for another one out of the same 20 foals, are candidates for DOD?

To evaluate this error in estimating pasture intake by difference, one should use sensitivity analysis by performing the same calculations for the mean and for the upper and lower limits of the 90% confidence interval of estimated DE intake. For example, subtract the known intakes of DE from hay and concentrate, say 7.2 Mcal, from the mean DE intake of 14.4 Mcal [1], to find that 7.2 Mcal are consumed in the form of pasture. Assuming 2 Mcal/kg DM, the pasture intake is 3.6 kg of DM, for this mean foal. Now if we have 20 foals, the DE intake on one is likely to be 7.5 Mcal (52% of the mean), and the pasture intake will be estimated by difference as 0.3 Mcal or 0.15 kg DM for this lean foal. Moreover, from the same 20 foals, another should have a DE intake of 21.3 Mcal, and a pasture intake by difference of 14.1 Mcal or 7.05 kg DM for this fine foal.

In summary, instead of evaluating only one mean ration, calculate also the upper and lower estimates. First, evaluate the mean, say 2 kg DM (6.6 Mcal DE) of concentrate, 0.6 kg DM (1.2 Mcal) of hay, 3.6 kg DM (7.2 Mcal) of pasture, as is the usual procedure [39, 40]. Then also evaluate another two estimates of the ration that represent the limits of the 90% confidence interval of total DE intake, by substituting 0.15 kg DM (0.3 Mcal) or 7.05 kg DM (14.1 Mcal) for the mean estimate of pasture intake. Finding these three results does not require three times the work; it takes only a moment to change one datum and re-run the computer program.

Proximate and mineral analysis

The feed samples are sent to a laboratory that analyses pasture, and the routine profile is likely to be suitable for ruminants (for dairy cattle in the US, reflecting the importance of the Dairy Herd Improvement Association). Routine profiles usually include DM, crude protein (CP), acid detergent fiber (ADF), neutral detergent fiber (NDF), non-structural carbohydrates (NSC, by difference), ether extract (EE or crude fat), ash, Ca, Mg, P, Na and K. Trace element assays are usually available and Cu, Zn and Se are often requested for the horse together with Fe, Mn, Mb, I and S, depending on cost.

The main inadequacy of ruminant nutrient profiles for the horse are the proximate assays for carbohydrates (Figure 3). For a hind-gut fermenter, the two main physiological groups would be hydrolyzed carbohydrates (CHO-H) and fermented carbohydrates (CHO-F), since CHO-H yields mainly glucose, whereas CHO-F yields mainly acetate, propionate and butyrate. Digestive and metabolic processes are much more efficient for CHO-H than for CHO-F [41]. Rates of fermentation of various carbohydrates form a continuum, but it is useful to split them into two groups, fast, in which lactic acid tends to accumulate, and slow, which yields mainly acetic acid (Figure 4).

The NSC includes the CHO-H (sugars and hydrolyzable starches) plus some CHO-F (oligosaccharides and resistant starches). Pending the ready availability

***Table 5.* Weighted averages (see text): The total diet can now be calculated on a DE or DM basis using weighted averages**

Nutrient	Conc.	Hay	Pasture	Total
	2.0 kg	0.6 kg	3.6 kg	6.6 kg DM
CP, g/kg	150 × 2 +	100 × 0.6 +	120 × 3.6 =	792 ÷ 6.6 = 12.0
Ca, g/kg	10 × 2 +	3 × 0.6 +	4 × 3.6 =	36.2 ÷ 6.6 = 5.5

of more accurate assays of CHO-H, arbitrary amounts of NSC may be shifted to the NDF [44], for example:

$$\text{CHO-H} = h \times \text{NSC}$$

$$\text{CHO-F} = \text{NDF} + (h \times \text{NSC}),$$

where h is 0.66 for roughness and 0.33 for concentrates.

Weighted averages are found for dry matter, energy and all measured nutrients. The diet (g/kg food) can be multiplied by its daily intake (kg/day. animal) to obtain the daily intakes of all nutrients, that is, the ration.

Some nutritionists assert that it is more correct to use the DE basis than the DM basis to calculate the diet, since food is consumed voluntarily to meet energy needs, and because many nutrients are involved in energy metabolism. On the other hand, the use of the DM basis may be preferable, because feedstuffs that have a lower energy density (Mcal/kg DM) usually have a relatively lower digestibility. Copper, for example, has a mean minimum requirement of 10 mg/kg DM [1]. A diet of hay and grain (1:1) has an energy density of 2.65 Mcal/kg DM, so the Cu requirement is 3.8 mg/Mcal DE. Hay and grain have energy densities of 2.0 and 3.3 Mcal/kg DM, so the Cu requirements are, respectively, 7.5 and 12.5 mg/kg DM in compliance with energy densities. However, if the bioavailabilities of Cu in hay and grain are 10 and 20%, respectively, then this difference counteracts the adjustment for energy density and the use of the DE basis instead of the DM basis is unwarranted. Nevertheless, in addition to using the DM basis, it is customary to calculate the proportions of protein, fat, CHO-H and CHO-F on a DE basis or a metabolizable energy (ME) basis, because these proportions powerfully influence the efficiency of metabolism [41].

The calculation of diets and rations by means of weighted averages is simple arithmetic, but it is tedious, time consuming and subject to errors that are hard to find because they are usually repeated. For these reasons, complete ration evaluations were seldom conducted by veterinary practitioners before the advent of the personal computer.

Ration evaluation programs

The mathematical drudgery of ration evaluation has been eliminated by the availability of inexpensive, user-friendly computer software. Spread sheets readily perform weighted averages.

Specifically designed dietetic programs calculate the total diet and the daily intakes of nutrients and also compare these sets of values with nutritional goals, such as the nutrient requirements of horses [1]. In addition, some programs will calculate diets and rations from combinations of feed ingredients, either from specified amounts or on a least-cost basis if the cost of each ingredient is entered into the program.

The relative merits of rival programs are arguable objectively and subjectively. I became familiar with *Animal Nutritionist*™ (Version 2.5, 1987, N-Squared Computing, Silverton, OR, USA) a decade ago and continue to use it. This software can be used to evaluate a ration, calculate a diet from specified amounts of ingredients (stored in an adjustable data bank), or calculate a least cost diet from a stipulated set of ingredients. Much simpler to use and very inexpensive is *Spartan* (Cooperative Extension, Michigan State University, East Lansing, MI, USA). A recent program for ration evaluation but not formulation is *Microsteed*™ (Kentucky Equine Research, Versailles, KY, USA). This software has several advantages: it is designed solely for the horse, it is simple to use, it is the subject of detailed explanatory articles [40], it is likely to be up-dated and expanded, and, most of all, it offers an option of using the minimum requirements of the NRC or Kentucky Equine Research's own set of nutritional goals.

Nutritional goals

Nutritional science is usually applied to the determination of minimal nutrient requirements, whereas practical nutrition really needs optimal ranges for specified purposes (Figure 2). The performance traditionally evaluated in farm animal nutrition is energetic efficiency, but other measures of interest would include reproductive efficiency, conformation, tractability, low disease incidence and competitive athletic ability. Optimal ranges have been determined for vitamin A during growth [42] and, less well, for dietary fat with respect to muscle glycogen concentration [43]. Also, the optimal range for dietary calcium for growth that has been determined for large dogs may apply equally well to the horse. Much remains to be done in equine nutrition to establish nutritional goals in the form of optimal ranges or target zones to be used in ration evaluation and formulation.

Minimal requirements

Three authoritative sets of requirements for energy and nutrient intakes are available for horses [1, 44, 45]. The three systems are reconcilable only with time, patience, detailed knowledge and a good calculator. One system uses DE in Mcal, another DE in MJ, the third net energy (NE) in Mcal (1 Mcal = 4.183 MJ, approximately). One system uses crude protein, another digestable protein and the third, available protein.

The most widely used nutritional standards for animals are the NRC series for many species. These requirements are performance-oriented for production animals, but they are mean minimums for companion animals. A common aberration in the design of horse feeds is the use of the NRC minimum standards for horses in the same way as the production standards for cattle, swine and chickens. Mean minimal nutrient requirements are sufficient for 50% of the population, hence have little practical value.

Practical allowances

Recognizing that the nutrient requirements for dogs and cats have little practical value, the Association of American Feed Control Officials created nutrient profiles for dogs and cats, that were nonsystematically about 1.3 to two times corresponding NRC values. The human recommended dietary allowances (RDAs) are two standard deviations above mean minimum requirements, thereby being sufficient for 98% of the population [46]. When the standard deviation is not known for a nutrient, the CV of 15% for energy is used; thus many RDAs are 1.3 times the mean minimum. Applying the same approach to horses, a set of equine RDAs would be about 1.3 times the NRC requirements for maintenance and up to 1.6 times the NRC requirements for more demanding nutritional situations. These equine RDAs are more likely than the NRC requirements to reach the lower regions of the optimal ranges for nutrients (Figure 2) and hence be useful guides for practical nutrition.

Most clients of professional nutritionists are seeking help to achieve a high level of performance of various kinds. Each nutritionally competent person or corporation in equine practice has their own set of nutritional goals or tentative target ranges, and these goals are usually regarded as proprietary and valuable intellectual properties. Thus, the inclusion of the nutrient standards of Kentucky Equine Research in the *Microsteed*™ program must be regarded as an unusual contribution to the welfare of horses and the horse industry.

Vitamin–mineral supplements

Researchers have recommended that horses should be fed two times the vitamin A requirement specified by the NRC [35, 42]. Others have recommended three times the Cu requirement specified by the NRC [17]. Both vitamin A and Cu interact with several other vitamins and minerals, so elevating them but not the others which is likely to induce imbalances.

The *Nutrient Requirements of Horses* [1] is a sound scientific document that achieves compromises on minimum requirements. Although these requirements may have less practical value than allowances, the proportions among the requirements are probably the best that can be devised with the available information. Consequently, if the vitamin A and Cu contents of the diet are doubled, prudence dictates that all of the other micronutrients should be doubled.

An examination of a dozen equine vitamin–mineral supplements, which were advertized in a popular equine magazine, revealed that none approximated the proportions stipulated by the NRC [47]. Several products contained potentially toxic levels of vitamin A, vitamin D, or cobalt. Three supplements were judged to be almost satisfactory but none was recommended.

Sick horses

Nutrient goals for sick animals are based mainly on studies of human patients and clinical experience with animals [3, 48]. The energy requirements in multiples of maintenance for hospitalized horses, as discussed above (hypo- and hyper-metabolism) are based on the mean estimates of DE of the NRC [1].

The nutritional management of anorexia, botulism, tetanus, weak neonates, gastric ulcers, diarrheas, colics, liver disease, pancreatic disease, kidney disease, pulmonary diseases, rhabdomyolysis, skeletal diseases and plant poisonings is peripheral to this chapter. A sound clinical assessment of nutritional status, however, should help to guide the managment of most of these cases.

Conclusion

The clinical assessment of the nutritional status of a horse or group of horses consists essentially of dietary information obtained in the history and an evaluation of water, energy and protein status in the physical examination. Further use of laboratory aids and ration evaluation can be extremely useful, but these procedures have numerous pitfalls in execution and interpretation that this review has attempted to bring to light and rectify. Several procedures, such as function tests, that are already being used in human clinical nutrition, have been summarized in the expectation of impending availability to equine practioners.

References

1. National Research Council. *Nutrient Requirements of Horses*, ed. 5. Washington, DC: National Academy Press, 1989.
2. Kronfeld DS. Starvation and malnutrition of horses: recognition and treatment. *J. Equine Sci.* 1993; **13**, 298–304.
3. Donoghue S. Nutritional support of hospitalized patients. *Vet Clin N Am/Small Anim Pract.* 1989; **19(3)**, 475–495.
4. Naylor JM & Kenyon SJ. Effect of total calorific deprivation on host defence in the horse. *Res Vet Sci.* 1981; **31**, 369–372.
5. Solomon SM & Kirby DF. The re-feeding syndrome: a review. *J Parent Ent Nutr.* 1990; **14**, 90–97
6. Naylor JM, Freeman DE & Kronfeld DS. Alimentation of hypophagic horses. *Comp Cont Ed Vet Pract.* 1984; **6**, S93–S94.

7. Porr CA, Kronfeld DS *et al.* Bone mineral density responses to conditioning and dietary calcium. *Proc Equine Nutr Physiol Soc* 1997 (in press).
8. Rothman KL. *Modern Epidemiology*. Boston, MA: Little, Brown and Co. 1986; 1–358.
9. Kronfeld DS & Donoghue S. Metabolic convergence in developmental orthopedic disease. *Proc Am Ass Equine Pract.* 1987; **33**, 195–199.
10. Kronfeld DS. Diet and performance of racing sled dogs. *J Am Vet Med Ass.* 1973; **162**, 470–473.
11. Green HC. *An Introduction to the Study of Experimental Medicine.* By C. Bernard, translated from French. New York, NY: Macmillan, 1927.
12. Kronfeld DS, Meacham TN *et al.* Dietary aspects of developmental orthopedic disease in young horses. *Vet Clin N Am/Equine Pract.* 1990; **6**(2), 451–465.
13. Jeffcott LB & Savage CJ. Nutrition and the development of osteochondrosis (dyschrondroplasia). *Pferdeheikunde.* 1996; **12**, 338–342.
14. Donawick WJ, Mayhew IG *et al.* Early diagnosis of cervical vertebral malformation in young Thoroughbred horses, and successful treatment with restricted diet and confinement. *Proc Am Ass Equine Pract.* 1989; **35**, 525–528.
15. Savage CJ, McCarthy RN & Jeffcott LB. Effects of dietary energy and protein on induction of dyschondroplasia in foals. *Equine Vet J.* 1993; Suppl **16**, 74–79.
16. Knight DA, Gabel AA *et al.* Correlation of dietary mineral to incidence and severity of metabolic bone disease in Ohio and Kentucky. *Proc Am Ass Equine Pract.* 1985; **31**, 445–461.
17. Williams MA, Stowe HD and Sickle RL. Relationship of nutrition and management factors to incidence of equine development orthopedic disease: a field survey.
18. Murray M. Gastric ulcers in adult horses. *Compendium.* 1994; **16**, 792–797.
19. Cohen ND, Matjeka PL *et al.* Case-control study of the association between various management factors and development of colic in horses. *J Am Vet Med Ass.* 1995; **206**, 667–673.
20. Sprouse RF, Garner HE & Green EM. Plasma endotoxin levels in horses subjected to carbohydrate induced laminitis. *Equine Vet J* 1987; **19**, 25–28.
21. Potter GD, Hughes SL *et al.* A review of research on digestion and utilization of dietary fat by the equine. *Pferdeheilkunde.* 1992; **1**(123), 119–124.
22. Kronfeld DS, Custalow SE *et al.* Acid-base responses of fat-adapted horses: relevance to hard work in the heat. *J Appl Anim Behav Ethol* (in press)
23. Gibson RS. *Principles of Nutritional Assessment.* Oxford, UK: Oxford University Press 1990; 1–691.
24. Detsky AS, Baker JP *et al.* What is subjective global assessment of nutritional status? *J Parent Ent Nutr.* 1987; **11**, 8–13.
25. Lawrence LA, Ott EA, *et al.* The mechanical properties of equine third metacarpals as affected by age. *J. Anim Sci.* 1994; **72**, 2617–2623.
26. Bellamy JEC. Medical diagnosis, diagnostic spaces, and fuzzy systems. *J Am Vet Med Ass.* 1997; **210**, 390–396.
27. Kronfeld DS, Donoghue S *et al.* Nutritional status of dairy cows indicated by blood analysis. *J Dairy Sci.* 1983; **65**, 1425–1433.
28. Naylor JM, Kronfeld DS & Johnson K. Fasting hyperbilirubinemia and its relationship to free fatty acids and triglycerides in the horse. *Proc Soc Exp Biol Med.* 1980; **165**, 86–90
29. Freeman DE, Ferrante PL, Kronfeld DS *et al.* The effect of food deprivation on D-xylose absorption test in mates. *Am J Vet Res.* 1989; **50**, 1609–1612.
30. Meyer H. Contributions to water and mineral metabolism of the horse. *Adv Anim Physiol Anim Nutr.* 1990; **21**, 1–102.
31. Kronfeld DS, Cooper WL *et al.* Supplementation of pasture for growth. *Pferdeheilkunde.* 1996; **12**, 317–319.
32. Greiwe-Crandell KM, Morrow GA & Kronfeld DS. Phosphorus and selenium depeletion in Thoroughbred mares and weanlings. *Pferdeheilkunde.* 1992; **1**(216), 96–98.
33. Bertone JJ, Hintz HF & Schryver HF. Effect of caffeic acid on thiamin status in ponies. *Nutr Rep Int.* 1984; **30**, 281–283.

34. Greiwe-Crandell KM, Kronfeld DS *et al.* Seasonal variation in vitamin A status of grazing horses is assessed better by the relative dose response test than by serum retinol concentration. *J Nutr.* 1995; **125**, 2711–2716.
35. Greiwe-Crandell KM. Vitamin A depeletion and repletion in the Thoroughbred horse. PhD dissertation, Blacksburg, VA: Virginia Polytechnic Institute and State University 1996.
36. Blythe LL, Craig AM *et al.* Serially determined plasma α-tocopherol concentrations and results of the oral vitamin E absorption test in clinically normal horses and in horses with degenerative myeloencephalopathy. *Am J Vet Res.* 1991; **52**, 908–911.
37. Mayhew IG, Brown CM *et al.* Equine degenerative myeloencephalopathy: a vitamin E deficiency that may be familial. *J Vet Int Med.* 1987; **1**, 45–50.
38. Kronfeld DS. Feeding on horse breeding farms. *Proc Am Ass Equine Pract.* 1978; **24**, 461–464.
39. Lewis LD. *Equine Nutrition, Feeding and Care.* Media, PA: Williams and Wilkins 1995; 1–587.
40. Pagan JD, Jackson S & Duren S. Computing horse nutrition: How to properly conduct an equine nutrition evaluation using Microsteed™ equine ration evaluation software. *World Equine Vet Rev.* 1996; **1**(2), 10–17.
41. Kronfeld DS. Dietary fat affects heat production and other variables of equine performance,, especially under hot and humid conditions. *Equine Vet J.* 1997; **22**, Suppl. 24–34.
42. Donoghue S Kronfeld DS *et al.* Vitamin A nutrition of the equine: growth, serum biochemistry and hematology. *J Nutr.* 1981; **111**, 365–374.
43. Kronfeld DS, Ferrante PL & Grandjean D. Optimal nutrition for athletic performance, with emphasis on fat adaptation in dogs and horses. *J Nutr.* 1994; **124**, 2745S–2753S.
44. Martin-Rosset W. *L'alimentation des Chevaux.* Paris: INRA 1990.
45. Meyer H. *Pferdefutterung.* Hamburg: Verlag Paul Parey 1993.
46. Food and Nutrition Board. *Recommended Dietary Allowances.* Washington, DC: National Academy Press, 1989.
47. Donoghue S & Kronfeld DS. Vitamin-mineral supplements for horses, with emphasis on vitamin A. *Comp Cont Ed Pract Vet.* 1980; **2**, S121–S125.
48. Donoghue S. Nutritional support of hospitalized patients. *J Am Vet Med Ass.* 1992; **200**, 612–615.

Index

Numbers in **bold** refer to main entries.